Osteopathy

Models for Diagnosis, Treatment and Practice

For Elsevier:

Senior Commissioning Editor: Sarena Wolfaard
Project Development Manager: Mairi McCubbin
Project Manager: Gail Wright
Senior Designer: Judith Wright
Illustrations Manager: Bruce Hogarth

Osteopathy

Models for Diagnosis, Treatment and Practice

Jon Parsons DO PGCE MSc Ost

Osteopathy Practitioner, Maidstone, Kent;
Senior Lecturer and Senior Clinical Tutor, European School of Osteopathy, UK

Nicholas Marcer DO MSc Ost

Osteopathy Practitioner and Teacher, Fribourg, Switzerland and Ischia, Italy
International Lecturer and Examiner

Forewords by

Simon Fielding OBE DO

Founding Chairman, General Osteopathic Council, London;
Director, Prince of Wales's Foundation for Integrated Health, London, UK

and

Renzo Molinari DO

Principal, European School of Osteopathy, Boxley, UK

Illustrations by

Amanda Williams

ELSEVIER
CHURCHILL
LIVINGSTONE

EDINBURGH LONDON NEW YORK OXFORD PHILADELPHIA ST LOUIS SYDNEY TORONTO 2005

ELSEVIER
CHURCHILL
LIVINGSTONE

Cover photographs © Kampfner Photography

First published 2006

ISBN 0 443 07395 3

British Library Cataloguing in Publication Data
A catalogue record for this book is available from the British Library

Library of Congress Cataloging in Publication Data
A catalog record for this book is available from the Library of Congress

Notice
Knowledge and best practice in this field are constantly changing. As new research and experience broaden our knowledge, changes in practice, treatment and drug therapy may become necessary or appropriate. Readers are advised to check the most current information provided (i) on procedures featured or (ii) by the manufacturer of each product to be administered, to verify the recommended dose or formula, the method and duration of administration, and contraindications. It is the responsibility of the practitioner, relying on their own experience and knowledge of the patient, to make diagnoses, to determine dosages and the best treatment for each individual patient, and to take all appropriate safety precautions. To the fullest extent of the law, neither the publisher nor the authors assumes any liability for any injury and/or damage.

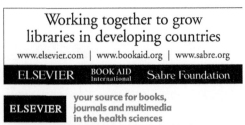
ELSEVIER   your source for books,
journals and multimedia
in the health sciences

www.elsevierhealth.com

Transferred to Digital Printing in 2011

Contents

Contents

Forewords

Having known both the authors as students it is a great privilege to be asked to write a brief foreword to this, their first book. Sadly, in spite of their both having been my students, I can make no claim whatsoever for any of the wisdom contained within these pages.

In the late 1970s I became aware that if osteopathy was to fulfill its potential in healthcare and achieve any form of recognition from conventional medicine there needed to be universal and credible standards of undergraduate training underpinned by the principles of conventional anatomy, physiology and pathology. At that time anyone, irrespective of their level of training, could set up and practise as an osteopath. Training courses ranged from 4-year full-time programmes to merely a few weekends' instruction in manipulation. This situation meant that neither patients nor conventional medical practitioners could rely upon the safety and competence of all members of the osteopathic profession.

Throughout the 1980s and early 1990s I was fortunate to be able to assist the profession in coming together to form a consensus on the needs of undergraduate training and proper regulation, which resulted in the passing of the Osteopaths Act 1993. The establishment of osteopathy as a statutory regulated profession along the same lines as medicine and dentistry is, however, only the beginning of the story. The profession now has a firm foundation from which to realize its full therapeutic potential and establish the coherent body of osteopathic knowledge and research essential for its future development. This book by Parsons and Marcer is a significant contribution to that much-needed body of knowledge, charting, as it does, the historical perspectives of osteopathy and its evolution into a healthcare profession that has a rational evidence base for its concepts and clinical practice.

As the chapters progress the reader is given an overview of the major concepts in osteopathic thinking. The book traces these concepts from their historical roots too and describes how these are relevant to current osteopathic practice and its emphasis on integration with emerging orthodox concepts such as psycho-neuroimmunology. The book also describes how concepts such as tensegrity can be applied to the science of osteopathy and are relevant to clinical practice.

The book manages throughout to achieve a sense of holism and consistency of thought, bringing together the different concepts and models of osteopathic healthcare that have arisen within the worldwide osteopathic community. What emerges is a total concept of osteopathy, not only in terms of somatic dysfunction but also integrating areas such as tensegrity and psychology. While destined to be a set text for all osteopathic students, this book also has much to offer all practitioners of the mind/body therapies. I look forward with eager anticipation to the next offering from these two innovative osteopathic thinkers.

Simon Fielding OBE DO
Founder Chairman of the General Osteopathic
Council and Trustee of The Prince of Wales's
Foundation for Integrated Health

This book is written at a crucial point in the still young history of osteopathy and for this reason it will remain as a milestone.

Osteopathy developed in the USA and was integrated progressively into the medical culture of that country. In its early infancy, JM Littlejohn brought this young and fragile approach to health and medicine to Europe, where it has developed and expanded independently. Today we have a duality in approach and understanding around Europe, but we must work together to create a forum in which the successes of our osteopathic efforts can be shared.

The dynamic growth of our profession in Europe and throughout the world can be summarized by a discussion that took place between Viola Frymann and myself in Colorado Springs, USA. She was arguing that when the `osteopathic seed' is planted in one country, there are always two trees that grow and fight for life. To my mind, when the osteopathic seed is planted in one country, the roots spread in different directions; it is only when these roots are able to accumulate enough energy that the trunk can grow.

We are at exactly this moment in the development of osteopathy. In every country various educational groups have formed and strengthened; on different continents diverse groups have structured the professional and educational aspect of our art and science. It is now time to work together on developing the core of our profession.

In the last decade, osteopathy has spread irresistibly around Europe, not only as a discrete approach to health and medicine for the benefit of patients but also academically. A number of different groups have been active in this growth and the European School of Osteopathy is considered to be one of the main protagonists.

From its inception, the School has had a European outlook, having a French, English and very quickly a Belgian branch. From 1994 the network expanded and academic links developed progressively so that new schools were helped to structure themselves. 1998 saw the foundation of the Osteopathic European Academic Network (OSEAN), which aims to link these institutions.

The two authors of this book, Jon Parsons and Nicholas Marcer, have been active internationally during the last decade and it is now a great privilege to see their ideas coming to light.

The real internationalization of osteopathy is just beginning and the next step will take place through cross-fertilization between the two sides of the Atlantic. Research will be the medium to expand this dialogue, as the research basis of our science needs to be developed.

Renzo Molinari DO
Principal of the European School of Osteopathy

Preface

The aim of this book is to attempt to explore some of the fundamental concepts to which an undergraduate student of osteopathy, or other manual therapeutic approach, will be exposed. We are relating these concepts to the treatment and support of human beings. This creates certain difficulties, as the rich complexities of the human form and function are not easily pinned down and so the attempts to interpret these complexities for a therapeutic purpose are often numerous and varied.

Within the osteopathic world specifically there are a multitude of varied interpretations and perceptions, and though it is a relatively young profession, over time osteopathic concepts have been subject to the interpretation and reinterpretation of many great thinkers, and some less great! Each has added their own perspective.

Different countries have also developed their understanding in subtly different ways. Within Europe there are shades of differences that occasionally appear so opaque that they severely limit communication: one simple example of this is the nomenclature utilized to classify somatic dysfunction. In the USA, the allopathic/osteopathic combination has further modified their contribution.

As a result of the above considerations, there are many differing perceptual and practical approaches utilized, often with tension arising between the apparently differing schools of thought. It is with this situation in mind that we draw in this book on founding principles in an attempt to facilitate understanding in a relative newcomer to osteopathy.

We were both trained at the European School of Osteopathy in Maidstone, England. As we are all influenced by the osteopathic paradigm in which we developed, it is almost certainly the case that many of the fundamental concepts that are expressed within this book are rooted in 'English' or perhaps even 'Maidstone' osteopathy; however, between the two of us, we have worked extensively in Europe and the USA, and have been exposed to many other osteopathic paradigms. Wherever possible, we have tried to incorporate or explain these varying views. We have also sought the advice of osteopaths throughout the osteopathic world. Any shortcomings are our own, however, and are apologised for.

The book has been structured in four sections:

Section 1 looks at the development of osteopathy, how we may define it, and then explores the idea of the osteopathic lesion (somatic dysfunction), as an entity itself and within a more holistic perspective.

Section 2 addresses some of the conceptual models that have been used, in an attempt to understand how functional or pathological problems may be explained from an osteopathic perspective.

Section 3 discusses some of the models of diagnosis and treatment, how they have arisen and (where known) their underlying physiological rationale.

Section 4 consists of several case histories that attempt to integrate the first three sections by demonstrating the processes involved in analysing several conditions from an osteopathic perspective.

Though there was a combined input in all sections logistics dictated that Sections 1 and 2 were predominantly written by Jon Parsons and Sections 3 and 4 by Nick Marcer. It is hoped that the slight difference in writing styles is not too off-putting, but it does allow us as individuals to express the concepts that are most important to each of us.

Throughout this book we have made much use of conceptual models. Many may feel that this is inappropriate, criticizing the fact that people are too varied to conform to models; or that a particular model is too reductionist in its conception with regard to the whole that is a person. Both these and the many other arguments that could be put forward have validity; however, it must be understood that these, as with all principles, are not to be followed slavishly but are there rather as a support designed to facilitate the comprehension of the complexities of the human form and its function for the neophyte body worker. Through application, the inherent strengths and weaknesses of each model will become apparent, and clinical experience will then remodel each individual's understanding.

We have also discussed models originated by some of the early osteopathic innovators which, with the advances in science, perhaps appear to be naïve or lacking in scientific gravitas or simply incorrect. We have done this as we feel that it is important to understand the concepts that underpin the foundation of osteopathy and that have been the springboard for development of the more recent interpretations, to gain a more complete understanding of osteopathy.

Though we have attempted to offer much information, as is so often the case with osteopathy the answers are not always obvious and it may be that in some sections you will come away with more questions than answers. That being said, we hope that you find this book helps you take the first steps on the exciting, confusing and rewarding osteopathic path.

Maidstone and Fribourg   *Jon Parsons*
                                        Nicholas Marcer

Acknowledgements

Our greatest thanks must go to my wife, Alison, for her patience, support and understanding (JP), and to Holly my daughter (NM).

Others who have contributed greatly, some both intellectually and emotionally, are Phil Austin, Christian Fossum, Celine Meneteau, Renzo Molinari, Lizzie Spring, Caroline Stone, Frank Willard, Jane Carreiro and Margaret Gamble.

For those brave souls who read the early drafts, Lynne Pruce, Hedi Kersten, Rob Thomas and Steven Bettles.

And all of the students and faculty and staff at the European School of Osteopathy for the last 20 years, who have nurtured us as individuals, as osteopaths and as teachers. Similarly, the students and faculty of all of the schools in which we have taught and learnt, notably College International d'Ostéopathie, St Etienne; College Ostéopathique Français, Paris; College of Osteopaths, London; The Academy of Children's Development, St Petersburg; Skandinaviska Osteopatskolen, Gothenburg; Norwegian Osteopathic School, Oslo; Instituto Superiore d'Osteopatia, Milano; Russian Academy of Osteopathic Medicine, St Petersburg; Wiener Schule für Osteopathie, Vienna; Osteopathie Schule Deutschland, Hamburg, Stuttgart, Bremen and Kassel; University of New England, College of Osteopathic Medicine, Maine, USA.

Heidi Harrison of Butterworth-Heinemann for commissioning us originally and with Elsevier, Mary Law and Mairi McCubbin for their patience and Gail Wright for quietly and efficiently making order out of the chaos.

Finally, we would like to thank Ewan Halley for jumping in at the eleventh hour and saving the day!

Abbreviations

AACOM	American Association of Colleges of Osteopathic Medicine
AC	anterocentral (anterior central)
ACTH	adrenocorticotropin hormone
ANS	autonomic nervous system
AP	anteroposterior
ASIS	anterior superior iliac spine
ASO	American School of Osteopathy
BLT	balanced ligamentous tension
C	cervical
BMT	balanced membranous tension
CAT	computer assisted tomography
CCP	common compensatory pattern
CNS	central nervous system
CRF	corticotropin-releasing factor
CRH	corticotropin-releasing hormone
CRI	cranial rhythmic impulse
CSF	cerebrospinal fluid
D	dorsalsyn thoracic
D/L	dorsolumbar
ECM	extracellular matrix
EEO	Ecole Européenne d'Ostéopathie
EFO	Ecole Française d'Ostéopathie
ESO	European School of Osteopathy
ERS	extension rotation sidebending lesion
ESR	electrical skin resistance
FRS	flexion rotation sidebending lesion
GOsC	General Osteopathic Council of Great Britain
GAR	general adaptive response
GAS	general adaptation syndrome
GAT	general articulatory treatment
GHRH	growth hormone-releasing hormone
GIT	gastrointestinal tract
GOT	general osteopathic treatment
GST	general systems theory
HPA	hypothalamic-pituitary-adrenal
HVLA	high velocity low amplitude
HVT	high velocity thrust
IBS	irritable bowel syndrome
IL	interleukin
IVM	involuntary mechanism
L	lumbar
LC	locus ceruleus
L/S	lumbosacral
LVHA	low velocity high amplitude
MET	muscle energy technique
MRI	magnetic resonance imaging
NIM	neuroimmunomodulation
NMDA	N-methyl-d-aspartate
NMT	neuromuscular technique
NO	nitric oxide
NSAIDs	non-steroidal anti-inflammatory drugs
NRS	easy normal rotation sidebending lesion
PA	posteroanterior
PC	posterocentral (posterior central)
PGI	paragigantocellularis
PMS	premenstrual syndrome
PNI	psychoneuroimmunology
PNS	peripheral nervous system
PSIS	posterior superior iliac spine
PSNS	parasympathetic nervous system
PRM	primary respiratory mechanism
PRT	progressive relaxation training
PVN	paraventricular nucleus of the hypothalamus

RTM	reciprocal tension membrane	SRR	stress resistance resource
S	sacral	T	thoracic
SAM	sympathetic adrenal axis	TBA	total body adjustment
SAT	specific adjusting technique	T/L	thoracolumbar
SBS	sphenobasilar symphysis	TMJ	temporomandibular joint
SCS	strain counterstrain	TOL	total osteopathic lesion
SI	sacroiliac	TRH	thyroid-releasing hormone
SNA	sympathetic neural axis	WDR	wide dynamic range (neurone)
SNS	sympathetic nervous system		

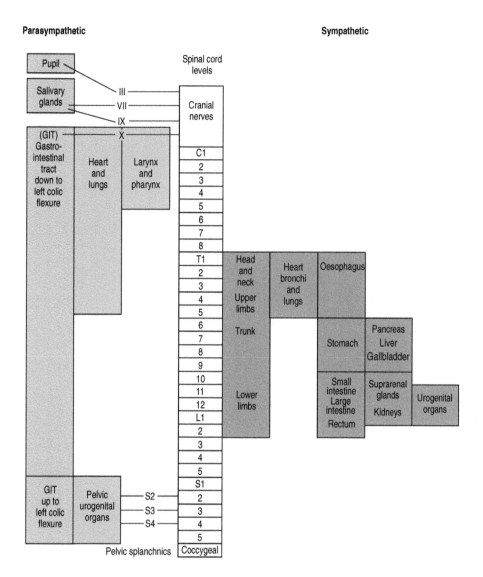

The autonomic nervous system: (left) parasympathetic outflow; (right) sympathetic outflow. The basis of osteopathic medicine lies in an understanding of the autonomic nervous system. All practitioners of osteopathy should have their own image of the autonomic nervous system firmly imprinted in their own central nervous system to refer to during every treatment. This converts the lay bone-setter into the osteopath.

SECTION 1

Osteopathy and the osteopathic lesion – a developing concept

This section introduces the term osteopathy and reviews some of the numerous attempts at the difficult task of defining what it actually is. It explores the precepts originally conceived by Andrew Taylor Still, the founder of osteopathy, and their role in underpinning and informing the practice of osteopathy. It also reflects briefly on the historical development of osteopathy itself.

The osteopathic lesion, or somatic dysfunction, is used as a vehicle to explore the variety of ways of perceiving osteopathy. This section also includes an attempt to draw some parallels between the varieties of models used, to minimize the confusion that can arise when communicating with osteopaths grounded in differing conceptual models.

Chapter 1

What is osteopathy?
Towards a definition

INTRODUCTION

The concept of osteopathy came to Andrew Taylor Still, the founder of osteopathy, at 10 o'clock on 22 June, 1874.[1] He describes it as a revelation; it is not uncommon for innovators or inventors to describe the moment of comprehension in this way and this is often referred to as the 'eureka principle'. After years of study and background work, the ideas suddenly coalesce at a particular point in time, a revelation so significant that the individual can recall the *actual time* that it occurred. Another interpretation is that it was more a 'point of decision' than a revelation. At this point, Still's cumulative experience enabled him to decide that he would 'reform' current medical practice by introducing a system of therapeutics which would utilise 'natural forces' in the process of healing, rather than 'poisonous chemical agents'.

Whether it was a eureka 'experience', or a point of decision, Still certainly possessed an appropriate background. He is reported to have had an interest in anatomy from his childhood, and he worked as a Frontier doctor during the American Civil War. This experience, combined with a deep dissatisfaction with the current practice of medicine, would have contributed to the development of his ideas.

His original conception was founded on the importance of anatomy and its relationship to the 'flow of natural forces' in the body. As he became more pragmatic, these 'natural forces' eventually developed into his ideas on 'the rule of the artery', 'venous liberty' and later 'nerve force'. The anatomical relationship matured into the theory that the normal workings of the body could be disturbed by anatomical abnormalities or displacements.

However, it was not until 1885 that he chose to name this new approach 'osteopathy'. In the intervening time, he experimented with several approaches. He continued to use his skill as a medical doctor (at the standards of his time), in combination with 'magnetic healing' (in 1865 he advertised himself as a 'magnetic healer' in Missouri) and bone setting (which he might have learned from the Shawnee Indians whilst working at Wakarusa Mission in Kansas in the 1850s). He gradually realized that, of all of these approaches, manipulative techniques were the most effective in working on 'anatomical abnormalities'. He therefore started to refine these techniques, so that they could be applied in disorders beyond the purely rheumatological and orthopaedic cases where the natural bonesetters did most of their work. In the early 1880s, manipulative techniques were the a priori of his practice, and, around 1882, he started advertising himself as a 'Lightening Bone-setter'.[2]

Thus in 1885 Still coined the term 'osteopathy'. It derives from two Greek words: 'osteon' meaning 'bone', and 'pathos' meaning 'suffering'. However, within medical literature 'pathos' is taken to mean 'disease', as in 'myopathy', a disease of the muscles. For this reason the name osteopathy has, in the past, and to this day, created some confusion, often being taken to mean 'bone disease' or more simply 'something to do with bones'. Early osteopathic writers[3,4,5] explain that this was not Still's intention, most notably Wilson and Tucker, who consulted with a Classical Greek scholar to find a true etymological root. He directed them to the root derivation of 'pathos' and the similar term, 'ethos'. The original meaning of 'pathos' was 'sensitive to' or 'responding to' incoming impressions, in contrast to 'ethos' which describes the same impressions, but their outgoing effects.

The name was created to contrast with allopathy and homeopathy. These terms arise, respectively, from 'allos' meaning 'another' or 'opposite', and 'homoios' or 'homeo' meaning 'the same' or 'similar'. Thus, allopathy involves responding to or being influenced by opposites, and homeopathy means responding to similars. Osteopathy involves sensitivity or responsiveness to bones, reflecting the concept that derangements of the musculoskeletal system can, via the various systems, lead to disease, and that disease can be diagnosed and treated via

the musculoskeletal system.[4] This is a subtle distinction for the layperson to appreciate, and the concept that osteopathy is just related to bones is one that generations have tried hard to escape. One such attempt is:

> Osteopathy, or osteopathic medicine, is a philosophy, a science and an art. Its philosophy embraces the concept of the unity of body structure and function in health and disease. Its science includes the chemical, physical and biological sciences related to the maintenance of health and the prevention, cure and alleviation of disease. Its art is the application of the philosophy and the science in the practice of osteopathic medicine.[6]

This tries to demonstrate that osteopathy refers to a complex interplay of concepts and bodies of knowledge, not just a bone out of place.

In the time since its conception 130 years ago many people have attempted to define osteopathy, though not without difficulty. Wolf stated, 'On many occasions members of our profession have tried to define the term 'osteopathy', but I doubt anyone has produced a definition which satisfies'.[7] Each attempt will have a validity, but as with any healthy areas of pursuit, osteopathy is continually advancing. As new developments arise, and thought processes change, the understanding and therefore the definition of osteopathy will subtly change.

It is of benefit to look at some of the definitions of osteopathy that have been utilized in the past: in so doing, it is possible to observe the range of interpretations. It is logical to start with two of Still's own definitions. The simplest was given in response to the question, 'What is osteopathy?'. Still replied: 'It is anatomy first, last, and all the time'.[8] A more complete attempt, cited in his autobiography, is:

> Osteopathy is that science which consists of such exact, exhaustive and verifiable knowledge of the structure and function of the human mechanism, anatomical, physiological and psychological, including the chemistry and physics of its known elements, as has made discoverable certain organic laws and remedial resources, within the body itself, by which nature under the scientific treatment peculiar to osteopathic practice, apart from all ordinary methods of extraneous artificial or medicinal stimulation, and in harmonious accord with its own mechanical principles, molecular activities and metabolic processes, may recover from displacements, disorganisations, derangements, and consequent disease, and regain

its normal equilibrium of form and function in health and strength.[9]

This is written in somewhat archaic language and is typical of Still's manner of writing, which can deter people from attempting to read his original texts. It is perhaps necessary to look beyond the words for the meaning within. However, the key element is the breadth of the description.

This broad ranging version contrasts with a somewhat later definition given by Edythe Ashmore.[10] Once the Professor of Osteopathic Technique at the American School of Osteopathy (ASO) in Kirksville, she wrote in 1915 that osteopathy is 'based upon the sciences of anatomy, chemistry and physiology' and that the 'central thought of the science of osteopathy is the lesion'. This focus on the lesion as central to osteopathy is reinforced by Jocelyn Proby,[11] a graduate of the ASO who wrote in 1937: 'It is by the bony 'lesion', and particularly the vertebral lesion that osteopathy as a school of practice must stand or fall.'

In essence there are similarities with Still's definitions, but it is possible to perceive the rationalization of the osteopathic concept and its reduction to the lesion and to a structural cause and effect. This continued throughout the 1930s and 1940s. Dr Leon Page wrote in the introduction to his book, *The Principles of Osteopathy*, in 1952:[12]

The practice of osteopathy consists of various prophylactic, diagnostic and therapeutic measures designed to maintain or restore structural integrity and thus ensure physiological function. The rational application of therapy requires a comprehensive knowledge of normal structure and function and familiarity with those structural and functional perversions that constitute disease.

It is interesting for contemporary osteopaths to note that neither the person nor the body is mentioned and, as for the environment and psyche (discussed below), he tends to refer to these as complications that will be encountered and that will need to be dealt with in the clinic, but not as part of the aetiological whole:

Therapy itself is an art and reflects the ability of the practitioner to utilize the combined experience of himself and others in dealing with the intricate clinical problems which are complicated by such intangible elements as human personality, unusual environmental circumstances, and many physical and psychic aspects which are, as yet, unknown to factual science.

Progressing to 1991, William and Michael Kuchera[13] employed a description of the founding principles of osteopathy in their definition:

Osteopathy is a total system of healthcare which professes and teaches the osteopathic philosophy:
1. The body is a unit.
2. It has its own self-protecting and regulating mechanisms.
3. Structure and function are reciprocally interrelated.
Treatment considers the preceding three principles. Osteopathy also encompasses all recognized tools of diagnosis and healing including osteopathic palpatory and manipulative treatment methods.

Osteopathy has developed so many facets in the intervening years since its creation that there is now a trend for many current authors to not even attempt to define it, as to encompass all of the potential aspects would make a lengthy and somewhat complicated essay; rather, there is a tendency to state the key principles in a manner similar to Kuchera's above. If a definition is attempted, the result is generally kept very simple, as illustrated by the following two examples.

One of the most recent definitions, and the one that the British osteopaths practise under, is that of the General Osteopathic Council of Great Britain (GOsC) which states that:

Osteopathy is an established recognised system of diagnosis and treatment, which lays its main emphasis on the structural and functional integrity of the body. It is distinctive by the fact that it recognises that much of the pain and disability which we suffer stems from abnormalities in the function of the body structure as well as damage caused to it by disease.[14]

The American equivalent, compiled by the American Association of Colleges of Osteopathic Medicine (AACOM), defines osteopathy as:

A complete system of medical care with a philosophy that combines the needs of the patient with current practice of medicine, surgery and obstetrics; that emphasizes the interrelationship between structure and function and that has an appreciation of the body's ability to heal itself.[15]

The latter attempt demonstrates the incorporation of osteopathy into the allopathic system of healthcare in America, which contrasts with the European approach, where it is still a distinct entity, working with, but not within, the allopathic system.

Over the last few decades there has been a gradual return to a more holistic approach to health, and more attention has been paid to the interdependence of the mind, the body and the spirit. The next definition is a recent reinterpretation by Philip Latey of Still's quote cited earlier. It demonstrates the subtle shifts in conceptualization that have occurred since Still's time, but also the relevance, to this day, of the originating concepts:

The goal of osteopathy is the regaining of the normal equilibrium of form and function that typifies good health. The osteopath helps achieve this by treatment methods that are in harmonious accord with the human organism's own biological constitution and organisation. The treatment methods are aimed to enable or help the organism recover from displacements, derangements and disorganisations. We do this without using or introducing any extraneous, artificial or medicinal intervention. So: we rely only on those remedial resources contained within the organism. We are able to do this through our knowledge and discovery of organic laws; through careful and exacting scientific research into the anatomical, physiological and psychological structure and function of the human being.[16]

Wolf is perhaps correct, in that there are no perfect definitions. This appears to frustrate some individuals, particularly since osteopathy is considered to be a profession and, as such, we should to be able to define our practice precisely. However, it is also possible to consider this as one of the great features of our profession: it has many facets, and refraining from the imposition of a rigid definition allows space for each individual to create their own. One of the aims of this book is to assist you in creating your own uniquely personal definition of osteopathy based on the sum of all your experiences, belief systems and contemporary and past paradigms of osteopathy specifically, and science and knowledge generally. This definition will inform your whole approach to the practice of osteopathy and, as we have seen with the above definitions, it will change as your experience and knowledge grow.

In this brief discussion it can be seen that these have been, and continue to be, major conceptual shifts within the practice and philosophy of osteopathy and it is perhaps useful to look at the development of osteopathy to get a clearer picture of what osteopathy is, and how we have arrived at our current understanding of it.

A BRIEF HISTORY OF THE ORIGINS OF OSTEOPATHY

Manual medicine, in its broadest conception, is as old as mankind itself; it has developed in a multiplicity of ways of which osteopathy is one. Many of these approaches have been passed down through the generations with little recorded rationale. Conceptualization of disease was originally rudimentary and often incorporated a supernatural element.

Modern Western medicine has its deepest roots in Mesopotamia and Egypt, but the critical site of development of the science of medicine is thought by many to be Ancient Greece, notably on the two neighbouring islands of Cos and Cnidos where two of the earliest medical schools exist. It was from these schools, whilst medicine was still in its infancy, that a perceptual schism arose as to how to view patients and their disease processes.

The ethos of the school on Cos from around 400 BC was developed by Hippocrates; often cited as the father of medicine, his principal achievement at that time was to develop a rational approach based on observation of medical factors.

Fundamental to Hippocratic teaching was that:

- effect must have a cause, and this cause may be in the internal or external environment;
- whether that cause is an internal or external factor, it could be explained by natural phenomena, (thus dispelling the mystical concepts of medicine, such as possession by evil spirits).

But perhaps more critically significant, and the root cause of the philosophical schism, are the concepts that:[17]

- the medical art has three terms: the sickness, the sick person, and the doctor. The doctor is the servant of the art, and, with the doctor, the sick person must combat the sickness; and
- the body will heal itself, and it is the role of the practitioner to assist the patient's body in achieving this.

However, these views were not shared by his contemporaries at the neighbouring school at Cnidos, where the opinions held were notably divergent. Here they concentrated on the internal structures of the body, dividing the contents into systems, and rather than believing that disease processes followed general 'rules', considered that each body system and disease required a separate philosophy and method of treatment. Treatment should, then, be aimed directly at that specific disease process rather than at assisting the patient in the resolution of the problem.

It is from this that the conceptual differences arose. Stated somewhat simplistically, allopathic medicine has tended to follow the Cnidian philosophy of the practitioner intervening in the disease process. This has become especially apparent over the last century with the discovery of the germ theory. Treatment has become more symptom specific and research is looking ever more microscopically for the specific pathogen or biochemical imbalance. Thus the disease process itself has become the principle. The individual is less and less the one who expresses health or ill health, but instead one who is afflicted by disease in the form of noxious pathogenic agents or phenomena and requires antidotal treatment (though it should be noted that, recently, allopathic medicine is shifting away from this reductionist approach).[18]

The Cos school, imbued by Hippocrates' ideas promulgating a more global concept of disease, acknowledging the body's ability to resolve problems, and seeing the role of the practitioner as supportive rather than interventionalist, has been pursued by the more holistic complementary approaches, and as such it is of no surprise that the legacy of Hippocrates was picked up by Still.

ANDREW TAYLOR STILL (1828–1917)

Still was born in 1828 in Lee County, Virginia. He was reportedly interested in anatomy from an early age and, as a teenager, was known to dissect animals that had been shot. Through a process of apprenticeship, some tuition and self-motivation he became a frontier doctor. During the Civil War, he was a captain in the Union Army. He used his medical skills to help the wounded and, by so doing, continued to develop his anatomical knowledge.

In 1864, after witnessing the death of his children from meningitis and being impotent to help them, he began searching for an alternative approach to healthcare. He experimented with magnetism and Mesmerism[19] but the final result of this search was the creation of osteopathy. On 22 June 1874 he proposed a different model of treatment and diagnosis that was mediated principally by the musculoskeletal system but recognized the great importance of the blood supply in human function or dysfunction, as well as the concept of natural immunity, or the body's inherent capacity to self-regulate and cure itself.

As we have seen, it was not until 1885 that he coined the term osteopathy, and it was not until 1889 that he actually called himself an osteopath. Prior to that, he called himself a 'magnetic healer' or 'lightening bone-setter'.[20] It is possible that the reason for this delay was that Still did not realize for some time that he had invented something different from healing and bone-setting.[21]

By 1892 he had founded the American School of Osteopathy (ASO) in Kirksville, where he taught philosophy and osteopathic treatment. Still was aware of the need to distinguish osteopathy as a separate entity from medicine, and though the charter of the school permitted the award of an MD degree, he insisted on awarding the distinctive DO, Diplomate of Osteopathy. He continued to work as an osteopath and teacher all his life and observed the gradual flowering of osteopathy until his death in 1917.

SUBSEQUENT DEVELOPMENTS

POLITICAL AND ACADEMIC

The first graduating year from the ASO consisted of just 14 students; included within this group were three of Still's sons and one daughter. The course was less than a year long for the first alumni. John Martin Littlejohn enrolled as a student in 1898 and graduated in 1900. At the same time as being a student he held the post of Professor in Physiology and later became Dean. There was an amazingly rapid growth in osteopathy. By the turn of the century, 12 other osteopathic schools had already been formed, and collectively they had some 700 students.

Osteopathy, as a subject, was introduced in the UK in 1898 through a lecture at the Society for Science, Letters and Arts in London by Littlejohn. These lectures were repeated in 1899 and again in 1900. The first osteopaths settled to practise in the UK in 1902: they were FJ Horn, Lillard Walker, Harvey Foote and Jay Dunham. The influx of American-trained osteopaths was so numerous that in 1910 the British Osteopathic Society was founded. In 1911 they changed their name to the British Osteopathic Association. The first school in Europe, the British School of Osteopathy in London, was founded in 1915 by Littlejohn, and incorporated in 1917. Migration of osteopaths continued into the rest of Europe. In 1923 Dr Stirling introduced osteopathy to a group of medical doctors in France, one of whom was Paul Geny, who went on to found the Ecole Française d'Ostéopathie (EFO) in Paris in 1951. This later moved, under the directorship of Tom Dummer, to Maidstone in England to become the Ecole Européenne d'Ostéopathie (EEO), later the European School of Osteopathy (ESO). Many of the first graduates of the EFO went on to found schools in other parts of Europe. Osteopaths trained in America moved to Australia in the early 20th century, and in 1909 several osteopaths were listed as practitioners in the Melbourne area. Canada and New Zealand followed a similar pattern of development.

CONCEPTUAL

Statutory recognition has not been straightforward. In America, Vermont became the first state to license DOs in 1896 but it was not until 1989 that Nebraska finally passed an unlimited practice law for DOs (the last of the states to do so).

In the UK, after several failed attempts at getting a Bill passed through Government, it was recommended that a voluntary register be set up. This was legally constituted in 1936 under the title, The General Council and Register of Osteopaths Ltd (GCRO). The GCRO, and particularly Simon Fielding, continued to pursue recognition but it was not until 1993 that they finally succeeded and The Osteopaths Act was passed to regulate the osteopathic profession in England, granting osteopaths a status equivalent to doctors of medicine and dentists. The wording of the Act is as follows:

> An Act to establish a body to be known as the General Osteopathic Council; to provide for the regulation of the profession of osteopathy, including making provision as to the registration of osteopaths and as to their professional education and conduct; to make provision in connection with the development and promotion of the profession; and for connected purposes.[24]

In 1994, the practice of osteopathy and osteopathic training became federally regulated in Finland. Belgium and France have draft propositions in place and Norway is poised to grant recognition. By the time this book has been published, other countries will almost certainly have followed suit.

Concurrent with the spread of osteopathy throughout the world was a gradual shift in the conceptual principles and means of applying osteopathy. Dummer[22] describes four evolutionary stages of the development of osteopathy. (These stages are an oversimplification, but have a use in describing trends, particularly in the material being taught within the osteopathic schools at the various stages.)

The first stage is essentially formative and developmental, starting with the origin in 1874 and passing through to 1900/1910. There is little clear idea of the true nature of Still's treatment approach as he wrote no books on technique, but it would appear that though he describes both maximal and minimal approaches, essentially it was based on a minimal structural approach and was rather intuitive and subjective. It is also clear that he was difficult to learn from; he demonstrated on actual patients and rarely repeated any particular treatment or technique. He felt that 'common sense applied in a mechanical way was the fundamental principle underlying the successful treatment of all disease of the human family'.[23] His students tried to imitate his treatment but, lacking his experience and understanding, ended up using a 'shot gun' type method of treatment, cracking every joint in the body to ensure that nothing was missed. This marked the start of the second stage of development.

Occurring between the years of 1900/1910 to 1950/1960, this was a structural-mechanical period. There was a tendency to objectivity and rational approaches. The osteopathic lesion became the focus of attention (as seen in the definitions of Ashmore and others; see p. 5). The treatment style was more maximal than that of the earlier 'find it, fix it' minimal approach. Much treatment was based on thrust techniques reversing the dysfunction of the osteopathic lesion. Littlejohn and Fryette were prime influences in this era, and it was Littlejohn that kept alive the early more maximal general treatment approaches by developing the 'general osteopathic treatment' (GOT), also now known as 'total body adjustment' (TBA).

It should be remembered that though these approaches dominated, other systems were developing concurrently. In 1915, FP Millard's approach was based on mobilization of the body fluids and particularly the lymph, and in the 1920s Sutherland and Weaver developed the concepts of cranial motion and the approaches later to be known as balanced ligamentous or membranous tension

(BLT and BMT). This reached fruition in the next era.

By the 1950s a new paradigm began evolving, further developing the cranial approach of Sutherland and spawning the emergence of the so-called 'indirect techniques'. CH Bowles and HV Hoover were responsible for developing the concept of functional technique, while TJ Ruddy and F Mitchell concentrated on muscle energy techniques, and LH Jones focused on counterstrain. This, the third stage of development, from 1950 to 1975, could be termed the cranial-functional phase.

Development has continued apace with each approach leading to further subtle developments, so that today we have a rich and varied armamentarium enabling us to modify conceptual and practical approaches to the needs of each individual, leading us to the fourth and present stage. This is described as the 'holistic return-to-the-source which gives (apparently in keeping with Still's original conception), equal emphasis to the dynamic structural/functional–functional/structural aspects both in diagnosis and technique'.[22]

Even though, as the above demonstrates, there have been marked changes in conceptualization and we now possess a great variety of approaches within osteopathy, it is possible to trace nearly all of these approaches back to the original principles espoused by Still. The following section will return to the roots of osteopathy and explore some of these principles.

STILL'S FOUNDING PRINCIPLES

Like Hippocrates, Still developed a 'person-specific' rather than disease-specific approach. His philosophy was based on the integrity of the individual as a unified whole, rather than a review of physiological processes occurring in individual and separate systems.

The earliest interpretation of Still's writings resulted in the formation of the four precepts of osteopathy, which can be stated as follows:

- The body is a unit.
- Structure governs function.
- The rule of the artery is supreme.
- The body possesses self-regulatory and self-healing mechanisms.

These are still utilized as guiding rules, but as is the case with most concepts, they have been gradually redefined. Thus in 1953 the Osteopathic Committee at Kirksville[25] restated the above as:

- The body is a unit.
- Structure governs function.
- The body possesses self-regulatory mechanisms.
- The body has the inherent capacity to defend itself and repair itself.

And later these four were supplemented[26] by the following:

- When the normal adaptability is disrupted, or when environmental changes overcome the body's capacity for self-maintenance, disease may ensue.
- The movement of the body fluids is essential to the maintenance of health.
- Nerves play a crucial part in controlling the fluids of the body.
- There are somatic components to disease that are not only manifestations of disease but also are factors that contribute to maintenance of the diseased state.

These simple precepts require some explanation to appreciate the depth of thought behind these few words.

THE BODY IS A UNIT

Still was a devout man who believed that the body was designed by God (whom he often described as 'the Architect'). Being divine, the design should be perfectly suited to its function, with each element contributing to the whole. In *Research and Practice*, he utilized the analogy of man as a city. 'Let us say that each person is a well organised city and reason by comparison that the city makes all the workshops necessary to produce such machinery as required for the health and comfort of its inhabitants. Each organ is a labourer of skill and belongs to the union of Perfect Work.'[1] All parts of the body are integrated. On an anatomical level, it can be observed that the entire body and its systems are united by means of the fascia. It is continuous throughout the body, uniting system to system and cell to cell, and by supporting and maintaining these structures enables them to work in harmony.

This phenomenon is also observed on a functional level. Each part of the body has its own specific function to achieve (e.g. temperature regulation or pH balance); however, each of these separate elements works as part of a 'team' to support the overall functioning of the individual. These are all regulated by the nervous system, the central nervous system controlling the musculoskeletal system whilst the autonomic nervous system oversees the visceral function; the endocrine system controlling hormonal balance; and the immune system defending the body. Once described as separate entities, it is now known that these work together in a complex harmony, termed the neuroendocrine-immune system.

Compensation and adaptation are also highlighted in this notion of unity. Change in one system will be accompanied by adaptation in another, always trying to maintain an integrated and functioning (homeostatic) system. Taken beyond the anatomical level, the concept of unity can incorporate the elements of the mind, the body and the spirit; this removes the locus of evaluation from the body alone and places it within the environment, expanding the osteopathic concept into a truly holistic arena. Thus a change in any one of the body's systems, whether caused by an internal or external agent, will have an effect on other areas, be they in the body, the mind or the spirit, and affecting one will affect all of the others.

STRUCTURE GOVERNS FUNCTION

This statement appears to be immediately understandable and on the simple level it is possible to conceive that if anything is designed for a purpose, change in that design will obviously affect the achievement of the purpose. For centuries, practitioners have been aware that if there is a pathological change in a structure, this naturally affects the way that the structure functions. So, for example, a ruptured ligament would lead to instability in the relevant articulation and thus affect its ability to function normally. Similarly, cirrhosis of the liver will have an effect on every function that the liver is expected to perform, such as detoxification of the blood, anticoagulant formation and so on.

Still's strength was taking these concepts into the non-pathological realm and looking at both local and distal consequences of such a disturbance. (It should be noted that in Still's original concept, because 'the rule of the artery is supreme', the function disturbed is that of circulation of the body fluids; either directly, or indirectly via the autonomic nervous system reflexes controlling vasomotor tone; this then affects all of the other tissues.[22]) As a doctor, Still had realized that certain disease processes had consistent reflection in the somatic structure.

Furthermore he discovered that by addressing the somatic structure he could beneficially affect the function of the local tissue/organ, and the general health of that individual.

We say disease when we should say effect; for disease is the effect of a change in the parts of the physical body. Disease in an abnormal body is just as natural as is health when all parts are in place.[1]

This concept of structure functional dependency is one of the fundamental tenets of osteopathic medicine; implicit within it are predictive or diagnostic possibilities. Thus by understanding in detail the anatomy of the body and the relation of one structure to another, it should be possible to predict the consequences that would arise when one structure is moved from its normal position, and what effects this would be likely to have on its contiguous and continuous structures. For example, with an aberrant position of a rib, there will be consequent disruption of the attached intercostal muscles. This will in turn have an effect on the structures passing within them, i.e. on the fluid exchange of the artery, vein and lymphatic system, and on the nerve conduction of impulses, both peripheral and centrally to its spinal segment, and on its neurotrophic function, having deleterious consequences on both somatic and visceral structures supplied. The inappropriate position of the rib will result in a compensatory pattern developing in other areas of the thorax or spine, which themselves will then create a similar disturbance.

As osteopaths we have access principally, and most obviously, to the body's structure, and it is by observing and palpating the structure of an individual that we can conceive the possible effects on function. By treating these structural problems we hope to improve both the local and global functioning of the individual, supporting the body in its homeostatic role.

With a correct knowledge of the form and function of the body and all its parts, we are then prepared to know what is meant by a variation in a bone, muscle, ligament, or fibre or any part of the body, from the least atom to the greatest bone or muscle. By our mechanical skill, preceded by our intelligence in anatomy, we can detect and adjust both hard and soft substances of the system. By our knowledge of physiology we can comprehend the requirements of the circulation of the fluids of the body as to time, speed, and quantity, in harmony with the demands of normal life.[27]

The intimate and inseparable relationship of structure and function has been recognized by subsequent authors, and this precept is more commonly stated as: 'Structure and function are reciprocally related'. Dr Viola Frymann is said to have taken this one step further when she stated that 'structure is solidified function'. Tom Dummer responded that 'function (motion) is de-solidified structure' and stated:

> Structure and function are indivisible and are simply two aspects of the one expressed bioenergy. There is no 'starting-point' – function and structure are in this sense continuous and relative in their expression of the life-process.[22]

So far in this discussion, we have focused on the larger tissue systems; however, 'one function of anatomy is the supplying of a framework, even to the remotest cell structure'.[28] The structural functional reciprocity process is easy to imagine when dealing with large organs or tissue structures, but envisaging the effects at the cellular level is perhaps more difficult. The system that best illustrates the micro-macroscopic relationship is the fascial system. This system is continuous throughout the body, creating an internal 'soft tissue skeleton' composed of connective tissue ranging from the dense tissue layers separating the body systems, down to the microfibrils uniting the internal structures of the cells. Affecting any part of this system will have a cascade effect on the continuous structures from macroscopic to microscopic, influencing the structures invested by the connective tissue and thus affecting the function of these structures, be they systems, organs or cells. The particular relevance of this system will be discussed further in Chapter 4 on tensegrity.

THE BODY POSSESSES SELF-REGULATORY MECHANISMS

Still believed that as well as possessing self-regulating mechanisms, the body also possesses self-healing mechanisms, often described as 'vis medicatrix naturae'. What Still ascribed to 'nature', we would now refer to as the homeostatic mechanisms.

The body always works towards homeostasis, and possesses mechanisms to control the function of the body, e.g. through hormonal mediation (hypothalamic–pituitary axis controlling the endocrine glands) and nervous mediation (baroreceptors, receptors to salt in the kidneys, etc.). These mechanisms are in constant interaction, thus enabling the body to achieve a constant state of balance (e.g. blood pressure control, acid secretion in the stomach). However, when dysfunction occurs, the body will have to work harder to maintain its balance; this additional work is referred to as the allostatic load (see Ch. 7). If great or sustained, this would lead to possible specific effects on the body as well as general fatigue or malaise. By removing the dysfunction, the allostatic load would be reduced, the body returning to 'normal homeostasis', and there would be both a local and a general improvement in the person's health.

Note that the practitioner's role is to remove the dysfunction: the body is then able to restore function.

This ability has, in the past, been ascribed to the life force, but more recently has been thought to be due to the body working as a tensegrous system. Implicit with tensegrity structures is the ability to self-stabilize once any opposing force has been removed.

THE BODY HAS THE INHERENT CAPACITY TO DEFEND ITSELF AND REPAIR

This could be seen, to an extent, as an extension of the previous precept. In Still's words, 'the brain of man was God's drugstore, and had in it all liquids, drugs, lubricating oils, opiates, acids, antacids, and every quality of drugs that the wisdom of God thought necessary for human happiness and health'.[29]

The body has several levels of defence against potential external or internal aggressors (the skin, and the various tissues and cells of the immune system and their relationships with the nervous and endocrine systems) and therefore is able to maintain health within the body. If damage does occur, the body has the capacity to repair itself.

Still's conception of disease is not focused on the invading pathogen, but rather on the body's attempts to resist it. This is in contrast to the allopathic concept which is based on Pasteur's Germ Theory which, stated simply, believes that the primary causal agent of a disease is an external pathogen which has gained access to the body. Disease can therefore strike anybody. To prevent disease, we have to build defences. Still's understanding is more akin to that of the Cellular Theory of Antoine Bechamp (1816–1908) and Claude Bernard (1813–1878) which states that pathogens are nearly always present in the body, and therefore the body's tissues, 'the terrain', are constantly exposed to them, but the body's inherent systems have a capacity to resist them. They only become pathogenic as the health of the individual deteriorates; this could be due to stressors such as somatic dysfunction, psychological or social problems, poor diet, other pathology, etc. Therefore disease or illness occurs when in unhealthy conditions the inherent systems are caused to fail and the terrain becomes vulnerable. The implication is that if the cause of the excessive demand is found and resolved, the body will be able once again to resist the effects of the pathogens. Thus, to prevent disease we have to create health; to create health, the body structure must be as near normal as feasible.

WHEN THE NORMAL ADAPTABILITY IS DISRUPTED, OR WHEN ENVIRONMENTAL CHANGES OVERCOME THE BODY'S CAPACITY FOR SELF-MAINTENANCE, DISEASE MAY ENSUE

This is essentially an extrapolation of the latter two precepts. Its relevance is to perhaps make more explicit the holistic nature of the stressor, and the inherent capacity of the body to deal with most pathogenic agents, as long as its capacity is not overwhelmed. The term 'environmental' can be interpreted broadly so that stressors that could overcome the body's defences may be from any source, somatic, functional or pathological, psychosocial or spiritual. Stress is also accumulative, thus several small stresses, perhaps from differing sources, can have the same effect as one large stress. The effects of a stressor may also have long-term consequences such as unresolved grief or anger, or deformity resulting from poor union of a fracture; both could be significant components of an individual's 'environmental changes', decades after their original occurrence.

THE MOVEMENT OF THE BODY FLUIDS IS ESSENTIAL TO THE MAINTENANCE OF HEALTH

This precept is a clarification of the often cited principle that 'the rule of the artery is supreme'. The clarification ensures that one is concerned not only with arterial flow, but rather with the flow of any body fluid, including arterial, venous, lymphatic and cerebrospinal fluids. It is through these fluid systems that physiological processes are mediated,

including immunity, nutrition and detoxification, all of which are essential to the maintenance of health. Thus, any disturbance of this flow, directly or indirectly, will have an effect on well-being. The flow of bioenergy could also be included within this section.

NERVES PLAY A CRUCIAL PART IN CONTROLLING THE FLUIDS OF THE BODY

This is perhaps aimed at removing the apparent primacy of the fluid systems in the earlier precepts. It addresses both mechanical or direct impingement, and that produced reflexively via vasomotor control.

The mechanical aspects are largely dictated by the somatic nervous system, which controls muscle tone and thereby the gross posture of an individual. Changes in muscle tone will have possible consequences locally, i.e. if the muscles become hypertonic this could possibly affect contiguous fluid systems. Contraction of muscle can create a relative pressure barrier, impeding fluid flow; hence if the pelvic diaphragm is hypertonic there will be impaired fluid return from the lower extremities. More systemic or global changes can occur as a result of muscle tone changes leading to a modification of the body posture and thus of the way that the body cavities relate to each other, affecting their function as a whole, including fluid exchange. (These are discussed more fully in Section 2.)

The reflex control of vasomotion is mediated by the autonomic nervous system (ANS), with many of the fluid systems having direct relationships with the ANS. Thus changes in the ANS will affect body fluids and therefore its general health. The ANS itself is subject to stressors of any source, be they physical or psychological. This offers one mechanism through which problems within any aspect of the total osteopathic lesion, whether arising in the mind, body or spirit, may have global systemic effects. This is discussed more fully in Chapters 6, 7 and 9.

THERE ARE SOMATIC COMPONENTS TO DISEASE THAT ARE NOT ONLY MANIFESTATIONS OF DISEASE BUT ALSO CONTRIBUTE TO THE MAINTENANCE OF THE DISEASED STATE

This precept attempts to address the concept of reflex relationships that will arise when structures are subject to somatic dysfunction or become diseased, and the reciprocal relationship that arises between them. The clearest example is perhaps that of a visceral disease and its somatic manifestation.

If, for the sake of this discussion, a viscera is in a diseased state, neural information will convey this information to the appropriate spinal segment, where it will synapse with visceral efferents in an attempt to rectify the problem. It will also synapse with alpha and gamma motor efferents which will cause aberrant muscle tone, perhaps around the vertebral segment, and result in somatic dysfunction in the 'soma' or body. Thus, a viscerosomatic reflex has been instated. Osteopathic terminology distinguishes hierarchically between the first dysfunctioning structures, in this case the viscera, which would be called the primary lesion, and the dysfunction that arises as a consequence of this primary lesion, in this example the somatic problem, which would be termed the secondary lesion. Thus the secondary lesion is the somatic manifestation of a disease.

However, the precept indicates that this is not a one-way relationship, primary to secondary; as the secondary lesion begins to become dysfunctional itself, it will have a deleterious affect on the primary lesion, thus setting up a vicious cycle. Clinically, this is pertinent as in order to achieve resolution of a problem both elements will need to be addressed.

This example is a simplification. There may be multiple somatic secondaries; there may also be the possibility of visceral secondaries.

Having addressed the precepts it is of interest to look at the 'political platform' that Still originally envisaged for osteopathy.

STILL'S POLITICAL PLATFORM

This is stated in his *Research and Practice*:[30]

- First: We believe in sanitation and hygiene.
- Second: We are opposed to the use of drugs as remedial agencies.
- Third: We are opposed to vaccination.
- Fourth: We are opposed to the use of serums in the treatment of disease. Nature furnishes its own serum if we know how to deliver them.
- Fifth: We realize that many cases require surgical treatment and therefore advocate it as a last resort. We believe many surgical operations are unnecessarily performed and that many operations can be avoided by osteopathic treatment.

- Sixth: The osteopath does not rely on electricity, X-radiance, hydrotherapy or other adjuncts, but relies on osteopathic measures in the treatment of disease.
- Seventh: We have a friendly feeling for other non-drug, natural methods of healing, but we do not incorporate any other methods into our system. We are all opposed to drugs; in that respect at least, all natural unharmful methods occupy the same ground. The fundamental principles of osteopathy are different from those of any other system and the cause of disease is considered from one standpoint, viz: disease is the result of anatomical abnormalities followed by physiological discord. To cure disease the abnormal parts must be adjusted to the normal; therefore other methods that are entirely different in principle have no place in the osteopathic system.
- Eighth: Osteopathy is an independent system and can be applied to all conditions of disease, including purely surgical cases, and in these cases is but a branch of osteopathy.
- Ninth: We believe that our therapeutic house is just large enough for osteopathy and that when other methods are brought in just that much osteopathy must move out.

SUMMARY

The precepts offer an insight into Still's perception of the body. He stressed the unity of the body, from the macroscopic level (mind, body and spirit within a given environment), through the continuity and interdependence of the human body on an organic, tissue and cellular level. There is a synergy between all of these elements, enabling the body to regulate and defend itself, to achieve homeostasis and when problems arise, to repair itself. It is nourished by the fluid system and overseen by the neurological system.

In stating this, Still makes explicit some of the significant features of the body and its function. These concepts are not unique to osteopathy, and would have been understood even by Hippocrates. Perhaps, however, what is fundamental to osteopathic practice (and to that of other holistic body workers) is the structure–function reciprocity. With a deep understanding of the structure of the human body, differences from the norm can be perceived and an understanding of the functional changes that may arise can be derived. With this understanding and an ability to differentiate subtle changes in the affected tissues, it is possible to discover problems and resolve them before they have become frank pathology. An allopathic diagnosis would generally be made by noting the collection of signs and symptoms of a disease process; but these will only manifest themselves when frank pathophysiological changes have occurred. Thus, it is by applying the above precepts that osteopathy can work with the subclinical, prepathological states and, as well as resolving complaints that a patient is aware of, it can also function as a preventive medicine.

However, if disease has arisen, osteopathy has the tools to remove elements that may have been precipitating or may be maintaining factors of the diseased state, and to help the body activate its own defence and repair systems to restore itself, eliminating or reducing the need for medication. Thus, osteopathy can be a complete therapeutic system. This having been said, when Still originated his osteopathic political platform, medication was haphazard, passing from the useless through to the extreme of poison and with every shade between. Current pharmaceuticals have advanced from those days and many have the ability to save lives. There are not many osteopaths who would argue against the use of antibiotics in the management of bacterial meningitis (and Still's children might have survived had these been available in his time).

Although osteopathy is a complete system and an osteopathic rationale could be devised for treating almost any disease state, one should not hesitate from recommending another approach should this appear to be the most effective treatment for any particular condition.

A separate point that has current value is that with an armamentarium practically bursting the doors of the 'osteopathic therapeutic house', it is perhaps pertinent to reflect on the ninth statement and, by thorough critical reflection and appropriate research, begin to dispense with some of the more redundant methods.

Finally, Still saw the body as a whole. He never demonstrated techniques, but rather whole treatments. He did not talk about lesions in the sense that the term 'osteopathic lesion' is used today, but rather used terms such as 'strains', 'sprains', 'twisted vertebrae', 'bony lesions', and even in a few cases 'hypermobility'. He promoted a very holistic approach. It has been said earlier that his students found it difficult to assimilate all that Still tried to convey. In their attempt to understand, and later to convey Still's ideas to their own students, they attempted to dissect his approach with rational thought and analysed the parts independently. This hailed the second stage, the structural–mechanical era. Of great importance in this period was the concept of the osteopathic lesion and its role in disease. This will be explored in the following chapter; however, before passing to that, it is germane to reflect that though the reason for the dissection of Still's concepts is understandable, and educationally it may be perceived that such disection does facilitate the learning of otherwise complex concepts, it carries with it an inherent danger. The danger is that the concepts, having been deconstructed, may later not be reconstructed, thus losing that which is arguably the most important principle of osteopathy, that the body is a whole and that the whole is greater than the sum of the parts.

References

1. Still AT. Osteopathy research and practice. Kirskville: Journal Printing; 1910.
2. Fossum C. Lecture notes. Maidstone: Unpublished; 2003.
3. Tucker EE. The word 'osteopathy'. Osteopath 1904; May:194–196.
4. Tucker EE, Wilson PT. The theory of osteopathy. Kirskville: Journal Printing; 1936.
5. Chila AG. Exposition of Still's thought: the word 'osteopathy'. J Am Acad Osteopath 2003; 13(2):2.
6. Warner MD et al. The osteopathic concept. Tentative formulation of a teaching guide for faculty, hospital staff and student body prepared by the special committee on osteopathic principles and osteopathic technic. AAO; 1954:57–59.
7. Wolf AH. Osteopathy – A state of mind. Colorado Scott memorial lecture – 1965. AAO; 1966:42–46.
8. Hoover MA. Some studies in osteopathy. AAO; 1951:55–72.
9. Still AT. Autobiography. Kirksville: Journal Printing; 1897.
10. Ashmore EF. Osteopathic mechanics. Kirksville: Journal Printing; 1915; 2.
11. Proby JC. Essay on osteopathy. Oxford: private printing; 1937:13.
12. Page LE. The principles of osteopathy. Kansas City: AAO; 1952:31–32.
13. Kuchera WA, Kuchera ML. Osteopathic principles in practice, 2nd edn. Columbus: Original Works; 1992; 2.

14. General Osteopathic Council. Online. Available: http://www.osteopathy.org.uk 3 Aug 2003.

15. Educational Council on Osteopathic Principles. Glossary of osteopathic terminology. Chicago: American Association of Colleges of Osteopathic Medicine; 2002.

16. Latey P. Still and osteopathy before 1900. Aust J Osteopath 1990; Dec:2–17.

17. Littre E. Oeuvres completes d'Hippocrates. Vol I:1839. In: Kulungian H. On the moral obligation of the medical profession according to Hippocrates. 1999. Online. Available: http://www.macrodiet.com/Contributors/Kulungian-Hippocrates.shtml 24 Aug 2003.

18. Lever R. An osteopathic orientation within a social context. J Soc Osteopath 1981; 10.

19. Abehsera A. Concepts of bo ne setting mesmerism. Israel: Unpublished lecture notes; 2002.

20. Trowbridge C. Andrew Taylor Still, 1828–1917. Kirksville: Thomas Jefferson University Press; 1991.

21. Abehsera A. The roots of osteopathic technique: healers and bone-setters. Israel: Unpublished lecture notes; 2002.

22. Dummer T. A textbook of osteopathy, vol 1. Hadlow Down: JoTom Publications; 1999.

23. Webster Jones S. Osteopathy as revealed in the writings of A T Still, Martin Littlejohn Memorial lecture 1954. London: The Osteopathic Publishing Company; 1954.

24. GOsC. Osteopathy in the United Kingdom. Online. Available: http://www.osteopathy.org.uk/goc/law/index.shtml 6 Sept 2003.

25. Special committee on Osteopathic Principles and Osteopathic Technic. An interpretation of osteopathic concept. Tentative formulation of a teaching guide for faculty, hospital staff and student body. Journal of Osteopathy 1953; 60 (October):8–10.

26. DiGiovanna EL, Schiowitz R, eds. An osteopathic approach to diagnosis and treatment. Philadelphia: JB Lippincott; 1991.

27. Still AT. Philosophy and mechanical principles of osteopathy. Kirksville: Journal Printing; 1902: 22–23.

28. Jordan T, Schuster R, eds. Selected writings of Carl Philip McConnell, D.O. Columbus: Squirrel's Tail Press; 1994:34.

29. Still AT. Autobiography, 2nd edn. Kirksville: Journal Printing; 1908.

30. Still AT. Osteopathy research and practice. Kirksville: Journal Printing; 1910: 14–15.

Chapter 2

The osteopathic lesion or somatic dysfunction

INTRODUCTION AND DEFINITION

Defining the osteopathic lesion, like defining osteopathy itself, is difficult. In a recent lecture, the author stated that one of the General Osteopathic Council's (GOsC) working definitions of osteopathy was 'Osteopathy is what osteopaths do'. When he later asked the students to define an osteopathic lesion one wit replied, 'That which osteopaths find!'

There is in fact much truth in this statement, as the definition appears to be dependent on one's perception or understanding of osteopathy. This chapter will attempt to discuss the commonly used models and underlying principles of the osteopathic lesion.

The expression 'osteopathic lesion' has tended to be superseded in more recent years by the term 'somatic dysfunction'.[1] This was defined as 'an impaired or altered function of related components of the somatic framework; skeletal, arthroidal, myofascial and related vascular, lymphatic and neural elements'.[2]

The principal reason for this change was the confusion that arose from the word lesion. Lesion has different meanings within the osteopathic and allopathic paradigms. In allopathic terms, lesion indicates a pathological entity or process. Osteopathically, it is indicative of a functional rather than a pathological problem, hence the more recent use of 'dysfunction'. Additionally, the 'osteopathic' descriptor tends to indicate exclusivity in diagnosis and treatment to osteopaths. This is relevant as, with the growing interest in manual medicine, these concepts are being shared and anything that permits ease of communication and breaks down barriers between the various disciplines is beneficial.

In this text, the terms have tended to be used interchangeably, the reason being that when discussing some of the early osteopathic concepts the word lesion is an integral part of the terminology (e.g. first degree lesion). It is felt that it would not be appropriate to retrospectively modify this to 'first degree dysfunction', and the same applies to other similar terms.

Thus, in this book, any usage of 'lesion' will mean a functional rather than pathological entity, unless clearly stated otherwise.

In an attempt to define what is meant by the term 'somatic dysfunction' the following chapter will offer several different perspectives and also trace some of the concepts from a historical perspective.

ANATOMICAL FINDINGS IN JOINT DYSFUNCTION

When attempting to understand joint dysfunction it is possible to analyse it from two major perspectives: quantitative and qualitative.

A *quantitative approach* addresses the range of movement that each structure is subject to. This applies to visceral and cranial structures as well as the musculoskeletal articulations discussed below.

Each articulation has a normal range of movement that, in the ideal situation, it is able to move through. This is governed by local articular factors, such as the type and shape of the joint itself and the nature of the supporting myofascial structures. It is possible to find the specific direction and expected ranges of movement of each articulation in relevant text books. However, there are often differences in the values cited by these texts. This may possibly be due to differing research methods employed or perhaps to the more individual or person-specific factors such as the gender, age, biotype and health state of the individuals assessed. For example women's articulations are generally slightly more mobile than those of men. Articular flexibility and range of movement usually reduces as age increases. The biotype of the person will have an effect, as will their state of general health and the degree to which they have exercised, or even overused, an articulation.

Osteopathically, it is necessary to be aware of the 'ideal' or expected range and planes of movement of each articulation, and then to have the flexibility to superimpose any of the above individual differences noted in the person being assessed and, by applying this, to arrive at some concept of what their actual norm is likely to be.

This process is an excellent exercise in understanding the musculoskeletal system and developing the concept of an individual's norm as opposed to the textual norm. In a clinical situation, it is also helpful to compare an articulation with its paired or similar articulation, though when differences in range of movement are found it is important to know whether the relative hypomobile or hypermobile range is the norm for that individual.

This approach is objective, permitting one to utilize apparatus, such as a goniometer, to record the actual differences in range of movement. Usually, however, it is the palpatory and visual sense of difference in range of movement that is used in daily practice.

The *qualitative approach* is a subjective perspective that is utilized in somatic dysfunction analysis. It assesses the quality of movement, assessing whether movement is free flowing or whether there is a disturbance in the quality of the movement. If there is disturbance, it is important to assess whether it is throughout the entire range of movement, or if it occurs at a specific point of movement. The nature of the disturbance is also relevant, be it fine or coarse, hard or soft, as well as the nature of the associated soft tissues: elastic, indurated, boggy, hot, cold, etc. The sensations noticed by the individual also contribute to the qualitative assessment of dysfunction, such as whether it feels tender or painful.

Being subjective, this approach is not verifiable by conventional analytical methods and utilizes terms that may sound naïve and unscientific, such as 'boggy' or 'sticky'. However, this qualitative palpatory sense is as critical to the understanding of somatic dysfunction as the quantitative, the two together combining to give the necessary information to make an initial diagnosis of that dysfunction. By the nature of its subjectivity, it is the responsibility of each individual practitioner to develop their own 'palpatory reference library' and to make the links to the underlying functional or pathophysiological changes that have caused the symptoms to occur.

These two perspectives will now be addressed more fully.

QUANTITATIVE CONSIDERATIONS IN ARTICULAR SOMATIC DYSFUNCTION

Each articulation has an active and passive range of movement. 'Active' means that the movement can be achieved by voluntary contraction of the muscles acting on the articulation. There is possible movement beyond this range, but this can only be achieved passively; that is, movement introduced by someone other than the individual being assessed, and this is therefore not under voluntary control. The end-points of these movements are termed 'barriers'.

Active movement is said to stop at the 'physiological barrier'. This is determined by the tension in the soft tissues around the joint (e.g. muscles, ligaments, joint capsule). The normal range of movement of a joint occurs within the physiological barriers of this joint. This range can be slightly increased if the individual regularly exercises, particularly with stretching type exercises, and generally decreases with age.

However, movement can be introduced passively beyond the physiological barrier, stretching the supporting soft tissues until the limit of tension in these tissues is reached. This is the 'anatomical barrier' (Fig. 2.1). If a movement is applied beyond the anatomical barrier, it will damage the surrounding soft tissues and disrupt the joint structure, and the resulting damage would be considered within the realms of pathology. The anatomical barrier can not be altered by exercise.

Somatic dysfunction occurs when there is a restriction of motion occurring within the normal range of movement. This restriction of movement is sometimes termed a 'restriction barrier'. Most osteopathic experts believe that true osteopathic dysfunction can only occur within the physiological barriers. This will certainly be the case with compensatory dysfunction, but in the case of traumatically induced problems it is felt that they can occur beyond the physiological barrier up to the anatomical barrier, and still be non-pathological and reversible. In the following discussion a somatic dysfunction will be considered to occur within the normal range of motion, i.e. within the physiological barriers.

In the case of pathological change in an articulation (such as osteoarthritis, fracture, cancer, oedema, etc.) there will be a 'pathological barrier'. As with the osteopathic lesion this can also occur within the physiological barrier, and generally there will be a limitation in all ranges of movement of the affected articulation.

When somatic dysfunction occurs (for the sake of this discussion in the absence of any underlying or secondary problems) there will be a restriction of movement before the physiological barrier in one or more of the possible planes of movement. In each affected plane of movement there will be one direction away from the neutral where the range of movement is less than full, whilst the range of movement in the other direction remains full. This is a useful finding to differentiate between a pathological problem and somatic dysfunction, as with pathological problems movement is generally limited in all directions, whereas with somatic dysfunction, as just stated, one direction of movement is limited but the other full.

Thus, to consider a vertebra that has a dysfunction in rotation, it would be possible to find, for example, that on passive testing, rotation to the right from neutral to the physiological barrier is found to be full, but when left rotation is attempted, restriction to this movement is found before the left physiological barrier is attained. The point of limitation is the restriction barrier (R). This would be termed a right rotated somatic dysfunction and is shown in Figure 2.2.

The naming of lesions is bound by certain conventions, to ensure that there is some accord amongst the profession. In Figure 2.2 there are two pertinent conventions:

1. The direction in which a vertebra moves is always named by the direction in which the vertebral body moves. In Figure 2.2, the body moves fully to the right but not fully to the left, so right rotation is greater than left. (This can occasionally create confusion, as, when performing passive vertebral movement testing, the spinous process of the vertebrae is the structure contacted, and it is possible to become focused on its movement, the findings of which would be opposite to that of the body; however, the body is always the point of reference.)
2. The lesion is always named by the direction of the ease of movement rather than the direction of bind. Thus, in Figure 2.2, this would be termed a right rotated (or rotating) lesion. The same logic will apply to any of the planes of movement in which the joint is capable of moving, and any or all of which may be affected depending upon the complexity of the lesion.

This concept often appears to be counter-intuitive to students. An oversimplified concept that may help with visualization of this convention is to

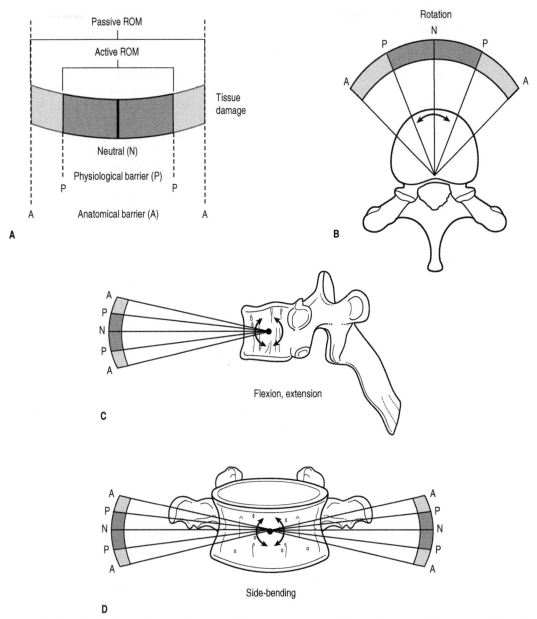

Figure 2.1 Anatomical (A) and physiological (P) barriers. Active movement occurs between the physiological barriers, the passive range of motion occurs between the anatomical barriers. Movement beyond the anatomical barriers will result in physical damage of the articulation and its supporting structures. **(A)** Schematic; **(B)** rotation; **(C)** flexion extension; **(D)** side-bending.

imagine a muscle, attached to the transverse process, as the initiating and maintaining factor in the dysfunction. To rotate the vertebra to the right, the muscle on the right transverse process would have to actively shorten, and to remain actively shortened to perpetuate it. If one attempted to rotate that vertebra to the left it would pull against the shortened right-sided muscle, limiting the range of movement in that direction. If, however, one attempted to rotate it to the right, the shortened muscle would further shorten and not impede rotation, thus moving more easily into the direction of the lesion. This is shown schematically in Figure 2.3.

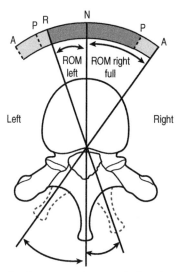

Figure 2.2 Passive segmental motion findings in rotation for a vertebra with a right rotated somatic dysfunction. Passively rotating the vertebra to the right results in a full range of movement terminating at the anatomical barrier (A). Passive rotation to the left is found to be limited, stopping before the physiological barrier has been reached. The point where this movement is limited by somatic dysfunction is termed the restriction barrier (R).

Please note that this is not a complete explanation of how lesions are maintained, but a simple illustration aimed to try to demonstrate how it is possible for the ease of movement to be in the direction of the lesion.

The principal active movements that joints are capable of are rotation, side-bending (lateroflexion), and flexion or extension. There are other often smaller accessory movements that can occur passively or as a consequence of, or coupled with, the greater movements. The most important of these is known as translation (gliding or shearing), which is movement of two contiguous parts of an articulation sliding relative to each other in a direction parallel to their plane of contact. This can occur in a lateral, anterior/posterior, or superior/inferior plane.

The above movements relate to dysfunction within the musculoskeletal system. Earlier it was stated that these concepts apply equally to the other structures in the body. The principles are the same, though it is not currently possible to look up the expected range of movement of a liver or a temporal bone! Every structure within the body is maintained in its position by the complex interplay of connective tissue (as has been described above with the articular structures). This tissue is divided into ligaments, capsules and tendons for ease of anatomical description, but osteopathically it is perhaps better to consider it as a connective tissue matrix (see Ch. 4 on tensegrity). Thus, in the ideal situation, there will be a range of movement that is permitted within this soft tissue matrix, within the equivalent of the physiological barrier, and if movement is encouraged beyond this point, stretching the supporting soft tissues, it will be possible to feel the point equivalent to the anatomical barrier. Dysfunction can be assessed on a quantitative level by palpating the permissible ranges of movement of any structure; where premature restriction of a movement occurs, dysfunction has been located. When the normal range of movement of that structure has been restored, then quantitatively that structure has been corrected. (Reflecting on the fact that the range of movement of any bodily structure is dictated by the supporting connective tissue matrix, it is perhaps possible to understand why there is such a wide variety of normal, as this matrix is as unique to an individual as their fingerprints and is an expression of all of the processes that are occurring within any individual at any time.)

The situation can become slightly more complicated when addressing the involuntary aspect of cranial, visceral or fascial osteopathic practice. In the above description it is the mobility of the structures that is being assessed. Within the involuntary field, one is assessing the motility as opposed to the mobility of the structures.

- 'Mobile' refers to an object's ability to have freedom of movement, to be moveable.
- 'Motile' refers to the inherent and spontaneous movement of a structure.

This is an important distinction to make; thus, rather than introducing a movement to assess mobility, the practitioner 'listens' to the inherent motility using a passive receptive hand.

Motility is usually described in terms of respiratory flexion and extension (as in primary respiration or cranial respiration, not the respiration of breathing which is termed secondary respiration). During respiratory flexion, the skull and body reduce in anterior posterior diameter and superior inferior diameter whilst increasing bilaterally laterally. This causes the midline unpaired structures to flex and the peripheral (paired) structures, which includes

Figure 2.3   A schematic demonstration to illustrate how it may be possible for a vertebra to move more freely into the direction of the lesion. **(A)** Rotation of the vertebra to the left will be resisted by the active contraction of the muscle on the right side. **(B)** Rotation to the right will further approximate the origin in insertion of the actively contracted right muscle, which will therefore offer no resistance to the movement. The left muscle will be stretched but as it is not actively contracting, it will offer limited resistance to movement. Thus, movement is easier into the direction of the lesion.

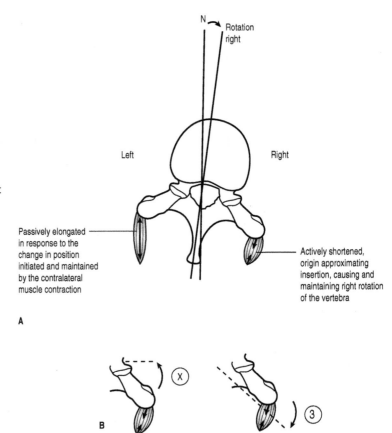

Left

Right

N — Rotation right

Passively elongated in response to the change in position initiated and maintained by the contralateral muscle contraction

Actively shortened, origin approximating insertion, causing and maintaining right rotation of the vertebra

A

B

the body extremities and viscera, to externally rotate. Respiratory extension is the reverse of this. Thus, unlike structural flexion or extension which describes movement of all structures with regard to the anatomical position, or approximation and separation of an articulation, respiratory flexion is more complicated and relates to the separate interactions of the articulations. More specific information on these movements will be dealt with in the relevant chapters in Section 3.

From a quantitative perspective, the basic criteria for assessing motile structures are amplitude and rate. Amplitude is the full range of movement from respiratory flexion to respiratory extension and the rate is generally described as the number of these cycles that occur in a minute.

QUALITATIVE CONSIDERATIONS IN ARTICULAR SOMATIC DYSFUNCTION

Qualitative assessment of articular movement is an important diagnostic tool for assessing both pathological and functional problems. Fluent movement is dependent on many elements, including articular integrity, 'correct' physiological processes and even the phenomenally complex interplay between the soft tissues and the neuroendocrine immune system. Absence of this fluency may lead one to suspect an underlying dysfunction.

This may be a minor disturbance, such as movement not feeling 'quite as free' as its paired articulation, perhaps indicating general soft tissue changes due to a local inflammatory response or, at the other end of the spectrum, the gross findings of coarse crepitus associated with articular degeneration from osteoarthritis, or cog wheel rigidity due to the neurological disturbance associated with Parkinson's disease.

There are numerous medical texts that discuss pathological qualitative findings, therefore the following discussion will focus principally on the non-pathological situation. Also as with the previous section, the concepts will first be explored with regard to a musculoskeletal dysfunction, and will then be applied to other systems.

Dysfunction in the supporting connective tissue matrix, as well as causing problems within the range of movement, will also have an effect on the quality of this movement. This will obviously be subject to the individual variation cited earlier, but it will also be subject to the changes that occur in the soft tissues over time. Initially, the body tries to resolve and repair any problems; if it is unable so to do, it will adapt. As time passes, the soft tissues progressively change and these changes are discernable through palpation. Thus the qualitative 'feel' of a dysfunctioning area can give information regarding both the nature of the underlying problem and an indication of how long the problem has been present. The range of qualitative changes are described in a variety of ways. These will be discussed below.

End feel

The quality at the end range of the movement is termed the 'end feel'. In a non-lesioned articulation it describes the quality of the movement between the physiological and anatomical barriers. As previously stated the physiological barrier is the end-point of active movement, where the articulations' periarticular soft tissues are engaged. Passively taking the joint beyond that range will stretch these tissues, thus in a normally functioning joint an elastic and progressive tissue tension should be felt towards the end-range of motion.

When an articulation is in lesion, it is observed that end feel is felt before the physiological range of movement. The end feel varies according to the articulation and on the tissues limiting the movement.[3,4]

- Muscles can cause a range of end feel, from soft and elastic to a relatively hard 'twangy' sensation, depending on the degree of protective spasm present.
- Ligaments or capsule limiting the movement create a firm and elastic end feel, as if stretching thick rubber.

- A springy block at the extreme range of movement would be suggestive of an intraarticular displacement, such as a meniscal tear.
- Fibrosis associated with the more chronic restrictions has a very rapid build-up in tension occurring close to the limiting barrier and with a firmer elasticity than felt with a hypertonic muscle or ligamentous problem.
- An abrupt stop to the movement short of the normal range of motion that is hard and inelastic would suggest a bony limitation.

Dysfunction may result in hypermobility as well as the hypomobility discussed so far. Hypermobility is difficult to appreciate by palpation: there is often a sensation of increased elasticity of the joint complex and increased range of motion, with a rapid build-up of tension and hardness as one reaches the end of the range of motion.

Additionally oedema is associated with an end feel that is 'boggy'. Pain often causes a sudden, jerky and at times inconsistent ratchet-like sensation, often due to guarding behaviour of the muscles associated with the joint. The relationship between the onset of pain and the resistance is also very useful diagnostically.

The onset of pain before any resistance is felt is indicative of possible pathology or extraarticular lesion, such as acute bursitis, abscess or neoplasia. The lack of resistance is due to the fact that pain has limited the movement before the articulation has been engaged (this is sometimes termed an 'empty' end feel).

If the resistance and pain are synchronous this would indicate an active dysfunction, and the nature of the end feel would reflect the degree of acuteness. Thus a hard, muscular end feel would indicate a more acute dysfunction, and a firm, elastic feel would be less acute.

If the resistance to the movement is felt before the onset of pain, this would be indicative of a more chronic dysfunction.

Tissue texture changes

The quality of the tissue surrounding a joint is perhaps one of the principal indicators of somatic dysfunction of that articulation. These tissues include the skin, muscles, ligaments, joint capsules and subcutaneous fat. Palpation of these tissues not only indicates the presence of dysfunction but can also give an indication of the age of the lesion, i.e. whether it is acute, subacute or chronic. These tissue changes are often referred to as 'tissue texture abnormalities'.

The changes are mainly driven by the action of the local tissue or humoral response and its interaction with the sympathetic nervous system.

In the initial acute stage of injury, the affected tissues release vasodilator substances (e.g. bradykinin). This leads to an inflammatory response and local oedema. The area will become hot, red, swollen and tender.

There is a simultaneous increase in sympathetic autonomic nervous system activity. The sympathetic system controls blood vessels, sweat gland activity and the erector pilae muscles. In the acute stage, the sympathetic action on the local blood supply is to cause vasoconstriction and therefore relative decrease in perfusion; however, in the early stages of dysfunction the action of bradykinin overpowers the sympathetic activity, thus there is a resultant vasodilatation and consequently local oedema is present. There will also be increased local sweat gland activity, and possibly raised hairs, where present.

As time passes the local tissue response decreases and the vasoconstrictive effects of the sympathetic system become more apparent. The area concerned consequently receives a reduction in blood flow. With greater time the reduction in perfusion becomes more apparent and in very chronic states the signs of relative hypoxia become marked. The area concerned will become cold and pale, the skin quality becomes poor with signs such as local skin dryness and flaking, increase in skin pore size, and spots. Sweat gland activity also decreases due to progressive fatigue of the sweat glands, further exacerbating the skin dryness.

Whilst the above relates particularly to the effects observed within the connective tissue, these changes are also observable within the muscle tissue. On a muscular level, what is first observed is a reactive muscle spasm (this being a protective mechanism). After about a week, this reactive spasm decreases but a hypertrophy of the muscle is observed, due to the continued neural output maintaining the muscle contraction, and the lesion pattern.

Later, the muscle begins to fatigue leading to progressive hypotrophy. As the muscle is still being required to contract, connective tissue starts to be deposited in the muscle fibres to maintain the muscle shortening with minimal energy expenditure to the body.

If the problem is not resolved, the fibrosing process continues and may lead to marked fibrosis of the muscle. There will also be associated atrophy of the muscle.

Louisa Burns[5] researched the changes that occur over time in somatic dysfunction. She identified at least eight stages:

1. Hyperaemia in the capillary bed, which will be evident in the first few minutes.
2. Congestion of blood in the precapillary arterioles, occurring in less than 10 minutes.
3. Oedema or the accumulation of fluid in the tissue space will be seen in 30 to 40 minutes.
4. In several hours, minute haemorrhages or petechiae will appear in the oedematous fluid.
5. In 3 to 7 days, organization of the petechiae will be seen.
6. Organization, which is the canaliculization of the petechiae by the infiltration of fibrocytes, will result in one of two changes: absorption of the petechiae, or continuing fibrocytic invasion with early fibrotic changes in the ground substance.
7. If fibrosis continues, it will shut off the capillary circulation and result in ischaemia over the next several months.
8. Ischaemia will eventually lead to atrophy of the periarticular tissues.

Part of these tissue changes will be mirrored in any tissues or organs that are segmentally related to the area of dysfunction via the embryological metameric divisions, i.e. that segment of the spinal cord supplied by one pair (right and left) of motor and one pair of sensory nerves including the:

- Myotome: all of the muscles supplied by the paired nerves exiting that spinal segment. (This will also involve the complex reflex balance between agonist and antagonists.)
- Dermatome: leading to areas of tenderness or dysthesia and nutritional changes on the skin due to impaired sympathetic supply to the superficial capillary beds, sweat glands and sebaceous glands of that dermatome.
- Sclerotome: leading to periarticular, ligamentous or periostial pain.
- Viscerotome (enterotome): causing disturbed visceral dysfunction (somaticovisceral reflex) as well as 'tender points' such as Chapman's reflexes or Jarricot's dermalgie réflexe (viscerocutaneous reflex).

This is summarized in Table 2.1.

Though the terms boggy, ropey and stringy sound rather unscientific, they are useful descriptors and have been defined in the *Glossary of Osteopathic Terminology*[2] as follows:

- Bogginess: A tissue texture abnormality characterized principally by a palpable sense of sponginess in the tissue, interpreted as resulting from congestion due to increased fluid content.
- Ropiness: A tissue texture abnormality characterized by a cord-like feeling.
- Stringiness: A palpable tissue texture abnormality characterized by fine or string-like myofascial structures.

Asymmetry

Due to the asymmetrical muscle tonicity associated with somatic dysfunction, asymmetry may be observable and palpable in comparison with its opposite if paired, or other similar joints if not. This is noticeable in the articulation itself and its associated soft tissues. There may also be consequent asymmetry in the whole body, as it attempts to adapt to the local dysfunction. This asymmetry may be noticed through positional change, changes in function or, as is more usual, both position and function. Static or observed asymmetry alone is not a reliable indicator of dysfunction as there are many bony and soft tissue anomalies that can occur in the absence of somatic dysfunction; a common example of this is the spinous processes of the thoracic vertebrae. They are often not straight, and the resulting deviation to one side could be interpreted as a rotation to the opposite side; however, when passively segmentally tested, it may be found to have an equal movement bilaterally thus indicating that there is no dysfunction and that the spinous process is anomalous. Therefore it is always important to first observe the body for asymmetry, then to test it.

Not all asymmetry is significant or needs to be 'corrected'. There are numerous genetic or postural asymmetries, such as those arising from right or left handedness, which one needs to be aware of but not necessarily attempt to resolve.

Tenderness

This is due to the humoral or inflammatory response, and the neurological response to the dysfunction. Generally, the more recent the dysfunction, the greater the tenderness. As the lesion becomes more chronic in nature the tenderness decreases and may disappear totally. Thus pain and tenderness is only useful in indicating the presence of an acute lesion. Tenderness appears to be becoming progressively more used as an indication of the significance of a lesion. This is incorrect; it is not possible through pain or tenderness alone to intuit any primacy or particular osteopathic significance to any underlying dysfunction.

Temperature

In the acute stage of dysfunction it is often possible to palpate a slight increase in temperature, either at the skin surface or by running your hand about 15 cm above the area (this is generally termed 'thermal diagnosis'). Again, this is caused by the initial humoral effect. As the lesion becomes older the temperature difference will become less pronounced. In very chronic lesions, where the blood supply has become reduced, the area may feel slightly colder. Thermal diagnosis is used by some osteopaths to indicate the relative state of the viscera as part of the somaticovisceral or viscerotomal relationship, the interpretation of the findings being based on the above logic.

Table 2.1 A comparison of tissue changes in an acute and chronic somatic dysfunction

	Acute	Chronic
Skin	Inflammatory response: oedema, vasodilatation, hot, red, increased sweat gland activity	Skin is pale, cold, dry with signs of trophic changes such as spots, increased skin pore size
Subcutaneous tissues	'Boggy' feel	Indurated and atrophied
Muscles	Acute reactive muscle spasm, contraction, leading to hypertrophy	Atrophy ± fibrotic insertions, leading to fibrosis 'Ropey' or 'stringy' feel
Neural reflexes	Initially may not be apparent	Somaticosomatic and somaticovisceral reflexes
Pain	Tenderness or acute pain	Slight or absent tenderness

With regard to non-articular structures and the qualitative assessment, mention has already been made concerning the soft tissue changes that occur. In addition, as they guide all movement in the body, the qualitative changes in mobility can be deduced. Regarding the qualitative changes expected within the motile structures, rhythmicity is an important factor (i.e. how the structure is moving with regard to its axes of movement and with regard to its contiguous structures). Rate, rhythm and amplitude are the basic criteria for assessing motility in any structure. Beyond rhythm there is a phenomenal and confusing range of qualitative terms used to describe the state of tissues. These are often idiosyncratic and often only truly meaningful to particular individuals or small groups of people who have worked together and have established a communicable palpatory language. But they are no less important for this. The different tissues all have a particular feel and this will change depending on their particular state; this cannot be learnt from a book but will require coaching with an experienced teacher and practitioner, and an ability for you, yourself, to accept and analyse what you feel to enable you to make these links for yourself.

SUMMARY

It is through the summation of both quantitative and qualitative findings that one obtains an indication of the nature and age of the underlying dysfunction. Several mnemonics have appeared over recent years that attempt to summarize the findings in somatic dysfunction; none of these is complete, but they are useful as aides-mémoire.

TART[2]
Tissue texture abnormality
Asymmetry
Range of motion abnormality
Tenderness.

STAR[6]
Sensibility changes
Tissue texture abnormality
Asymmetry
Restricted range of motion.

PRATT
Pain
Range of movement abnormality
Asymmetry
Tissue changes
Temperature.

These offer the main diagnostic criteria for a somatic dysfunction, most particularly an acute dysfunction. There is insufficient mention of the end feel of an articulation; however, if that can be incorporated, they are reasonably complete.

The term 'restricted movement' is often used in the mnemonics TART and STAR. The reason that range of motion and abnormality (from PRATT) has been utilized in this text is because the dysfunction may have hypermobility associated with it, rather than hypomobility.

STAR has the advantage of including sensibility changes rather than pain or tenderness, allowing for the full range of sensation changes that can accompany any dysfunction.

INTRODUCTION TO CONCEPTS OF LESIONS

There are several different ways to conceptualize somatic dysfunction or the osteopathic lesion. Many were devised early in the genesis of osteopathy, and have been modified by subsequent generations, and none is without its detractors. The main models will be presented to enable you to obtain an overview of the various concepts, to help you to challenge them yourself. Inherent within these models are concepts related to:

- causation of the lesion – traumatic, postural or compensatory;
- temporal considerations – reflecting the changes that may have occurred in the lesion with time;
- hierarchical concepts – which is the first or most significant lesion, which are compensatory; and
- physiological aspects – proposed models of spinal movement and aspects of the distal effects mediated largely via the nervous system.

The term lesion is being used in this discussion as the models are early and predate the use of dysfunction.

Conceptualization and the description of lesions is an area where much confusion exists. Paradoxically, it appears generally that what is being said is the same, but it is being said in differing ways. Where possible this section will draw parallels between these apparently differing concepts.

FIRST AND SECOND DEGREE LESIONS

One of the means of classifying somatic dysfunction in the UK is by utilizing the terms first or second degree lesions. Inherent within these terms are the possible causative factors, and the response of the segments over time. The causative factors in fact relate to Fryette's theories of spinal motion, though this aspect is often lost in the UK. As Fryette's nomenclature is used widely in Europe, included at the end of each section is the equivalent Fryette nomenclature for ease of cross reference. A fuller explanation of Fryette's nomenclature is presented later in this chapter.

Causative factors

A first degree lesion is considered primarily to be due to a traumatic event, usually affecting a single vertebra at one of the pivotal areas of the spine, occurring whilst the spine is out of neutral position. The subsequent coupled movements of rotation and side-bending occur to the same side (ipsilateral), i.e. if rotation is to the right, side-bending will also be to the right. (In early osteopathic texts this lesion is known as a 'Still lesion'.)

In Fryette's terms it would be described as an extension, rotation, side-bending lesion, abbreviated to an ERS lesion.

A second degree lesion is thought to be principally adaptive or postural, thus tending to occur when the spine is in neutral. These lesions tend to occur as group lesions, which are several vertebral segments moving as one complex in the direction of the lesion. The rotation and side-bending occur in opposite directions (contralaterally). Thus, if rotation is to the right, side-bending will occur to the left. Occasionally this pattern of contralateral rotation and side-bending may not occur, due to the direction of the forces applied by the faulty repetitive postural or occupational changes overriding the anatomical 'logic'.

In Fryette's terminology the second degree lesion is termed a flexion, rotation, side-bending lesion, the flexion referring to the 'easy normal flexion', Fryette's term for the neutral position of the spine. This is abbreviated to an FSR or sometimes NSR (the F and N representing the easy normal flexion).

Where UK nomenclature differs from much of the rest of Europe is that both first and second degree lesions can occur in either flexion or extension. This is in contrast to 'pure' application of Fryettian concepts of ERS and FRS.

To name these lesions, the convention is to state whether it is first or second degree, and then to cite the direction of the rotation. By understanding the principles of first and second degree lesion and knowing the direction of the rotation, the direction of side-bending should be understood. The appropriate flexion or extension component is then added at the end.

It can be seen that in this system of nomenclature the lesions are named by the rotation.

For example, a first degree right lesion (abbreviated to 1°R or 1st °R) is:

- First degree – this would mean that rotation and side-bending will occur ipsilaterally.
- The right relates to the rotation, in this case being to the right.
- As it is in first degree and rotation and side-bending are ipsilateral, the side-bending will also be to the right.
- Flexion means that the lesion is also in flexion.

A second degree left flexion would mean left rotation and right side-bending in flexion.

As will be seen later, this is a somewhat flexible interpretation of Fryette's principles.

As well as the causal element inherent within these terms there are also considerations relating to anticipated changes with the passage of time.

Temporal considerations

As stated, a first degree lesion generally arises as a result of a traumatic event, thus it is an acute episode with all of the consequent local tissue changes (see the discussion on tissue changes in acute lesions earlier in this chapter). At this stage the effects are purely local and functional.

If the body is unable to resolve the resulting lesion and the individual does not seek treatment, the lesion then tries to 'stabilize' itself. It can do this by creating compensations with other vertebrae in the spine, and/or by adapting at the lesioned segment itself.

Other vertebrae, either local to the site or distal to it, will begin to compensate, and this can often involve a group of vertebrae adapting to the original dysfunction. These compensating lesions will be second degree lesions with rotation and side-bending occurring in opposite directions. This may be sufficient to create adequate balance within the spine. The whole process of establishing a compensatory pattern that results in postural balance may take weeks or months. This will have an effect on the tissues local to both the initial area of dysfunction and those areas compensating for it, thus the joint capsule, overlying muscles, associated nerves and blood vessels, all tending to a chronic state. It will also begin to have an effect on those associated distal structures, such as segmentally supplied viscera, via the somaticovisceral reflex. The longer the dysfunction has been present the more marked the tissue changes will be, both locally and distally, resulting in progressively greater functional or even pathological tissue changes; and proportionately the longer the expected prognosis and duration of treatment.

Also, there will be changes occurring at the site of the original lesion, starting usually within a few days. The process often involves a counter rotation from the original position, heading towards a slightly more stable position. As the vertebra is in lesion and by definition is not able to resolve itself fully, the counter rotation may be slight, and the resulting lesion positionally will still appear to be a first degree lesion, but if the segment is motion tested there will be limitation in *both* directions of rotation. This is because the initial rotation, say for example to the right, would by definition result in left rotation being limited. However, as the vertebra attempts to rotate to the left, right rotation will be limited, hence the bilateral limitation. This is often quite difficult to diagnose, as the rotation may be approximately equal (but limited) at the segment, therefore it will be picked up by comparison with its adjacent vertebral segments. There will also be chronic tissue changes at the affected segment which will also be indicative.

Another feature of this lesion is that as it is 'actively' counter rotating, when assessing the vertebrae functionally it will be positionally rotated one way, but functionally rotating in the opposite direction, going in the direction of the lesion.

(*Note on terminology*: Because of the dynamic nature of this process the terms rotating or side-bending as opposed to rotated or side-bent are preferred, thus differentiating the dynamic adapting/compensating situation that is occurring in this physiological model from that of the static non-adapting situation that is inherent in the positional model where the term 'rotated' is sufficient.)

THIRD DEGREE LESIONS

There are occasionally situations that are slightly more complex, where even the adaptations described above fail to achieve satisfactory balance.

As a consequence, the body may overcompensate and a subsequent imbalance occurs on the contralateral side of the body. This may potentially evoke the next level of adaptation, whereby the body *as a whole* compensates. The pelvis reverse tilts in an attempt to shift the entire spine and body back into the midline, resulting in a third degree lesion. Dummer[7] states that this is obvious to the naked eye, as with first and second degree lesions the high side of the pelvis is ipsilateral to the concavity in the lumbar spine, but in third degree lesions it is on the opposite side. This is, by its very nature, a long-standing and slowly evolving process. The functional element progressively diminishes and the consequences become more structural and pathological, resulting in long-term and profound physiological and tissue changes both locally and distally.

The above is the definition with which many osteopaths in the UK will be familiar; however, there are several other interpretations of the third degree lesion. The features that they have in common are the profound and chronic nature of the lesion and its inherent complexity. Other versions include:[8]

- a counter rotating first degree can be described as a segmental third degree lesion
- a first degree superimposed on a second degree, or more simply, one lesion superimposed on another
- a lesion that does not 'obey' the osteopathic conventions (described by Fryette[9] as an 'off the rails' lesion)
- a 'complicated lesion' as described by Hoover,[10] being the total summation of two or more simple lesions
- in Europe it is often described as a side-shift lesion, this occurring as it tries to 'escape' from the coupled rotation side-bending
- a hyper mechanical and hyper physiological lesion.

Table 2.2 summarizes the key features of this model.

Many osteopaths have made the conceptual link between the temporal aspect of this model and the gradual but progressive tendency towards chronic tissue changes, hypofunction and ultimately pathology, and the physiological triphasic stages of Hans Selye's General Adaptation Syndrome.[11] Table 2.3 indicates this proposed relationship.

Table 2.2   A summary of the key features of the first, second and third degree lesions

	Onset	Affecting	Rot/SB	State
First degree	Traumatic	Single vertebrae	Ipsilateral	Acute
Second degree	Compensation	Group vertebrae	Contralateral	Chronic
Third degree	Compensation	Whole body (+/- single vertebrae)	Side shift/complex	Very chronic

Table 2.3   A proposed relationship between the stages of dysfunction and the General Adaptation Syndrome

Dysfunction	General Adaptation Syndrome
First degree lesion	Alarm phase
Second degree lesion	Resistance phase
Third degree lesion	Exhaustion phase

FRYETTE'S TYPE I AND TYPE II LESIONS

It would be logical to discuss these at this point; however, as they form an integral part of a complex biomechanical principle, they are discussed as part of Fryette's spinal mechanics later in this chapter. Having read that section it would be of benefit to reread the first and second degree lesion section (p. 26) and contrast these with Type I and Type II lesions (p. 32).

HIERARCHICAL CONSIDERATIONS

PRIMARY AND SECONDARY LESIONS

Any attempt to unravel the complex patterns of dysfunction found in the average person merits a related attempt to establish what has initiated the problem, and then what areas have compensated or are secondary to this. The terms primary and secondary lesion are used to describe this hierarchy.

The primary lesion is defined by Mitchell[12] as 'one that causes an adaptive or compensatory change to occur in the body or directly causes some other part of the body to malfunction or undergo trophic changes'. Dummer[7] is more succinct, defining primary lesions as 'those basic disturbances of structure which eventually cause secondary and compensatory disturbances of other related structures' and secondary lesions as 'the secondary and compensatory disturbances of structure which eventually arise from basic distur-

bances of structure'. Thus, essentially, the primary lesion leads to a secondary lesion. This does not just apply to problems occurring within the body. If one is thinking holistically, it is possible to imagine the primary lesion being *out of the body*, such as a major psychological stress which will result in a cascade of secondary consequences; similarly the secondary lesions may be somatic, visceral or psychic.

These terms are often confused with first and second *degree*. This is not altogether surprising as there is some overlap. In the recent or acute situation the primary lesion is often also a first degree lesion, but with time the first degree lesion may progress to a second or third degree lesion, but still be primary. Whatever similarities they have it is important to realize that they are based on different premises, and to avoid confusion it is better to treat the two concepts as separate entities.

Implicit within this concept is the premise that if one treats the primary lesion then the secondary compensations should resolve. This is possibly the case with short-standing patterns that have not become subject to chronic tissue changes, but with longer-standing problems this will often not be the case, as with time the associated tissues become progressively fibrosed, preventing spontaneous recovery.

For example, if a trauma had induced a lesion at C2/C3 approximately 2 years previously, there would have been an attempt to stabilize the situation locally by the C2 counter rotating. If this was insufficient to stabilize the body it would then be required to involve another area or areas of the spine to fully compensate. This would be a secondary lesion and, for the sake of this discussion, let us say this occurred at T4. This process may occur almost immediately or take weeks to occur. After the acute stage has passed, both areas will be subject to the process of stabilizing: the fibrosis, hypoperfusion, muscle hypertrophy then hypotrophy and generalized reduction in mobility. This will become progressively more marked in the intervening time between the onset of the lesion and the time when treatment is to be attempted. The concept of treating the primary lesion and the secondary resolving itself is clearly unlikely to occur in this situation; in fact if the primary alone were treated, the 'old secondary' could potentially become the 'primary' and reinstate the 'old primary' as a secondary!

This process can be continued throughout the body via reflex connections. Continuing the above situation, T4 will have had an effect via the somaticovisceral reflex on its segmentally related viscera and their supporting structures, creating possible disturbances in the viscera's mobility, motility and internal physiology, with all the consequent problems. As the T4 is now relatively chronic the structures likewise will be in a chronic state. This may set up a self-perpetuating somaticovisceral–viscerosomatic reflex loop. Thus there are cascading levels of primary and secondary lesions which may themselves be interchangeable.

There is thought, by some, to be a sole primary lesion within an individual's pattern, resolution of which will lead to resolution of the whole pattern of compensations. Whilst this may theoretically be the case, it fails to acknowledge the temporal elements discussed above – should the pattern of dysfunction and compensation have been present for any more than a few weeks, the subsequent tissue changes will prevent the 'unravelling' of the entire pattern. Perhaps more significantly, no person is without layers of dysfunction; this starts as a fetus with possible birth trauma and then is overlaid by every subsequent unresolved insult to the body, creating a complex pattern of compensation not easily unravelled.

The term 'most significant dysfunction' is used by many osteopaths to indicate the key dysfunction within a particular pattern, in a particular person at a particular time, and to an extent obviates the need for primary or secondary terminology. This having been said, it is still of great benefit (some would say essential) to attempt to analyse the complex superposition of lesion patterns in each individual to be treated.

THE OSTEOPATHIC LESION ACCORDING TO POSITIONAL FINDINGS

Osteopathic lesions are often described by their position, e.g. T4 right rotated, left side-bent flexed; extension of the sphenobasilar symphysis; or the liver is anterior and medially positioned. The positional findings do not have to be incorporated into the models of first and second degree or Fryette's Type I and II lesions, and as these models are used for describing articulation, they do not apply to viscera – which therefore will utilize just the stated positional findings for a positional diagnosis (functional findings are also used to describe the functional aspects of these lesions). Inherent within these statements of position are implications of expected relative ease or bind of movement. As noted earlier in a simple osteopathic lesion, for each plane of movement where there is restriction, there will be relative ease of movement in the opposite direction of that plane of movement. Convention decrees that the lesion is named according to the direction of ease of the movement. The same logic applies to any structure, including visceral, fascial and cranial.

The positional findings are thought by many osteopaths to be essential for accurate correction of the lesion, as it is believed that to effectively correct a lesion it is necessary to reverse all of the components of that lesion. This, however, is not the case with all practitioners; many feel that it is sufficient to note that an articulation is restricted, and will mobilize it successfully without previously assessing the specific positional findings. In this situation they are guided more by the feel or function of the articulation. Both approaches have merit, though there does currently appear to be a trend to move away from the positional findings model. Being able to understand and apply both models is perhaps the ideal.

OSTEOPATHIC LESION WITH REGARD TO THE UNDERLYING PHYSIOLOGICAL MECHANISMS

The previous models give us useful tools for diagnosing and naming positional lesions, but perhaps do not pay much attention to the maintaining factors, i.e. the neuromusculoskeletal, and fascial elements, or their more distal consequences.

The earliest osteopaths were well aware that it was not the facet lock alone that maintained the restriction of movement within somatic dysfunction. At its simplest they were aware of the role of the muscles in perpetuating the lesion and, obviously, linked with that, the role of the reflex arc. These tentative steps into the understanding of the neuromusculoskeletal basis of the osteopathic lesion were supported by the findings of John Hilton.

John Hilton's findings in the early 1860s were of great significance to the early osteopaths. These were summarized in what became known as Hilton's Law, and although it is stated in various forms, in essence it is: 'A nerve trunk which supplies any given joint, also supplies the muscles which move the joint and the skin over the insertion of such muscles'. The importance to the early osteopaths was the implication of an accurate and physiological harmony in the various cooperating structures, intra-articular, periarticular and the skin.[7] It seems naïve now to invest much significance in such a finding as this is now tacit knowledge, but it enabled the early practitioners to start to construct a rational basis for their practice.

Head's studies in the early 1890s are summarized as Head's Law, which states: 'when a painful stimulus is applied to a body part of low sensitivity (e.g. viscus) that is in close central connection with a point of higher sensitivity (e.g. soma), the pain is felt at the point of higher sensitivity rather than at the point where the stimulus was applied'.[2]

This means that sympathetic nerves which supply internal organs have, via their central connections (reflex arc), a relationship with spinal nerves which supply certain muscles and areas of skin. By applying Head's Law, as viscera are relatively insensitive to pain, sensation created by a noxious stimulus in the viscus is transferred to the area of greater sensitivity, i.e. the related muscles and skin. Through this, early practitioners established a relationship between a somatic problem and its related viscera. Of particular note was J.M. Littlejohn, who created a table of 'osteopathic centers' relating vertebrae to their physiological and visceral function. Early osteopathic texts refer to dysfunction created by this process as a reflex lesion; a primary reflex lesion if the origin of the dysfunction is in the soma reflexly affecting a viscus, and a secondary reflex lesion when the reverse is true, with a dysfunction in a viscus affecting a somatic structure.

These early concepts continued to be developed but it was not until the late 1950s that a relatively complete and rational model of the neurophysiological mechanism of the osteopathic lesion was proposed. Professor Irvin Korr, a physiologist working in the field of osteopathy proposed that the articular dysfunction, arising from either trauma or postural adaptation, is maintained by the complex interplay of the motor system via the afferent input from the muscle spindles and Golgi tendon organs and the sensory efferents controlling the muscle length and degree of contraction and thereby controlling the articular position and function.

Somatic afferents also synapse with the nuclei of the autonomic nervous system (ANS). This system has an effect on local blood supply, sweat gland activity, smooth muscle and visceral function. Much of this was thought to be organized at a spinal segmental level, though it is now known to be ultimately under the control of the higher centres of the central nervous system (CNS).

As much of this activity is organized at a spinal segmental level, Korr proposed that where there is somatic dysfunction there will be an increase in neurological activity at the appropriate spinal segmental level and therefore 'facilitation' at that level. The facilitation of that segment makes it more 'reactive' in response to both local or distal neurological input, causing a preferentially greater effect on all those structures supplied by that segment, via the somatic and autonomic nervous systems (be they muscle, viscera or blood vessel) than the non-facilitated segments.

The spread of excitation from the vertebral lesion to a viscus by the above mechanism, known to the early osteopaths as a primary reflex lesion, would currently be described as a somaticovisceral reflex. The reverse, where a problem arising in a viscus would be conveyed to the relevant spinal segment leading to local spinal facilitation, would be termed a viscerosomatic reflex (Fig. 6.5), or in earlier terms, a secondary reflex lesion. Korr's theories offered a coherent rationale for these various types of dysfunction that had been noted by osteopaths.

Korr's concepts are explored more completely in Chapter 6.

More recent models have expanded on Korr's concepts and on the functional consequences of somatic dysfunction, most notably the role of nociception and centralized sensitization (see Ch. 6).

The role of the psyche in this process cannot be overstressed; it is the overseer of all aspects of life, consciously and unconsciously. It is possible for the psyche to be 'facilitated', in a similar way as the spinal segment, by the stresses of the underlying condition, especially if the problem is chronic in nature, causing a somaticopsychic reflex. The converse may also occur, where general stresses (to which we are all subject, to a greater or lesser extent) may facilitate the higher centres, causing inappropriate responses in the body via psychosomatic reflexes. This will perhaps lower the overall resistance of that individual and facilitate more somatic disturbance (as in Bechamp's Cellular Theory of disease). See Chapters 6 and 7 for more detail.

FRYETTE SPINAL MECHANICS

HH Fryette, DO (1878–1960) wrote widely on osteopathy in general but is now perhaps best known for his work on spinal motion published in 1918 in a paper, 'Physiological Movements of the Spine'.[13] This was the first organized approach to the investigation of spinal motion that involved the three axes of motion. It has been condensed into Fryette's three laws of spinal motion and the associated lesion patterns. Fryette's other major contribution is that of expanding Dr AD Becker's 'total structural lesion' into the Total Osteopathic Lesion, thereby reintroducing holism at a time when the approach had a reductionist tendency (the 'total osteopathic lesion' will be explored in Ch. 9).

This chapter will look at the laws of spinal motion, which more correctly are now termed Fryette's principles. It will also address the concepts and nomenclature of the somatic dysfunction related to these principles. The lesion nomenclature devised by Fryette is widely used in Europe and America, but less so in the UK, so an attempt has been made to look at the various systems of lesion nomenclature and, where possible, draw equivalents in an attempt to ease communication.

THE PRINCIPLES OF PHYSIOLOGICAL MOTION

Fryette expanded on the work of Dr Robert A Lovett[14] published in *Lateral Curvatures of the Spine and Round Shoulders* (1907). Lovett based his studies on the movement of the whole spine, whereas Fryette applied these findings to individual vertebrae.

It would appear that, for Fryette, the critical feature of Lovett's work was an experiment in which he divided a human spine into two by sawing through the pedicles. This resulted in one column consisting of the anterior structures, the vertebral bodies and the intervertebral discs, and another consisting of the posterior elements, the articular facets and the posterior arch.

On experimenting with these two columns he found that in attempting to side-bend them under load they behaved differently. The anterior column tended to collapse toward the convexity. He described this as occurring in the same way that a pile of bricks would behave. The posterior column was unable to side-bend until it had first rotated to some degree; his analogy in this case was that 'they behaved like a flexible ruler or a blade of grass'.[9]

The difference in the manner in which these two columns behaved underpins Fryette's concepts. Essentially, these concepts are based on whether the spine is in easy normal flexion (neutral), at which time the spine will be supported by the discs and vertebral bodies, the facets being free to move in their permissible ranges of movement and thus acting as the anterior section of the spine in Lovett's experiment; or whether the spine is out of the neutral in either flexion or extension, and thereby the facets are engaged and as such are responsible for guiding the movement and acting as the posterior section, requiring rotation before side-bending can occur.

Fryette's conclusions from the analysis of this at a segmental level have now become known as his 'laws of spinal motion', or perhaps more correctly Fryette's principles of spinal motion.

There are three major principles of physiological motion, being:[15]

- First principle: When the thoracic and lumbar spine is in a neutral position (easy normal), the coupled motions of side-bending and rotation for a group of vertebrae are such that side-bending and rotation occur in opposite directions (with rotation occurring toward the convexity).
- Second principle: When the thoracic and lumbar spine is sufficiently forward or backward bent (non-neutral), the coupled motions of side-bending and rotation in a single vertebral unit occur in the same direction (with rotation occurring toward or into the concavity).
- Third principle: Initiating motion of a vertebral segment in any plane of motion will modify the movement of that segment in other planes of motion. (This is also sometimes stated as 'introduction of motion to a vertebral joint in one plane automatically reduces its mobility in the other two planes', sometimes called Beckwith's law or Nelson's law.)

The first and second principles are summarized in Table 2.4.

It will be seen that the first two principles are written only in regard to the vertebrae of the thoracic and lumbar spine. Due to the shape and orientation of the articular facets and the modified vertebral body shape (the uncinate processes) of the

Table 2.4 A summary of Fryette's first and second principles. (After Simmons SL. The cram pages. Online: http://pages.prodigy.net/stn1/Cram%20Pages.pdf 19 Sept 2003)

Spinal position	Direction
Neutral first principle	$S_X R_Y$ or $S_Y R_X$
Non-neutral second principle	$R_X S_X$ or $R_Y S_Y$

typical vertebrae of the cervical spine, side-bending and rotation will occur in the same direction regardless of whether the vertebral unit is in easy normal flexion, flexion or extension, behaving in accordance with the second principle of motion.

The atypical vertebrae are also exceptions to the above principles, most notably the C1 and C2, these having their own particular motions and lesion classification. This will be discussed later in this chapter.

The principles can be applied to somatic dysfunction that may arise. The lesions are named according to the principle that describes their motion, thus the first principle will result in a Type I somatic dysfunction.

Type I somatic dysfunction

The first principle applies when the thoracic or lumbar spine are in the neutral position. Thus, for a Type I somatic dysfunction to occur, the spine must be in the easy normal position at the time of the induction of the somatic dysfunction. That being the case, the side-bending and rotation will occur in opposite directions ($S_X R_Y$ or $S_Y R_X$ in Table 2.4).

So, if the spine is in neutral and side-bending occurs to the right at the T9 vertebra, it will then rotate to the left. This example would be written as T9NS$_R$R$_L$, or T9NSR$_L$, meaning:

T9 – the T9 vertebra in relation to the T10
N – neutral, or easy normal
S$_R$ – side-bending right
R$_L$ – rotating left.

In the second, more paraphrased, example the 'N' indicates that the spine is in the neutral position and therefore the first law applies. Thus by naming the direction of rotation, and applying the first law, the side-bending will be assumed to be opposite to that of the rotation.

The naming of the lesion gives an indication as to the sequence of movement that is likely to occur in

normal movement. According to the first principle, when the spine is in neutral and a compound movement of rotation and side-bending is initiated, the side-bending will occur first, followed by rotation to the opposite side. Hence, when naming lesions obeying the first principle, the side-bending component is stated first, i.e. NSR.

It is also possible to make some generalizations about Type I dysfunctions. They occur only when the spine is in the neutral position or, more importantly, when the articular facets are unable to guide the movement of the vertebral unit. There is a range of movement in which this can occur (which accounts for the rather bewildering number of names relating to Fryette's neutral position, see the note below), but this range is very small. It is rare for the spine to be within this range during activity, but not uncommon when the body is at rest. Thus Type I lesions are more commonly lesions of compensation or adaptation than of traumatic origin. They also more frequently occur in groups rather than individually.

Possible causes of a of Type I dysfunction include:[16]

- as a compensation to Type II dysfunction (nonneutral): either ERS or FRS
- cranial and/or upper cervical spine dysfunctions
- rib cage dysfunction (structural or functional)
- visceral and fascial dysfunctions in abdominal or thoracic cavities
- three-dimensional asymmetrical tightness – looseness in the myofascia
- viscerosomatic reflexes
- idiopathic scoliosis
- sacral base unlevel (sacroiliac or iliosacral dysfunctions)
- anatomical or functional short leg syndrome
- uncoordinated and faulty movement patterns and muscular imbalances.

Notes on nomenclature of the neutral position: 'Easy normal flexion' is the term used by Fryette to indicate that the spinal curve is in its normal resting position or neutral position. It is often abbreviated to 'easy normal', 'easy flexion' or simply 'normal' (hence the N in NSR).

In some texts the term 'easy normal extension' is also used. This is often coupled with 'easy normal flexion' to indicate the neutral range of movement of the spine, within which range the facets will not be engaged and thus the vertebrae will respond according to Fryette's first principle.

Type II somatic dysfunction

The second principle applies when the thoracic or lumbar spine are sufficiently out of the neutral position for the articular facets to direct the movement, i.e. in flexion or extension. Thus for a Type II somatic dysfunction to occur the spine must similarly be out of neutral at the time of the induction of the somatic dysfunction. That being the case, the side-bending and rotation will occur in the same direction, R_XS_X or R_YS_Y.

So if the spine is in (for example) flexion and side-bending occurs to the right, the vertebra will rotate to the right. Shorthand for this example would be FR_RS_R or FRS_R. In this case the initial F, flexion (or E, extension) indicates that this is to obey Fryette's second principle, hence in the later, shorthand, example only the direction of the side-bending is supplied, the ipsilateral rotation being implied. The vertebral level would precede the description.

The second principle derives from the observation Lovett made of the posterior column, described by Fryette as behaving like a flexible ruler or a blade of grass in that before it could side-bend it had to rotate. This is the sequence of movements that are thought to occur. Thus when naming lesions obeying the second principle the rotation is stated first, i.e. FRS and ERS.

Type II dysfunction is thought often to be due to trauma rather than postural adaptations or compensation, as the spine must necessarily be out of neutral at the time of the induction of the dysfunction.

They are also thought to occur quite commonly as individual rather than group lesions.

THE CERVICAL SPINE

The cervical spine, as previously stated, is an exception to the first and and second principles, due to the nature of the facet orientation and body shape. The cervicals are divided into the typical vertebrae, C3 to C7, and the atypical vertebrae, C1 and C2. These will be discussed separately.

Typical cervical vertebrae

The cervical spine is the most mobile area of the spine. This is due to the particular structure of the typical cervical vertebrae, the intervertebral discs and the facet orientation. As a result of this they act in accordance with Fryette's second principle regardless of whether they are in easy normal, flexion or extension. Thus cervical lesions tend to exist

with rotation and side-bending occurring to the same side. Possibly as a consequence of the cervical mobility, there is a tendency for the vertebrae to side-shift (translate) to the opposite side.

Thus if the vertebra is in extension with right rotation there will be an associated right side-bending and left side-shift.

Many utilize this side-shifting tendency to classify typical cervical lesions.

Thus if the vertebra side-shifts more easily to the left, the vertebra will be in right side-bending rotation, and if more easily to the right it will be in left side-bending rotation. All that remains to complete the diagnosis is to assess for flexion or extension.

Atypical cervical vertebrae

The anatomical structure of the upper two cervical vertebrae is sufficiently different from that of the rest of the cervicals to necessitate a separate method of classifying lesions of this area.

This can be done in two ways, with regard to Fryette's Principles of Physiological Motion or by the possible positional findings.

According to Fryette, whereas the typical cervical vertebrae respond to the second principle of physiological motion (ERS, FRS), the C0–C1 follows only the first principle (NSR), and the C1–C2 exhibits primarily rotation (with a very small amount of side-bending).

The possible positional findings or the potential lesion patterns anticipated are:[7, 17,18]

- posterior or anterior occiput, left or right
- bilateral anterior or posterior occiput
- occiput side-shift right or left
- posterior or anterior atlas, left or right
- side-shift of the atlas, left or right
- right or left rotation of the axis.

COMPLICATED OR 'DERAILED' LESIONS

Fryette utilized the term complicated or 'derailed' lesions for those lesions that have gone beyond his principles, or perhaps more precisely, lesions that have a non-physiological movement complicating the dysfunction. The clearest example that he states is that of the inclusion of side-shift or translation in an articulation where it is not within its normal physiological range of movement, the main possible sites for this being the L5, the T11 and C2 to C6 vertebrae. Before one can address the dysfunction, the non-physiological movement must be resolved, to put the vertebra 'back on the physiological track,[9] and then treatment can occur as normal. This approximately equates to the complicated lesion or third degree lesion.

A NOTE ON FRYETTE'S NOMENCLATURE RELATING TO FLEXION AND EXTENSION

Those of you wanting to read Fryette in the original will need to be aware of his occasionally confusing nomenclature around flexion and extension.

For Fryette, the terms flexion or extension have different meanings depending on whether one is discussing spinal curves or individual vertebrae.

Spinal curves

When referring to the spinal curves Fryette utilizes the mechanical or anatomical definition for the movements. Thus, flexion is defined as an increase in the normal existing curve, or the approximation of the two ends of a curve. Extension is the reduction, straightening or even reversal of the curve so the ends of the curves become more distant; this is sometimes referred to as 'flattening' of the curve. As the individual curves differ in their anteroposterior orientation they will be described as moving in different ways. Therefore, if applying Fryette's nomenclature, when an individual forward bends fully, the cervical and lumbar curves will have extended and the thoracic spine flexed.

Vertebral segments

When discussing individual vertebral movement the position of the vertebral body is always used as the reference point. Therefore in spinal flexion the vertebral body approximates that of the vertebra below (forward bending), and vice versa for vertebral extension.

Table 2.5 summarizes the above and includes what would be described, according to Fryette, as occurring at each of the three spinal curves as the whole body progressively bends forwards or backwards.

As often mentioned, it must be appreciated that the principles of physiological motion are in fact only intended as guidelines to give an indication as to what may happen in the perfect situation. There will be exceptions. An obvious example would be that of trauma, with either macro- or microtrauma creating the lesion; should the force be sufficiently large or sufficiently constant then the anatomical principles can be overcome. Or, in osteoarthritis, as the disc degenerates, the role of the facets changes, thereby modifying the expectations inherent in the first principle. It also becomes more complex when lesions become layered, such as when an existing lesion is subject to another lesion-inducing force; again, the rules will no longer be obviously applicable.

Fryette's principles also have been questioned by more recent researchers. Since Fryette proposed the principles of physiological motion they have been subject to some further research to assess their veracity. In summary[19,20] Stoddard demonstrated radiologically that side-bending in the cervical spine is *always* accompanied by rotation to the same side regardless of cervical posture. His observations in relation to the cervical spine are consistent with Lovett's findings and Fryette's laws. These findings are further supported by research undertaken by Mimura et al.[21] However, no consistent pattern of coupling behaviour has been demonstrated in the lumbar or thoracic spine.[22–25] Therefore in the cervical spine, Fryette's second principle is consistent and verified by research, but in the lumbar and thoracic spine, the coupled motions are inconsistent and Fryette's second principle may or may not apply here. So, as with all models, it offers a hypothesis and it is then up to the practitioner to test whether that hypothesis is consistent with the findings in a patient.

Table 2.5 A summary of Fryette's nomenclature for segmental and spinal movement. (After Dummer T. A textbook of osteopathy, vol 1. Hadlow Down: JoTom Publications; 1999:129)

Movement	Individual vertebrae	Spinal curve	Fryette's description
Flexion	Forward bending	Ends of the curve approximate increasing the curve	Cervical extension. Thoracic flexion. Lumbar extension
Extension	Backward bending	Ends of the curve separate reducing the curve	Cervical flexion. Thoracic extension. Lumbar flexion

CONVERGENT AND DIVERGENT LESIONS

This is another model of somatic dysfunction used by many manual therapists. It is based on Fryette's concepts but relates only to Type II dysfunctions which are described as being convergent or divergent. It helps with the creation of a 'mental picture' of the articulation following the somatic dysfunction, thereby clarifying the methods and directions used to correct the dysfunction. The convergence and divergence relate to the state of the facets as to whether they are 'open' or 'closed': convergence means closing of the facet joints or extension, divergence means opening of the facet joints or flexion.

This is illustrated by the following examples[26] with regard to Type II lesions to the right in first extension, rotation, side-bending lesion (ERS) and then flexion, rotation, side-bending lesion (FRS).

ERS RIGHT DYSFUNCTION (TYPE II)

The superior vertebra is in extension, rotation and side-bending to the right, causing the right facets to approximate, and thus this facet will be convergent or will not open (or go into flexion or diverge). If the vertebra is moved into extension the dysfunction will neutralize and if it is moved into flexion the dysfunction will become more prominent and asymmetrical, as the right facet will remain 'fixed' while the left opens. See Figure 2.4.

FRS RIGHT DYSFUNCTION (TYPE II)

For an FRS dysfunction it is essentially the opposite: the superior vertebra is in flexion, rotation and side-bending to the right causing the left facet to separate, thus this facet will be divergent or will not close (or go into extension or converge). If the vertebra is moved into flexion the dysfunction will neutralize and if it is moved into extension the dysfunction will become more prominent and asymmetrical. See Figure 2.5.

SUMMARY

In an ERS dysfunction the facet joint in trouble is on the same side as mentioned in the dysfunction, e.g. in ERS right, the right facet will not go in flexion or divergence. In an FRS dysfunction the facet joint in trouble is opposite to the side mentioned in the dysfunction, e.g. in FRS right, the left facet will not go into extension or convergence.

Flexion

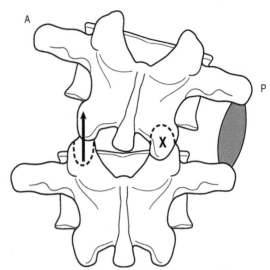

Figure 2.4 ERS dysfunction (Type II) ERS right or right convergent. In an ERS dysfunction the facet joint in trouble is on the same side as mentioned in the dysfunction, e.g. in ERS right, the right facet will not go into flexion or divergence. If the spine moves into flexion, the right transverse process will not move anteriorly and the right transverse process will be more prominent to palpation in flexion. In extension the movement will be symmetrical.

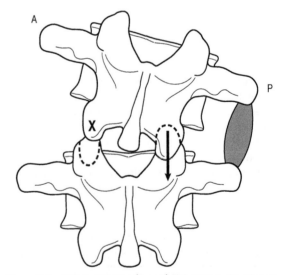

Figure 2.5 FRS dysfunction (Type II) FRS right dysfunction or left divergent: In an FRS dysfunction the facet joint in trouble is opposite to the side mentioned in the dysfunction, e.g. in FRS right, the left facet will not go into extension or convergence. If the spine moves into extension the left facet joint will not close which means that the right transverse process will be more prominent by palpation when the patient is in extension. In flexion movement will be symmetrical.

This can be utilized as a diagnostic tool. When a patient with an ERS right dysfunction moves into extension, both transverse processes will become symmetrical with respect to the frontal plane; they will become 'even'. If this patient then moves into flexion, the right transverse process will not move anteriorly as it should in flexion under normal circumstances. This means that the right transverse process will be more prominent to palpation in flexion.

Similarly, when a patient with an FRS right moves into flexion, both transverse processes will become symmetrical. But in extension, the right transverse process will not move anteriorly (in this case the left facet joint will not close, and the right transverse process becomes prominent when moved into extension). This means that the right transverse process will be more prominent by palpation (when the patient is in extension).

COMPARISON WITH OTHER MODELS OF DYSFUNCTION

The nomenclature and method of classifying lesions differs from country to country, creating much confusion. In fact, a large portion of all of the classifications derive from the same source (i.e. Fryette), with slight differences in interpretation creating the confusion. In much of mainland Europe Fryette's principles are applied more stringently and, as such, could correctly be called rules. This has some significance. If one is to be true to Fryette's principles, the rules apply only to the thoracic and lumbar spine; the cervical spine is only able to exhibit Type II lesions. It is interesting to note that within the degree type classification (first, second and third degree) no distinction is made between the three spinal curves, each being able to demonstrate lesions of all three degrees, thus the equivalent of a Type I could exist in the cervical spine according to this model (though this opposes recent research [20,21]).

Another aspect of Fryette's principles that creates some confusion is that Type I (NSR) dysfunctions are always compensations and do not involve the articular facets. As the facets are not restricted they do not need to be adjusted on an articular level, but rather are treated by addressing the causative dysfunctions and then the soft tissues maintaining the compensation. Thus, the only true vertebral dysfunctions are the Type II (FRS and ERS).

The Type II dysfunctions are sometimes, for descriptive purposes, also described as convergent or divergent, as discussed above.

Table 2.6 Common classifications and their equivalents

Type I	Type II
NSR	FRS
Second degree	First degree
Contralateral rotation side-bending	Ipsilateral rotation side-bending Convergent/divergent
Usually group dysfunction	Usually segmental dysfunction

Additionally, for the cervical spine there is also a model that utilizes the side-shift element to name the lesion. The side-shift results from the ipsilateral rotation and side-bending and occurs in the opposite direction to these movements. Thus a side-shift right dysfunction would be the equivalent of left Type II or possibly a 'derailed' Type II, or a first degree left dysfunction!

The array of different classification of somatic dysfunction is somewhat baffling; Table 2.6 illustrates some of the common classifications and their equivalents.

There appears to be a myriad of ways to qualify and quantify somatic dysfunction. Each has a particular relevance to certain conceptual approaches, e.g. defining a dysfunction by its positional findings is essential to the Specific Adjusting Technique (SAT) approach. The models of dysfunction are not necessarily interchangeable between treatment approaches, so that the positional findings necessary for SAT are not helpful in conceptualization of dysfunction within a functional approach. In this approach the critical factor is movement and not position, the ease or bind of the articulation.

Many osteopaths do not even feel the need to make specific diagnoses of dysfunction, diagnosis in the sense that is utilized in both Fryette's Type I and II lesions and the first and second degree lesions, believing that it is unnecessary to reverse the components and impossible to get a positional change, and simply aim to improve the function.

A HISTORICAL PERSPECTIVE

One can chart the history of osteopathy by its approach to the osteopathic lesion. Still did not talk about lesions but more about adjusting the abnormalities which interfered with the normal activities and function of the patient. Of prime importance was the relationship between structure and function, and though there have been attempts to base treatment rationale and approach on Still's practice, too little is known of the manner in which he treated to make supportable statements. However, this concept is perhaps in keeping with many of the current schools of thought that are interested in the harmony of structure and therefore function in contrast to the more mechanistic approach that followed.

As time passed, a rational approach was implemented and a search for the scientific basis of osteopathy caused the emphasis to pass to the structural cause of disease, which became known as the 'osteopathic lesion'. The focus was on its effect on local and distant tissues, to the extent of analysing the histopathological changes induced by artificially producing lesions in animals. Lovett developed the 'physiological' movements of the spine resulting in positional findings for lesions. The 'whole patient' became somewhat forgotten. This was a period where the aim of treatment was to reverse the components of the lesion, to 'retrace the vectors of force' and thus reinstate the normal neuromusculoskeletal harmony. Allied with this was the tacit assumption that, in so doing, the pathophysiological process that had been observed in experimental situations to be associated with the lesion would also be reversed.

This slightly linear interpretation of the lesion as a focus of disturbance which, via various reflexes, creates local and remote effects, caused the osteopathic approach to be rather reductionist. The lesion became the single target for osteopathic technicians, and an array of structural techniques were refined to address the lesion specifically and produce the desired clinical results.

In the 1920s, the trend began to change. Arthur Becker introduced the idea of the 'total osteopathic lesion', which was later expanded upon by Fryette. This is described as being 'the composite of all the various separate individual lesions or factors, mechanical or otherwise, which cause or predispose to cause disease from which the patient may be suffering at the moment. These factors may vary from corns to cholera, from "nervousness to insanity"'.[9]

This reintroduced the holism that had been temporarily lost. Somatic dysfunction was included as one of the many stressors to which a person may be subject. Stressors from both internal and external sources summate and detract from the individual's well-being. Depending on the extent of the stressors they will contribute to the aetiology and maintenance of disease. By treating those elements amenable to osteopathic treatment, the total load will be reduced, along with the tendency to disease.

At approximately the same time, WG Sutherland began applying Still's concepts to the cranium. He addressed its function rather than the positional changes. This reestablished the idea of exaggerating the lesion rather than reversing the components. From this arose the approaches later known as 'balanced ligamentous tension' or 'ligamentous articular strain'. Hoover and Bowles further developed this approach to establish 'functional technique'. Within these models, the aim is not to oppose and impose on a static site of dysfunction, but rather to move in the direction of ease, working with the body's inherent self-healing abilities, permitting it to resolve the problem. The combination of a more holistic approach, a more dynamic concept of somatic dysfunction, and the aim of working with the body rather than doing something to it, represented a radical conceptual shift from the earlier approaches. As such, the positional concepts of dysfunction are not applicable within these models.

The 1950s saw the arrival of approaches that were less spinally focused, taking the concept of dysfunction further into the body as a whole.

Carl Kettler and Thomas J Ruddy utilized the muscles as a corrective force, inspiring Fred L Mitchell Senior to develop 'muscle energy techniques'. William Neidner and George A Laughlin directed their attention towards the fascia and manipulative procedures designed to normalize it (Neidner used 'fascial twist techniques' of a more direct character, and Laughlin integrated Sutherland's 'involuntary mechanism' to release the fascia). Frank P Millard had since the 1920s emphasized a routine for evaluating and working on the lymphatic system of the body, possibly influencing Gordon Zink in his development of the 'respiratory-circulatory model of disease'.

Each of these approaches will have borrowed concepts of dysfunction from earlier models, but will understandably have had to create new concepts where these were lacking. It is for this reason that there is a rather bewildering array of concepts and models relating to somatic dysfunction or osteopathic lesion. An awareness of the principles behind each of these should enable you to be able to apply a wide range of treatment approaches, selecting the most appropriate one for each individual patient rather than making the patient fit an approach.

Many students have asked why the earlier approaches are still taught, as they believe that the more recent approaches have superseded them. This is a very pertinent question; the answer ultimately rests with each individual. The authors feel that no model has truly superseded any other; they all have a relevance to clinical practice, though the older concepts will require tempering in light of current research. It is possible for an osteopath to employ direct and indirect approaches, use positional and functional findings and work with structural, fascial, cranial, visceral and functional approaches. To do this as effectively as possible it is necessary to have some level of understanding of all of the concepts discussed in this section. If the practitioner's desire is to practise within just one area (such as structural, cranial or visceral) only those concepts related to that area need to be known, but it is difficult to understand why anyone would want to limit themselves in this manner.

Having explored the idea of the somatic dysfunction in such depth, it is perhaps pertinent to clarify one point.

'The contemporary definition of the somatic dysfunction is not exclusive to the osteopathic profession, but used in manual medicine and physiotherapy as well. We, as osteopaths, can not claim its ownership but trace its historical development to the profession, and chart the progression of the profession by it. The osteopathic identity, however, does not rest upon the somatic dysfunction as an identifying feature, but rests upon our ability to identify with the original philosophy of Still, Littlejohn and others, and to express this clinically through our evaluation and management of the patient. The somatic dysfunction didactically has a value, but philosophically only as part of the whole.'[8]

The next section will address the more global models that take the somatic dysfunction, in its abstract sense, and place it within its physical, mental and emotional context.

References

1. Rumney IC. The history of the developmental term 'somatic dysfunction'. Osteopathic Annals 1979; 7(1):26–30.
2. Educational Council on Osteopathic Principles. Glossary of Osteopathic Terminology. Chicago: American Association of Colleges of Osteopathic Medicine; 2002. Online. Available: http://www.aoa-net.org/Publications/glossary202.pdf.
3. Cyriax J. Textbook of orthopaedic medicine, vol I. London: Bailliére Tindall; 1978.
4. Isaacs ER, Bookhout MR. Bourdillon's spinal manipulation, 6th edn. Boston: Butterworth Heinemann; 2002.
5. Mitchell FL. The muscle energy manual, vol I. East Lansing: MET Press; 1995.
6. Dowling D. S.T.A.R.: A more viable alternative descriptor system of somatic dysfunction. AAO Journal 1998; 8(2):34–37.
7. Dummer T. A textbook of osteopathy, vol 1. Hadlow Down: JoTom Publications; 1999: 97.
8. Fossum C. Personal communication. 2003.
9. Fryette HH. Principles of osteopathic technic. Carmel, CA: Academy of Applied Osteopathy; 1980: 37.
10. Hoover HV. Complicated lesions. In: Barnes MW, ed. 1950 Academy Yearbook. Michigan: Academy of Applied Osteopathy; 1950: 67–69.
11. Selye H. The stress of life. New York: McGraw-Hill; 1976.
12. Mitchell FL. Towards a definition of 'somatic dysfunction'. Osteopathic Annals 1979; 7(1):12–25.
13. Fryette HH. Physiological movements of the spine. J Am Osteopath Assoc 1918;XVIII (1).
14. Lovett RA. Lateral curvatures of the spine and round shoulders. London: Rebman; 1907.
15. Mitchell FL. The muscle energy manual, vol II. East Lansing: MET press; 1998.
16. Fossum C. Lecture notes. Maidstone: Unpublished; 2003
17. Stone C. Science in the art of osteopathy. Cheltenham: Stanley Thornes; 1999: 155.
18. Littlejohn J. The occipito-atlantal articulation. Maidstone: Maidstone College of Osteopathy.
19. Gibbons P, Teheran P. Spinal manipulation: indications, risks and benefits. JBMT 2001; 5(2):110–119.
20. Stoddard A. Manual of osteopathic practise. London: Hutchinson; 1969.
21. Mimura M, Moriya H, Watanabe K et al. Three-dimensional motion analysis of the cervical spine with special reference to the axial rotation. Spine 1989;14: 1135–1139.
22. Pearcy M, Tibrewal S. Axial rotation and lumbar sidebending in the normal lumbar spine measured by three-dimensional radiography. Spine 1984; 9:582–587.
23. Plamondon A, Gagnon M, Maurais G. Application of a stereoradiographic method for the study of intervertebral motion. Spine 1988: 13(9):1027–1032.
24. Panjabi MM, Yamamoto I, Oxland T et al. How does posture affect coupling in the lumbar spine? Spine 1989; 14(9):1002–1011.
25. Vicenzino G, Twomey L. Sideflexion and induced lumbar spine conjunct rotation and its influencing factors. Aust J Physiother 1993; 39:299–306.
26. Fossum C. An introduction to spinal mechanics. Maidstone: unpublished; 2003.

SECTION 2

Osteopathic conceptual (perceptual) models

This section will look at some of the ways that osteopaths have attempted to perceive the human body and how it functions. For the purpose of this discussion certain elements of the body have been selected as the basis of conceptualization. The paradigms selected are:

1. The structural or musculoskeletal model
2. Tensegrity
3. Biotypology
4. Neurological models
5. Psychological considerations
6. Fluid model
7. The total osteopathic lesion

This reductionist approach of selecting certain aspects with which to analyse the human is anathema to the holistic concept of osteopathy. It is important to remember that in the reality of osteopathic practice, the total understanding is by the application of a mixture of these models. The reason that they have been separated out here is for ease of understanding.

It is also important to realize that while these models are useful to begin to understand a person, they are only concepts and are not prescriptive. No model is able to fully describe the rich variety that exists in humankind.

SECTION 2

Osteopathic conceptual (perceptual) models

Chapter 3

Structural concepts

CHAPTER CONTENTS

INTRODUCTION

This section will look at some of the concepts that relate to an understanding of how the structure of the body generally, and the spine specifically, have been interpreted osteopathically. It begins with some general concepts and concludes with a review of certain of the key elements of the biomechanics of JM Littlejohn. Nearly all of this material is founded purely in empiricism. From the fact that these concepts have survived, and are used daily in osteopathic practices throughout the world, it could be said that they have been thoroughly tested clinically. This does not of course prove their veracity; however, that is not the task of this book. They are presented here as possible interpretations that may enable you to develop your own way of seeing and understanding the body. Some of the models are purely conceptual or 'visual' and do not even attempt to have a rational scientific basis. An example of this is the section on 'areas under a curve', and how balance is achieved. Mathematically and biomechanically, there is no truth to it. However, if it is taken, as it is intended, as a visual comparison, with the numerical formulae there only to illustrate the point, it offers a useful tool to aid the initial interpretation of spinal curves.

Initially, the segmental relationships between the spinal curves will be explored and then the biomechanical concepts of JM Littlejohn.

DEVELOPMENT OF THE SPINE

It is of interest to reflect on how spinal curves develop from fetus to maturity. In utero the baby is floating in amniotic fluid. Its spinal curve is kyphotic, convex posteriorly, from occiput to sacrum. Its similarity in shape to the letter 'C' has led to this shape being termed the 'primary C curve' (Fig. 3.1).

At birth this fluid support is lost; it is at this point that the human starts its long and arduous battle against gravity. At birth the baby should be developed to the point of independent function. Naturally, it still relies on its mother for its nutritional needs, but anatomically the organ systems are fully functional. The nervous system has to begin the process of learning and the laying down of neural connections to complete its circuitry. From a structure/function viewpoint, the baby's movements of arms and legs are training the muscles and making connections that will allow the child to later perform coordinated tasks. Even at birth, the baby has a number of 'preloaded' reflexes present that allow it to survive, e.g. the rooting reflex in order to search for the nipple and gain sustenance, and the neck righting reflex which allows the baby to lift and turn its head from side to side in the prone position, preventing suffocation.

The natural progression from this stage is for the baby to lift its head and begin to interact with its new world, and thereby increase its visual knowledge of its whereabouts. This is not an easy task, considering the relative size of a baby's head and its body, compared with those of an adult. It also has to lift it against gravity. However, by about week eight, it has begun to raise its head. In doing so, the baby has begun to create the neurological circuitry to the cervical erector spinae muscles, initiating movement and muscle strengthening. The cervical erector spinae muscles become strong and introduce the first lordotic curve in the cervical region. This curve is often termed a secondary curve, to distinguish it from the primary C curve. This further develops as the baby sits and later crawls. See Figure 3.2.

The crawling position still limits one's interaction with the world, so the baby then tries to stand up. This means balancing on two potentially mobile ball and socket joints, the hips. To enable this to occur there needs to be some degree of dynamic fixation of the pelvis to permit the spine to rest stably on it. This is achieved by a complex interaction of the iliopsoas, pelvic floor, hip extensors and erector spinae muscles. For the baby to stand up it is also necessary for the hip to extend further than it ever has before. This will oppose the action of the hip flexors, the iliopsoas muscles. As these are attached to the anterior aspect of the lumbar spine, stretching the iliopsoas will cause a pull on their attachments on the lumbar spine. This and the strengthening of the lumbar erector spinae muscles cause the lumbar spine to be drawn anteriorly, creating the second secondary curve. See Figure 3.3.

As with the cervical spine this curve is largely maintained by the erector spinae muscles performing an 'antigravity' role, but from the above it can be understood also to be dependent on the interplay between the iliopsoas, pelvic floor, hip extensor and abdominal muscles, or in fact by anything else that could affect the degree of pelvic tilt.

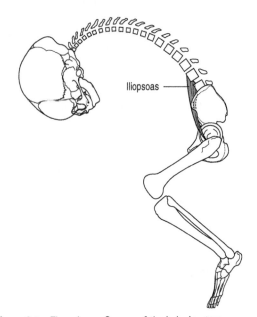

Figure 3.1 The primary C curve of the baby in utero.

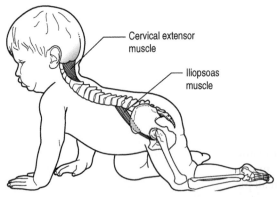

Figure 3.2 The development of the cervical lordosis as the baby crawls.

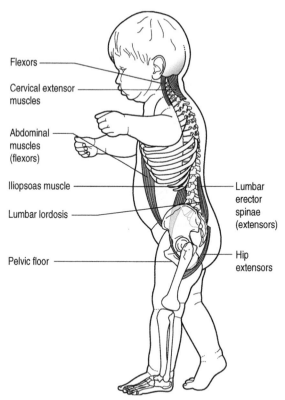

Flexors

Cervical extensor
muscles

Abdominal
muscles
(flexors)

Iliopsoas muscle

Lumbar lordosis

Pelvic floor

Lumbar
erector
spinae
(extensors)

Hip
extensors

Figure 3.3   The erect posture.

tain the vital organs, the brain, the heart and lungs; and our means of reproduction. They are protected in stable bony cages, therefore mobility has to come from other areas of the spine. The thorax is a perfect example of function affecting structure: the ribs create a bony box and to an extent these limit the mobility of the thorax, but their arrangement is such that they permit the box to expand and contract in response to respiration, whilst at no time leaving the vital centres within vulnerable.

The balance between the roles of protection and mobility is also demonstrated within the spine itself as a whole. The vertebrae may be considered to be comprised of two major components: an anterior part, which consists of the vertebral bodies and intervertebral discs, and a posterior part comprised of the bony vertebral arch and its superiorly and inferiorly projecting articular pillars. Thus the spine as a whole can be seen to consist of three pillars: a massive one anteriorly, designed for weight-bearing, and two much smaller ones, created by the articular pillars, designed to permit movement. The posterior arches, with the ligaments passing between, then create the spinal canal, designed to protect the spinal cord. It is this combination of the three bony columns that provides an intricate balance of stability and mobility whilst at the same time still achieving protection of the delicate central nervous system.

SOME CONSIDERATIONS ON THE FUNCTIONS OF THE SPINE

By looking at the spinal curves with regard to the developmental primary C curve, it is possible to see that the vestiges of this kyphotic curve are still present in the sacrum, thoracic curve and the cranium (the occiput can be considered to be a modified vertebra[1]). Intervening between these are the secondary curves. These are lordotic and are the areas where the body has adapted to enable upright posture, thus they are sites of adaptation. This ability to adapt may in part account for the finding that often individual segmental lesions are found within the secondary curves, whereas in the thorax this is rare, with most lesions occurring as group lesions.

Looking at their mobility it can be noted that the two lordotic curves represent areas that are mobile transitions between relatively hypomobile areas. (Lumbar mobility is greater than that of the thoracic in all planes except for rotation.[2]) This arrangement can, to some extent, be explained by the body's functional requirements. The hypomobile areas con-

THE ROLE OF THE CURVES IN THE RESISTANCE TO AXIAL PRESSURE AND THEIR ROLE IN MOBILITY

Another important function of the spine is that of resisting axial compression forces. The resistance of a curved column has been shown to be directly proportional to the square of the number of curves plus one, or $R = N^2 + 1$ (where R is the resistance and N is the number of curves).[2]

For a straight spine, or no curves, N = 0
$R = 0^2 + 1$
Therefore R = 1

For three curves, N = 3
$R = 3^2 + 1 = 10$
R = 10

Thus the introduction of three dynamic curves increases the resistance to *ten times greater* than that of a straight column.

Figure 3.4 The Delmas index. This is defined as the extended length of the spine divided by its actual height. Thus for the three spines illustrated this will give a low Delmas index for the increased spinal curves and a high index for the decreased curves. The index has a relation to the function of the spine, thus the greater the A/P curvature, the lower the Delmas index and the more dynamic the spine. A reduction in the A/P curvature leads to a higher Delmas index and therefore a more static spine. (After Kapandji IA. The physiology of the joints, vol 3: the trunk and vertebral column. Edinburgh: Churchill Livingstone; 1974.)

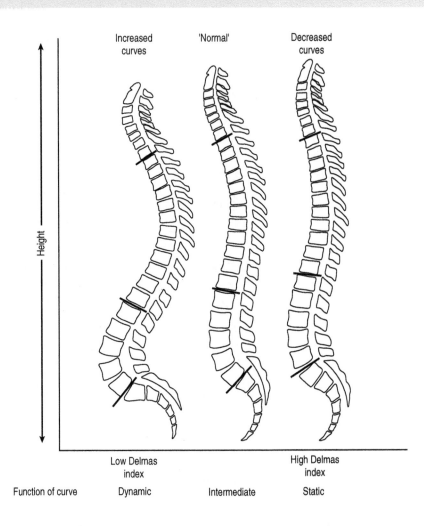

The nature of the curves has also been shown to have an effect on their function in terms of mobility, see Figure 3.4. This is quantifiable by applying the Delmas index.[2] This is established by dividing the height of the spinal curves in the upright individual by the length of the spine were it to be fully extended or straightened. Thus a spine with increased curves will be slightly shorter than one with 'normal' curves in the upright posture. If both had the same potential length when fully extended, the Delmas index would be lower for the increased curve spine. He concluded that the spinal column with augmented curves (and therefore a lower Delmas index) is more that of a dynamic type, whilst reduced AP curvature (and a higher Delmas index) leads to a more static type. (Perhaps it is fanciful to extrapolate from this concept to personality types, but reflect on your acquaintances and think of the mentally inflexible people:

how frequently are they also rigid in body, with a marked upright, straight spine appearance? This is verging on the point of stereotypical, but perhaps the body and mind are just different expressions of the same thing.)

THE ROLE OF THE SOFT TISSUES

We have talked about the functions of the bony structures, but of equal significance are the soft tissues. In the diagrams of the mature upright posture (such as Fig. 3.3) the extensor or antigravity muscles are generally illustrated by thick lines; this is to indicate their strength. Working against gravity has caused them to become strong. The flexor muscles in the anterior throat and abdomen are illustrated with thin lines, indicating their relative weakness. There is a tendency for osteopaths to be more focused on hypertonia of the strong antigravity muscles, and therefore the posterior aspect of their patient. However, it is important to remember that upright posture is achieved by a *balance* between the flexors and the extensors, and that though the extensors appear to be able to exert a greater effect, weakness or hypotonia of the flexor groups can have dramatic effects on posture.

For example Hides et al[3] have demonstrated that the abdominal container also has a role in the stabilization of the trunk on the pelvis. They defined this container or cylinder as being comprised of the pelvic diaphragm, the transversus abdominis muscle, the thoracolumbar fascia and the respiratory diaphragm. If someone has lost tone in any of these muscles, the consequence is that the lumbar lordosis increases. In Newtonian terms the flexor and extensor muscles can be imagined as opposing but balanced pulley systems: if the flexor pull is reduced there will be a dominance of the extensor pull, hence the increase in the lumbar curve.

Another way of perceiving this is based on the knowledge that the body cavities are an important part of the body's support structure. The abdominopelvic cavity is filled with viscera and fluid. They are constrained by a muscular 'container'. If the container is firm, the whole structure is relatively rigid, and can therefore offer support. When the container becomes lax, as in this example, with the abdominal muscles becoming hypotonic, the fluids are no longer compressed and the support offered is reduced. The viscera then ptose anteriorly, pulling on their posterior fascial attachments and causing an increase in the lumbar curve. (Another way of looking at this is to note that an increase in the lumbar curve may relax the peritoneum, to which organs are attached, and because they lose support they ptose.)

In each situation the hypotonic state of the weak anterior muscles is the cause. The consequent lumbar curve change, and any other compensations that may occur as a result of this, are secondary. It is possible that symptoms may arise as a result of the secondary problems, for example the L5 becoming symptomatic because of hyperextension. Treatment applied to the L5 or the lumbar curve will at best offer only temporary relief. True resolution will occur only when the primary problem of the weak abdominal muscles has been addressed (see Figs 3.5 A and B).

In actuality, upright posture and correct body functioning is maintained by a complex interplay of all of the elements of the body, bony and soft.

They act synergistically, that is, they work interdependently; dysfunction in one element will be conveyed to all elements. This concept is perhaps better explained by tensegrity mechanics rather than those based on Newtonian concepts and this will be discussed in Chapter 4.

THE BALANCE OF THE CURVES

In Figure 3.3 the relationship between the spinal curves is that which one would expect to find in the 'ideal' posture. Looking at people in general it is easy to see that this is not always the 'normal' posture. There are a great many variations from this ideal.

Osteopaths and others have spent much time trying to look for trends that would aid general understanding. Some of the commonly used models

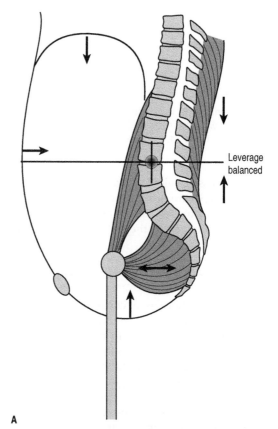

Leverage balanced

A

Figure 3.5 (A) A stable dynamically balanced situation. The 'container' (thoracic and pelvic diaphragms, transversus abdominis, thoracolumbar fascia and the erector spinae) is gently compressing the viscera creating a stable structure (like a football when fully inflated). The muscles are tonic, but generally are just fine-tuning the balance.

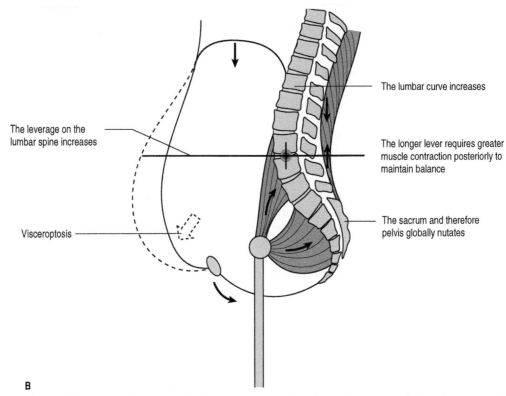

The leverage on the lumbar spine increases

The lumbar curve increases

The longer lever requires greater muscle contraction posteriorly to maintain balance

Visceroptosis

The sacrum and therefore pelvis globally nutates

B

Figure 3.5 cont'd   **(B)** The abdominal muscles have become weak, creating a less stable container for the viscera, which then ptose anteroinferiorly. This increases the leverage on the lumbar spine causing it to move anteriorly and the pelvis to nutate. The posterior muscles contract to resist the forward pulls spine.

will be discussed below. (Please note that the following concepts are not 'mathematically' accurate: they are conceptual models to aid in the visualization of the changes in the balance of the spinal curve.)

THE INTERDEPENDENCE OF THE CURVES

Stated simply, there is a constant relationship between the three dynamic curves. If one curve is changed, the others change to maintain this relationship. Figure 3.6 represents this principle. In this illustration the change in the curves is due to a change in the lumbosacral angle, causing an ascending pattern change. If the cervical curve was increased for any reason, this would theoretically also cause an increase in the other two curves; this would be a descending pattern of change. The thoracic curve, obviously, is able to affect the other two curves as well.

This is one possible model or pattern of spinal adaptation.

AREA UNDER A CURVE

A slightly simplistic view of why this occurs can be demonstrated by considering the area under a curve. If you were to draw the three mobile spinal curves and take a line through the length of the spine at the midline position, you would arrive at two small curves anterior to the line, the cervical and lumbar, and one longer curve posterior to the line, the thoracic (see Fig. 3.7A).

If the area anterior to the line was to be thought of as positive and the area posterior as negative, in order to achieve balance the summation of the anterior and posterior curves should equal zero.

Reflecting on the interdependence of the curves, if one curve is increased the area under the curve would be similarly increased. This would disturb the balance until the other two curves were equally increased (Fig. 3.7B). Thus it would be possible to say that we achieve a sense of balance throughout the spine by maintaining the balance underneath the curves.

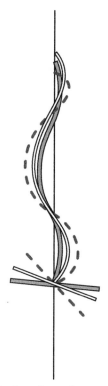

Figure 3.6 The interdependence of curves. If the lumbosacral angle is increased from the normal all three curves will be similarly augmented. The reverse will occur with reduction of the lumbosacral angle. This demonstrates the interdependence of the curves.

The interdependence is certainly not the only way that the spine can adapt. As long as the net result is zero, it is possible for the curves to behave dissimilarly. Figure 3.7C demonstrates one example of this. It would, however, have been equally effective for the cervical curve to have remained unchanged and the thoracic curve to have increased sufficiently to balance the increase in the lumbar curve.

BALANCE WITHIN THE CURVES

Still thinking of spinal curves and how they achieve balance, we can look at balance achieved *within* the curves, as opposed to the previous example of balance *between* the curves.

Let us take just one curve, for example the lumbar, and imagine that for the moment it is without its neuromuscular ligamentous support system. It does not take too much imagination to compare its structure, in a supine position, to that of a bridge. The bridge maintains its integrity by equal and

opposite forces acting on a central point, the keystone. Looking at the lumbar spine the keystone would be the L3 vertebra. As there are equal numbers of similar sized vertebrae either side of this keystone it seems a fair assumption to say that the L1 and L5 vertebrae are performing equal and opposite tasks, as are the L2 and L4. See Figure 3.8.

The significance, osteopathically, of this, is that if there is a specific dysfunction that occurs in a particular vertebra of a curve, to maintain balance, one of the (many possible) ways to adapt would be to have the equal and opposite vertebra perform the counter movement.

An example would be that if the L2 vertebra were to be rotated left, to maintain balance the L4 vertebra might rotate to an equal degree in the opposite direction (Fig. 3.9A).

Another very common adaptation is for the immediately neighbouring vertebra to counter the imbalance (Fig. 3.9B).

This would be one method of resolving problems within a curve, without requiring any adaptation from the other superimposing curves, as the area under the curve (in this case lumbar) has been maintained.

Resolution within a curve does not always occur, and the compensation therefore may occur across the curves. This is best explained diagrammatically (Figs. 3.9C and D).

The discussion so far has only indicated single vertebrae adapting to single vertebral dysfunction. This does not have to be the case: as long as the laws of equal and opposite are considered to apply, there is a seemingly infinite number of possible ways to ultimately achieve balance. Some basic concepts should help you in deconstructing compensation patterns in your patient.

If a vertebra has rotated 4° to the right (the figures are purely to illustrate a point), it may be adapted for by one vertebra rotating 4° to the left. Equally it may be by two vertebrae rotating 2° each to the left. Or four rotating 1° each; or one rotating 2° and two rotating 1° etc. This applies similarly to all planes of movement.

It is also possible to utilize the 'area under a curve' analogy to look at the possible adaptation patterns as just discussed, but from a visual perspective. This is best illustrated diagrammatically (Fig. 3.10).

So far, the discussion has principally been with regard to the anteroposterior (AP) balance of the curves. The previous concepts are equally applicable in the lateral plane, with the balance tending to occur

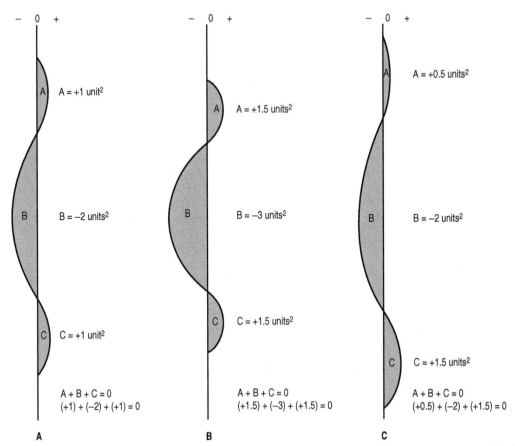

$A = +1 \ unit^2$

$B = -2 \ units^2$

$C = +1 \ unit^2$

$A + B + C = 0$
$(+1) + (-2) + (+1) = 0$

A

$A = +1.5 \ units^2$

$B = -3 \ units^2$

$C = +1.5 \ units^2$

$A + B + C = 0$
$(+1.5) + (-3) + (+1.5) = 0$

B

$A = +0.5 \ units^2$

$B = -2 \ units^2$

$C = +1.5 \ units^2$

$A + B + C = 0$
$(+0.5) + (-2) + (+1.5) = 0$

C

Figure 3.7 **(A)** Area under a curve. A, B, and C correspond to the areas described by each curve. To achieve balance A+B+C must be equal to zero. **(B)** This demonstrates the interdependence of the curves. An increase in one curve will lead to a similar increase in the other two, so that A+B+C still equals zero. **(C)** As long as the total equals zero, balance can be achieved in various ways.

across the same pivotal areas as in the AP examples. The same visual analogy of the areas also applies, the curves being in the lateral plane rather than AP.

The preceding concepts create what is perhaps one of the most basic of models with which to interpret patterns within a spine. There are numerous more

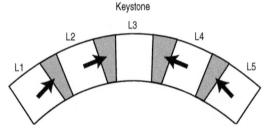

Figure 3.8 It can be seen that the vertebrae are acting around the central keystone of L3. As such, the L5 and L1, and the L2 and L4 can be hypothesized as performing an equal and opposite role around the keystone.

complex ones, some of which will be discussed later in this chapter. However, with these tools it is possible to start analysing superimposed spinal adaptation patterns and to begin to establish what is related to what. The key point within this model is to look for similars. The concept of 'similars' is frequently utilized in osteopathy, and as the word implies, similars are entities that are nearly or sometimes exactly the same. When analysing adaptation patterns the similar may be an opposite pattern but similar in its degree or extent. For example, there may be a shallow right side-bending group passing over three vertebrae. Its similar would be a shallow left side-bending group passing over three vertebrae, or, bearing in mind the previous material, a slightly deeper left side-bending group passing over two vertebrae, etc.

Many dysfunctions will have a major component to them, be it rotation, side-bending or flexion/extension. By looking for its 'similar but opposite' and making an assessment as to whether it is suffi-

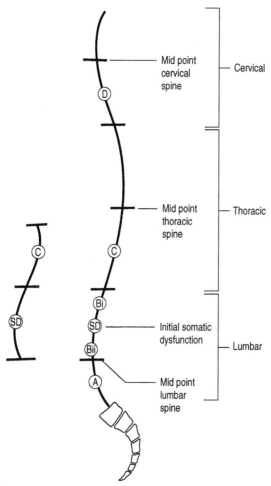

Figure 3.9 Several possible areas of compensation for a somatic dysfunction (SD). **(A)** Is equal and opposite within its curve. **(Bi and ii)** Either of its immediately neighbouring vertebrae. **(C)** Across the transition between the curves. The section is drawn out to reveal the similars across the central point. **(D)** With its reflection across the mid axis of the spine (T9).

cient to balance the original problem, you will have established a relationship hypothesis. This hypothesis will be repeatedly tested by the subsequent physical examination before it is acted on, but it is the starting point of a diagnosis.

Tissue feel is an extremely useful tool in helping you analyse these problems. As mentioned in Chapter 2, tissue changes associated with somatic dysfunction are proportional to the time that the dys-

function has been present. As compensation to dysfunction occurs relatively rapidly, the initiating problem, and any compensations to it, will have the same tissue feel. Other patterns in the body, which may be older or more recent, will have different tissue feels. Thus tissue feel can assist in identifying the relationships between specific dysfunction and its compensatory pattern. This all appears to be very simple; however, lesion patterns will often overlie each other, somewhat obscuring the patterns. But, with experience, and the will and interest to explore these ideas practically, their interpretation becomes progressively more easy. The advantage of understanding the layers of patterns is that it should be possible to remove a pattern with the minimum of disturbance to the rest. This is critical when treating someone who is about to do something important shortly after the treatment (take part in an athletic competition, get married, go on holiday), when they will not thank you for leaving them unbalanced and possibly suffering worse symptoms than before.

This approach has many detractors: osteopaths who feel that such ideas are unnecessary at best and fallacious at worst. However, it is often better to explore ideas first and then, if they do not work, discard them, rather than discarding them from a point of ignorance.

Figure 3.11 is a schematic attempt at illustrating these concepts within the whole spine.

The preceding information offers some insight into certain features of the spinal structure and function. However, for a truly complete structural system one has to look at the work of JM Littlejohn.

LITTLEJOHN'S BIOMECHANICS

John Martin Littlejohn (1865–1947) was one of the great early osteopathic thinkers. He refined and developed systems that encompass both segmental and global biomechanical analysis, and he was instrumental in bringing a sound physiological basis (based on contemporary knowledge) to the prevailing osteopathic concepts. He approached the spine as an articulated whole, looking at the osteokinematics, or its position in space in relationship to its different parts. He then approached the arthrokinematic level, the movement of the zygapophyseal joints, using the tripod concept outlined by George Webster and himself. The tripod theory has been superseded by Fryette's

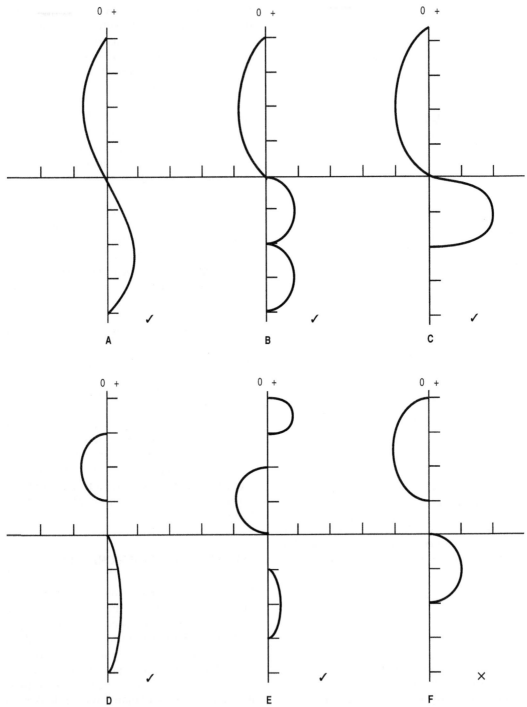

Figure 3.10 A selection of examples illustrating how balance may be achieved utilizing the 'area under a curve' analogy. The spine has been represented as a straight line to facilitate its interpretation. Note that the example F fails to achieve balance.

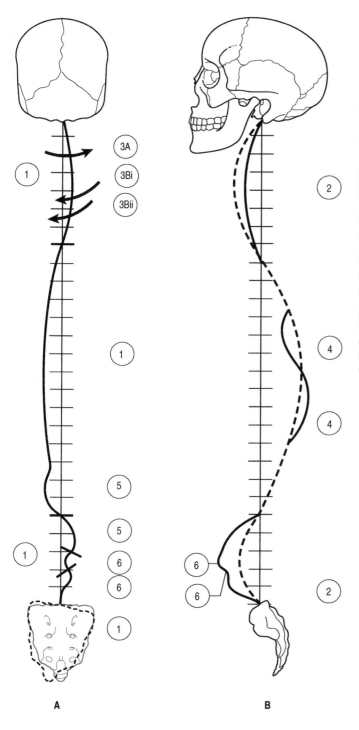

Figure 3.11 An example of the analysis of complex patterns of dysfunction. **(A)** Posterior view; **(B)** Lateral view. Note on the lateral view the dotted line is the theoretical 'normal'. A possible hypothesis of the relationships between the areas of dysfunction is: 1. The right side-bending sacrum leads to a scoliotic pattern arising in all three curves, demonstrating the interdependence of the curves. 2. The increase in the lumbar curve is compensated for by a decrease in the cervical curve, maintaining a balance with regard to the total spinal area under a curve. 3. Segmental balance of rotational dysfunction, one vertebra (3A) being compensated for by two lesser rotated vertebrae (3Bi and 3Bii). 4. A simple group flexion lesion compensated for by an equal extension group lesion. 5. A side-bending lesion being compensated for across the transition point of one curve and the next. 6. A side-bending curve or vertebra compensating with its immediately neighbouring vertebra within the same curve. Associated with this is a flexion and extension pattern (seen on lateral view). Note how patterns are superimposed on each other i.e. the lateral curve in (1) is overlain with the side-bending pattern of both (5) and (6). This makes interpretation less obvious; however, palpation of the associated soft tissues to 'age' the lesion will aid in repeating the various layers.

arthrokinematic observations, stated in his precepts. For this reason, the tripods will not be discussed here. Littlejohn's biomechanical principles underpin many of the osteopathic models that are in use throughout Europe, and though his ideas are almost synonymous with 'classical osteopathy', it can be demonstrated that his principles also underpin many of the more recent approaches.

The systems that Littlejohn developed in fact appear rather intimidating in their complexity and, perhaps for this reason (and perhaps their relative antiquity), have lost favour in certain osteopathic quarters. Those that do utilize the concepts generally fall into two camps: the traditionalists, who attempt to interpret the material as Littlejohn intended it, and those who utilize the concepts as a foundation and attempt to integrate them with new concepts as they arise.

There appears to have been a trend over the last few years to dismiss Littlejohn's work as non-scientific and inaccurate. A prime example that has given rise to this opinion is that he cites the L3 vertebra as the centre of gravity for the body, whereas most contemporary studies demonstrate that it is anterior to the body of the S2 vertebra. It is, however, perhaps worth reflecting on the source of his theories. They arose from close observation of individuals in a clinical setting and were tested in the treatment of these individuals. The construct of lines and pivots he created was his attempt to define what he saw. By contrast, the S2 level was discovered utilizing complex analytical equipment. Most osteopaths utilize the same assessment tools that Littlejohn used: our eyes, hands and intellect. Perhaps the models that he inspired still have a relevance to the practising osteopath. Ultimately, each individual practitioner must come to their own conclusions on this matter.

In this chapter, no attempt has been made to encompass Littlejohn's whole *oeuvre*, due to the confines of space, but the key elements are introduced as well as their more contemporary interpretations. For those interested in Littlejohn's original concepts there is a list of recommended reading at the end of this chapter.

THE ARCHES

Littlejohn analysed the spinal curves in a series of different ways. He based these interpretations on a wide range of criteria, including the morphology of the vertebra such as their facet orientation and body shape, the origins and insertions of muscles attaching to the spine, sites where the perceived lines of force (AP, PA, AC, PC and central gravity line) section the spine, the centre of the arc of individual vertebral movement (oscillatory centre), the embryological development of the spine, and observable function – to mention a few. This resulted in a series of 'arches and keystones' for each analysis. The term 'keystone' was used by Littlejohn to mean the most important vertebra in the arch, in relation

to its mechanics and the central gravity line and not necessarily the point of maximum curvature.[4] He excluded the C1 vertebra as he considered it to be little more than a connecting ring between the occiput and the cervical arch. He, and later Wernham, have drawn an analogy between its role and that of the L5, particularly in the 'functional arches', and as such it could be thought of as a pivot between the occiput and the C2.

Littlejohn described four types of arches:

- the structural arches
- the functional arches
- the central or double arch, and
- the physiological arches.

Each classification is based on a particular role or criteria, as implied by their names. A brief description of each follows.

The structural arches

This is essentially the manner in which the spine has been described by anatomists, based on regional anatomy. Thus the neck passes from the skull to the thorax, therefore the spine in that region is the cervical spine, and similarly for the other curves. Though it is possible to distinguish which group most of the vertebrae belong to by looking at their structure, it is not based principally on the morphology of the vertebrae. The arches are illustrated in Figure 3.12.

The arches	The keystones
C2–T2	C2/3
T2–T12	T5/6
T12–L5	L3
L5–Coccyx	

The functional arches

As the name implies, this classification is based on the way the curves function as units. Function is dictated by structure, in this case the structure of the vertebrae and their supporting muscle groups. Morphologically there is a gradual transition as the spine is descended. Some of these changes dictate the movements that are possible, such as the orientation of the articular facets of the vertebrae. The attachments of the spinal musculature can be interpreted as dividing the spine into functional units. Thus it is possible by observing the manner in which the spine functions and by analysing the nature and position of the above structures, to create a series of

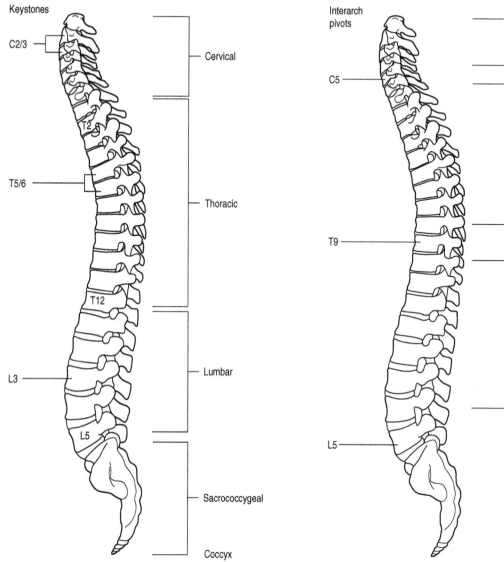

Figure 3.12 The structural arches.

Figure 3.13 The functional arches.

arches defined by the function (and structure) of the spine. This does not comply with the regional approach utilized conventionally in anatomical descriptions, such as that described above in the structural arches. The arches so defined are termed the functional arches. The key features are:

- The C5 and the T9 are cited as points of transition of facet orientation and therefore represent transitional points for movement.
- The L5 is envisaged as the linkage point between the lumbar spine and the sacrum, in an analogous role to that of the C1.

Thus these points – C5, T9, L5 (C1) – represent the pivots between the arches. One type of movement is permitted above and another type is permitted below. It is clear that these pivots will be subject to a lot of strain.

Complex analysis of the origins, insertions and directions of action of the surrounding spinal musculature reveals that though working as an integrated unit, it is possible to observe a functional division into groups, the position of which further supports the structural observations leading to the functional curves. See Figure 3.13.

The arches	The interarch pivots
C2–C4	C5
C6–T8	T9
T10–L4	L5
Sacrum–Coccyx	

The central (double) arch

The key element of analysis in this arch is that of support of the spine and body. The central arch is thought to represent the strongest unit of the spine. This is based on several concepts:

- The thorax is a primary curve; it has retained its embryological kyphotic curve into adulthood and is therefore stable and strong. The cervical and lumbar curves are secondary, and therefore almost by definition are areas of compensation rather than support, adapting to both the primary curve and to gravity.
- The T4 represents the point where the compressive forces of the head and neck are supported by the primary curve.
- The L3 represents the centre of gravity of the body with everything below being suspended from this point.
- Both of the above points are also major pivotal areas. The T4 is the point of articulation between the upper and lower triangles and the L3 is the apex of the little triangle (see p.64). These represent points of mobility either side of a relatively hypomobile stable thoracic group.

Thus the central arch supports the spine: the cephalad end of the arch is a foundation for the compression originating from the head and neck, and the caudad end is also the point of suspension from L3 and below for the pelvis and lower extremities. Thus the central arch runs from T5 to L2. It is sometimes referred to as the double arch as it is comprised of both a kyphotic arch and a lordotic arch (Fig. 3.14).

The arches	The keystone
C2–T4	
T5–L2 The central arch	T9
L3 below	

The physiological arches

This is based on a rather complex analysis of the lines of force, the osteopathic centres, autonomic nervous system control, and centres of oscillation (the central point of a circle described by the orientation of the facets).

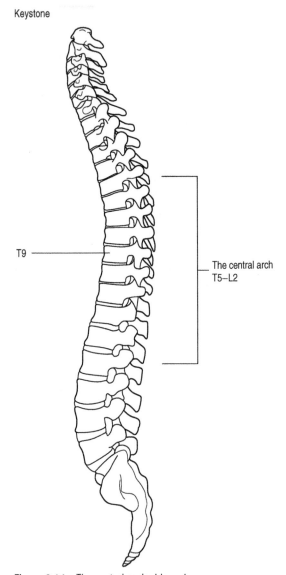

Keystone

T9

The central arch
T5–L2

Figure 3.14 The central or double arch.

The key points are that C7 and T9 are the oscillation centres for the cervical and thoracic and the thoracic and lumbar regions respectively and it is these that define the cephalad pivot of the two curves. Analysis of the osteopathic and autonomic centres within each region would enable one to predict the type of physiological dysfunction that might occur. See Figure 3.15.

The arches	The keystone
C7–T8	T9
T10–Coccyx	

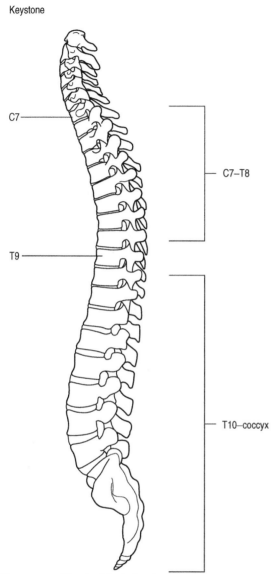

Keystone

C7

C7–T8

T9

T10–coccyx

Figure 3.15 The physiological arches.

- occiput/C1
- C5
- T4
- T9
- T12/L1 (thoracolumbar junction)
- L3
- L5/S1.

The C5, T9 and L3 are sometimes referred to as mid-arch pivots and the others are termed interarch pivots. This is not consistent with Littlejohn's usage of these terms, but has a practical use.

The spinal curves are thus described as follows:

- The cervical curve passes from C1 to T4 (often cited as C2 to T4 due to Littlejohn's ideas on the C1).
- The thoracic curve passes from the T4 to the T12.
- The lumbar curve passes from L1 to L5. See Figure 3.16.

Variations on this are often seen, the most common of whch are:

- Rather than occiput/C1, the occiput/C3 is used. This is based on Fryette's logic that the upper cervical complex should be perceived as one unit functioning as a universal joint, permitting all planes of movement within the group, enabling it to adapt to any postural changes in the body and still maintain the correct alignment of the head.
- The thoracolumbar junction is sometimes not included as a pivot.
- The L5/S1 junction is sometimes stated as the sacrum, presumably to allow for consideration of the sacroiliac articulations as well as the lumbosacral.

This reductionist interpretation of the arches and pivots has created a very useful model that can be used to underpin methods of diagnosis and treatment, e.g. the treatment models of specific adjusting technique (SAT) and general osteopathic treatment (GOT) (see Section 3) are discussed in the next two chapters. Below are two examples of how this model may be applied as a diagnostic tool. Though they could not be described as originating directly from Littlejohn, they have arisen from an interpretation of his concepts. On returning to the more classical views of Littlejohn, more uses of this model will become apparent.

'Functional' pivots

It must be appreciated that the pivots and curves are cited for the 'ideal' posture. In reality the

Analysis of each of these arches and their pivots enabled osteopaths to understand the patterns of dysfunction that might arise and how to treat them, but with passing time it became progressively simplified to what is nowadays sometimes referred to as a 'pivotal model', this being a synthesis of all four of the 'arches'.

THE PIVOTAL MODEL

This contemporary interpretation cites the pivots as being:

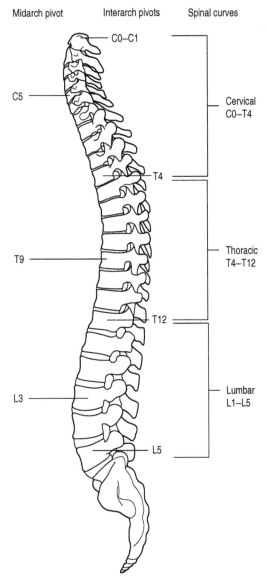

Midarch pivot   Interarch pivots   Spinal curves

C0–C1

C5

Cervical
C0–T4

T4

T9

Thoracic
T4–T12

T12

L3

Lumbar
L1–L5

L5

Figure 3.16 The pivotal model. Please note that the terms midarch pivot and interarch pivot used in this diagram are not consistent with Littlejohn's usage of these terms.

positions will vary, often markedly from that stated. Where there is this difference from the ideal the name of the pivot can be utilized as a functional descriptor. Thus if someone has a long lumbar curve extending up to the T10, the actual T9/T10 vertebrae will be acting as the transition between the thoracic and lumbar curves and it could be termed the 'functional T/L pivot'. The functional L3 pivot may be the actual L1 or L2 vertebra. See Figure 3.17A.

This is clinically useful if one accepts this pivotal model, and has an understanding of the interplay between the pivots, because by analysing an individual's pattern, one can interpret what areas of the spine are fulfilling each role. At the simplest level of treatment rationale, should the patient be relatively healthy and, with treatment, be able to adapt fully, the patient's pattern as analysed in relation to the functional pivotal model is the starting point and the 'ideal' model can be used as the ultimate aim of the treatment (Fig. 3.17B). It may only be possible to get the person to a certain point along the continuum from their current posture to the 'ideal', but it serves as a guide. A simple treatment rationale for Figure 3.17 may be that the lower thoracics are extended, causing the elongation of the lumbar lordosis and the shortened but deeper thoracic and cervical curves. If the low thoracics were the primary in this pattern, mobilization into flexion of this group would allow the thoracic spine to 'drop down' to its more ideal position. Similarly, the lumbar spine would be normalized, as would the cervical spine (assuming that the problem was relatively recent and no chronic tissue changes were present to prevent it from reestablishing balance). The pivots would thus pass to their more appropriate situations and the 'ideal' would have been achieved. *Note.* We as osteopaths are not always aiming for the perfect posture. In some individuals this may, for many reasons, not be possible, but a concept of where one would ideally 'go' with treatment is of benefit.

This is a very simple example of how one might apply this concept.

The application of the concepts of balance within a curve and across the curves to the pivotal model

Earlier in this section the means by which balance may be achieved within the curves and across the whole curves/spine was discussed. These concepts can be applied to the dynamic and functional patterns that are modelled using Littlejohn's pivotal model. Again, it should be pointed out that these are oversimplifications and therefore open to criticism; however, they do create a simple model with which to attempt to understand the complex interplay of spinal mechanics and thence the functioning of the body. From this level of understanding it is possible to pass to the next level of understanding.

One of the most important elements in the understanding is that the pivots will move, they are not static. However, the role of the pivot is still the same regardless of the vertebra acting as one. Littlejohn

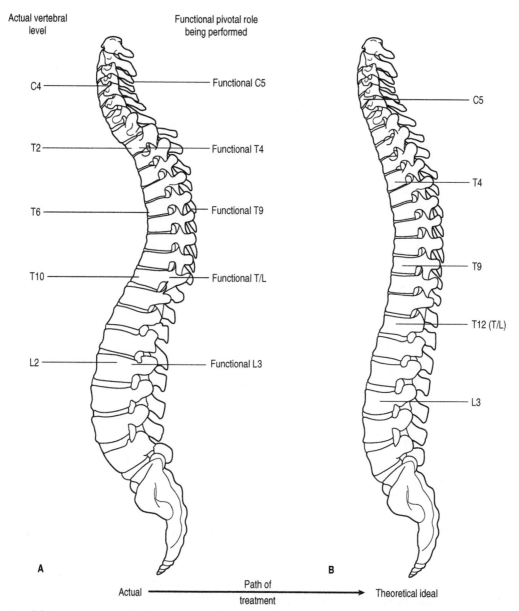

Actual vertebral level

Functional pivotal role being performed

C4 ——— Functional C5

T2 ——— Functional T4

T6 ——— Functional T9

T10 ——— Functional T/L

L2 ——— Functional L3

C5

T4

T9

T12 (T/L)

L3

A

B

Actual ——— Path of treatment ———→ Theoretical ideal

Figure 3.17 **(A)** The long lumbar curve has caused the pivots to be 'shifted' up, therefore vertebrae not designed to be junctional are forced into the role (and a greater chance to dysfunction). These new pivots are sometimes termed 'functional pivots' (in the sense that they are functioning as a pivot). Thus for example the T10 vertebra is the functional T/L. **(B)** This shows the theoretical 'ideal'. If the patient is fit and has the ability to adapt, this may be the end result of treatment. If structural changes have occurred it may be possible to go only so far along this route; it is then necessary to balance them around that pattern.

used the analogy of a keystone from architecture, this being the point where the forces are acting equally and in opposition, maintaining the integrity of the curve. Thus for the lumbar curve it could be supposed that the L3 is the logical keystone (Fig. 3.8). However, as shown in Figure 3.17 the role can be taken by L2. The lumbar spine from Figure 3.17 is shown schematically in Figure 3.18. From this it is possible to see that the T10 is the functional cephalad end of the lumbar curve, and the L5 the caudad end. Thus if dysfunction occurs at the L4, one of the places to expect compensation would be

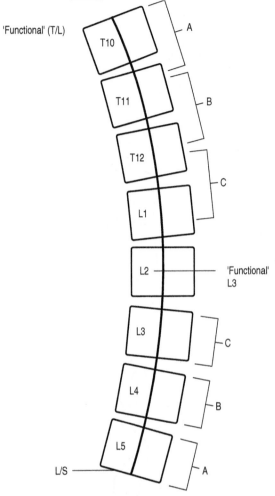

'Functional' (T/L)

T10

T11

T12

L1

L2 — 'Functional' L3

L3

L4

L5

L/S

A

B

C

C

B

A

Figure 3.18 Balance is still achieved within the curve in the same manner, even though the pivots have moved. This example demonstrates that the areas of balance may include more than just one vertebra; in this instance either may adapt, or both.

T11/T12. Balance within the curve is achieved in the usual way.

In the ideal situation, the keystone of the cervical curve is C5, of the thoracic curve is T9 and of the lumbar curve is L3. These three vertebrae serve the same function in their respective curves. As they have the same function, it is possible to imagine that dysfunction in one may be compensated for by one or both of the other keystones. This is equally true regardless of what actual vertebra is acting as each of the pivots. It is the role performed by the structure that is important, not its actual name. With this understood, it is possible to apply the simple concepts of balance within the curves and across the curves and establish hypothetical patterns of interdependence in any spine. Then, by utilizing palpation skills to assess tissue changes (the primary lesion and its compensation, after the acute period has passed, will have very similar tissue changes), and applying an understanding of the causative factors and how the particular individual's body will respond to these forces, further confirm or refute that hypothesis. The resulting hypothesis will then be further tested in the gross and segmental examination of the whole spine.

The significance of T9

Osteopathically, the T9 is of great significance, with many experienced osteopaths recommending caution when addressing it. Some of its significance can be understood when it is realized that the T9 can be perceived as being the keystone of *all three curves*; this is possible to envisage if the spinal curves are drawn as the person is prone (Fig. 3.19). This does not mean, however, that it should not be mobilized, but an awareness of its possible mechanical role in the entire spine is advantageous.

Now we return to the more 'classical' concepts of Littlejohn.

THE LINES OF FORCE, CENTRAL GRAVITY LINE, AND THE CENTRE OF GRAVITY

Littlejohn wanted to establish some means of discovering the central gravity line and the centre of

Figure 3.19 T9 can be thought of as the keystone of the whole spine, hence its great significance osteopathically.

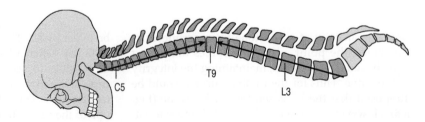

C5

T9

L3

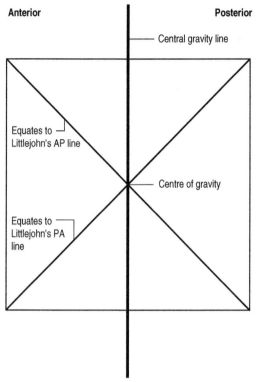

Anterior   Posterior

—— Central gravity line

Equates to
Littlejohn's AP line

—— Centre of gravity

Equates to
Littlejohn's PA
line

Figure 3.20   The method used to find the centre of gravity of a square, and the central gravity line, by resolving the two oblique lines.

gravity of the body. This is a relatively straightforward process if working with a square piece of wood, as shown in Figure 3.20.

However, applying this to the human body is not as straightforward. The human body is a dynamic structure, and the centre of gravity is constantly shifting. As well as the musculoskeletal element being dynamic, there is a constant change in the internal physiological and fluid dynamics which will have an effect on the whole body. On this, Campbell[4] succinctly states:

> *given these considerations the importance of the centre of gravity as the centre of mass of body tissue ceases itself to be of vital importance and gives way to the idea of a centre of balance between the internal forces, gravity and environmental factors. In the balanced and integrated body there will be a unique relationship between this 'centre of balance' and the centre of gravity.*

This makes explicit those concepts that are so often lost when discussing this aspect of Littlejohn's work.

It also helps to take some of the emphasis off one of the apparently major stumbling blocks for the acceptance of this work, namely the L3 being cited as the centre of gravity. However, in the orthograde position, the model that Littlejohn originated has helped numerous generations of osteopaths gain some understanding of the biomechanical relationships of the body, and what may be anticipated if the central gravity line shifts from the ideal.

Undeterred by the complexity of the human form, Littlejohn adapted the model in Figure 3.20 to the human body. He devised the anteroposterior (AP) and posteroanterior (PA) lines as mirrors of the lines crossing to give the centre of gravity of the piece of wood. He also, however, complicated this slightly by attributing a particular role to each line. He describes the AP line as a line of force uniting the spinal curves and the PA as a line to balance the cavity pressures.

The anteroposterior line

The AP line begins at the anterior-most point of the superior part of the spine, variously described as the anterior margin of the foramen magnum at the base of the skull, or the anterior tubercle of C1. It then passes inferiorly and posteriorly through the bodies of T11 and T12, to the posterior junction of L4/5 and then through the body of S1 to arrive at its most distal posterior point, the tip of the coccyx.

The stated role of this line is that it is a 'line uniting the entire spine into one articulated mechanism … and is the chief point of mechanical resistance to the loss of the normal arches of the spine'.[5]

Another way of looking at it is that it resolves the forces in the spine. Again, a simple analogy may help explain this, that of the bow, as in a bow and arrow. The bow's arch is maintained by the string running from tip to tip. It is in a state of balance, thus it is possible to say that the forces in the bow are balanced, equally and in opposition, by the tension in the string; or that the vector represented by the string resolves, or opposes and balances, the forces within the bow. This logic could be extended to systems that consist of more than one arc, as seen in Figure 3.21.

To balance this, Littlejohn described the posteroanterior line.

The posteroanterior (PA) line

This begins at the posterior-most point of the superior part of the spine, generally taken to be the midpoint of the posterior margin of the foramen magnum. It then passes anteroinferiorly to the

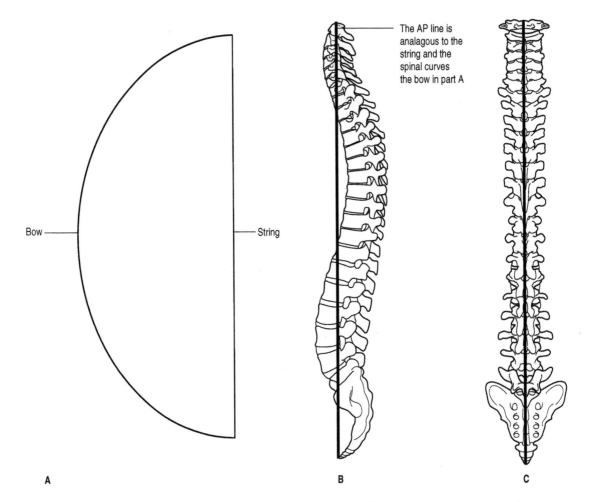

A **B** **C**

Figure 3.21 The bow and string analogy to illustrate how the AP line may unite the entire spine into one articulated mechanism. **(A)** The string can be perceived as resolving the forces present in the bow, or as the force maintaining the bow in its stable position. **(B,C)** This analogy can be taken further to address more than one curve. Thus the AP line represents the string and can be seen as resolving the forces in the spine or binding the curves into 'one articulated mechanism'. (B = lateral view; C = posterior view.) (After Campbell C. A brief review of the mechanics of the spine. Maidstone: Maidstone College of Osteopathy.)

The AP line is analagous to the string and the spinal curves the bow in part A

anterior margin of the articulation of L2/3 where it bifurcates and passes to the most anterolateral part of the spine and pelvis, the acetabulae. (In some texts it is shown as continuing anteriorly around the pubic ramus, encompassing the pelvic cavity, to meet at the symphysis pubis.)

This is a much more complicated line, with several functions. Figure 3.22 shows the areas of the PA line which particularly serve the functions stated. Wernham states that the functions are that it:[5]

- is complementary to the AP line. (Though it is complementary, Campbell warns that 'the lines are not mutually independent, thus while a particular function may be attributed to each line, the other line will have a component of force in that direction also'[4])
- represents a line of pressure binding the posterior occipitoatlantal articulation to T2 and the second rib to maintain the integrity of neck tension (see 1 on Fig. 3.22)
- strengthens the line of abdominopelvic support (see 2 on Fig. 3.22)
- directs tension from the articulation of L2/3 to the femoral heads (via the psoas muscle and the deep abdominopelvic fascia, which are repre-

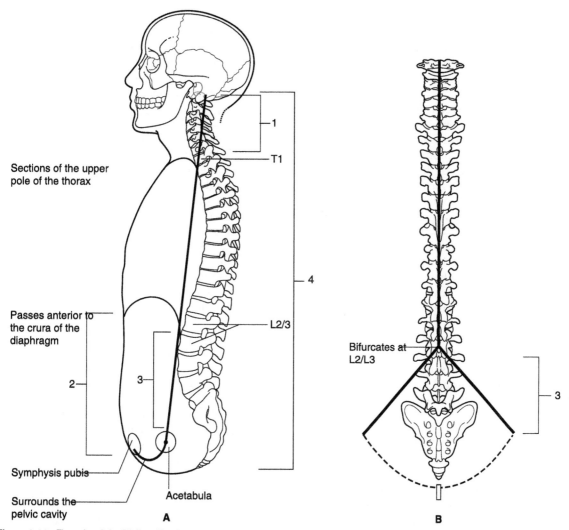

Sections of the upper
pole of the thorax

Passes anterior to
the crura of the
diaphragm

Symphysis pubis

Surrounds the
pelvic cavity

Acetabula

A

Bifurcates at
L2/L3

B

Figure 3.22 The role of the PA line. The figures refer to the stated functions of the PA line, please refer to the text for the details. This Figure shows that the line traverses key points of each of the cavities and its role in coordinating the pressures in the internal cavities of the body is more easily understood. **(A)** Lateral view. **(B)** Posterior view. (After Campbell C. A brief review of the mechanics of the spine. Maidstone: Maidstone College of Osteopathy.)

sented by the lines as they bifurcate at the L2/3 and pass laterally to the acetabulae; see 3 on Fig. 3.22)

- maintains tension of neck, trunk and legs coordinate with the pressures in the internal cavities of the body via the T/L ligaments which oppose the hip and leg movements in relation to the abdominal muscles and pelvic organs (see 4 on Fig. 3.22).

It can be seen that this line serves more of the elements balancing the internal forces, gravity and

environmental factors. Its role in balancing the cavity pressures can be understood by being aware that the PA line passes through the upper pole of the thoracic cavity at the level of T1. It then passes inferiorly through the junction of the abdominal and thoracic cavities and anterior to the crural attachments of the diaphragm at the level of the L2/3 vertebrae. There it bifurcates, passing anteriorly, laterally and inferiorly through the abdominal cavity to the acetabulae bilaterally. It finally passes around the pubic ramus to reunite at the symphysis. Thus it is present at key points throughout each of the cavities.

The central gravity line

As with our original piece of wood in Figure 3.20, if a line is drawn between the two oblique lines, the AP and PA, the resultant line should be the central gravity line.

This passes 'between the two condyles of the occiput, at the odontoid process', inferiorly to pass through the centre of the body of the L3, 'through the anterior promontory of the sacrum, medially to the centre of the hip, knee and ankle, thence anteriorly to the metatarsal head and posteriorly to the tuberosity of the calcaneus'.[5]

The centre of gravity of the body

As the central gravity line passes through the body of the L3 vertebra, this is cited by Littlejohn as the centre of gravity of the body. Thus the body above L3 is supported on it, whilst the spine, pelvis and lower extremities are 'suspended' from it.

This process has so far assessed the human body as if it were a two-dimensional object, resolving it only in the sagittal plane. To assess it in three dimensions it is necessary to perform the same procedures in the coronal plane. The lines used to do this are termed the anterior and posterior central lines.

The anterior central (AC) and posterior central (PC) lines

The same major role is apportioned to the AC as the AP line (much to the confusion of students), that is, maintaining articular tension; and similarly with the PC being assigned the same major role as the PA, namely integrating cavity pressures. This creates a slight problem in that as articular tension has only 1° of freedom, it can be represented in three dimensions as a single line – therefore there is only one AC line, but as cavity pressure is a volumetric concern, it cannot be represented in three dimensions by one line, so two PC lines are used. This is not a critical point but can sometimes further confuse students.

Thus the AC line passes from the anterior midpoint of the spine in the coronal plane and passes inferiorly and posteriorly to the coccyx. In fact, it is exactly the same as the AP line. See Figure 3.23.

The PC lines attempt to encompass as much of the coronal aspect of the spine and torso as possible. They therefore originate one from either side of the lateral-most aspect of the posterior border of the foramen magnum, passing medially across the body, crossing anterior to the T4 level and then continuing to the acetabulae opposite to their side of origin. (See Fig. 3.24.)

Resolution of the AC and PC lines will also give the central gravity line.

With these two sets of lines it is now possible to see how certain concepts have arisen.

The three triangles of force and the three unities

If the two PC lines and the PA line are superimposed on each other, three triangles appear. These are termed, rather descriptively, the little, lower and upper triangles. See Figure 3.25.

The little triangle has its base at the femoral articulations of the acetabulae, and its apex anterior to the body of the L3 vertebra. The lower triangle shares the same base as the little triangle, but the apex passes up to the anterior aspect of the T4. The upper triangle has its small base at the posterior margins of the foramen magnum, and its apex at the level of the T4, meeting the apex of the lower triangle.

For Littlejohn these triangles were another way of observing the interrelationships of the body. The L3 being the centre of gravity of the body and the T4 arguably the second most important pivot in the body (possibly in contest with the T9 for this position), this allows one to observe how the body may function around these significant pivots. A simple example of this is the 'gossip' or drop knee test. The knees are alternately bent and the effects observed. As the base of both the lower triangles is affected there should be movement noted at both the L3 and the T4. There also should be a smooth transition of side-bending curves throughout the spine; failure in any of these will indicate dysfunction. To find out where this dysfunction is occurring would involve further tests. In fact, there is a whole diagnostic routine based on these three triangles to establish the sites of various dysfunctions, which is termed 'unity testing'.

The three unities and unity testing

Unity testing is a complete series of tests based on the three triangles, which examines the whole body osteopathically. It was devised by Tom Dummer[6] 'based on an original concept of Still, i.e. that the body is made up of a triad of pelvis and lower extremities; cranium, neck, shoulder girdles and upper extremities; both articulating with the thorax and trunk, and all three being functionally independent'. The unities are just as described in the above section on the three triangles, though the unities also include

Figure 3.23   The AC line when viewed from the sagittal plane can be seen to be identical to the AP line. **(A)** Posterior view. **(B)** Lateral view.

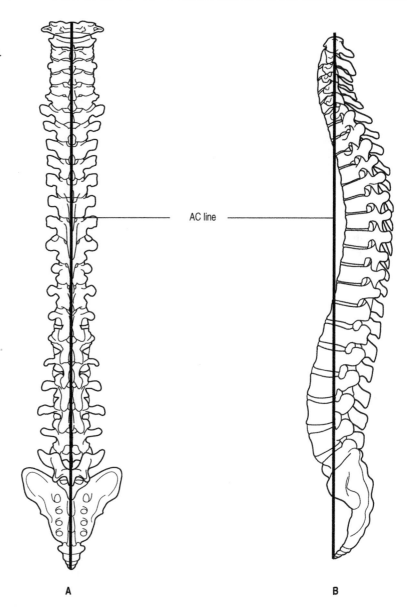

AC line

A

B

the limbs (this is implicit in the triangles but often not stated). As the body is an integrated structure there will be an overlap anatomically and functionally, and therefore some overlap when assessing the unities; however, essentially the boundaries of each unity are as for the triangles, thus:

- Unity 1 relates to the small triangle, thus it passes from the L3 and includes the pelvis and the lower extremities. Anatomically the whole lumbar spine is generally included and thus also in the assessment routine. (It is possible that this

was chosen as the first unity because of the prime importance placed on pelvic balance within 'classical' osteopathy.)
- Unity 2 is the same as the upper triangle, passing from and including the cranium to the T4. It also includes the shoulder girdles and the upper extremities. (The shoulder girdles and the upper extremities are functionally and anatomically related to both Unities 2 and 3. Generally, conceptually, they are related to Unity 2, but for the convenience of testing they are included in the testing routine of Unity 3.)

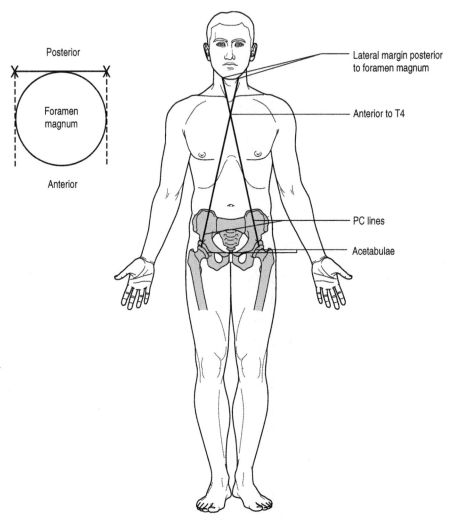

Figure 3.24 Superior origins of the PC line. **X** indicates the cephalad origin of the PC lines.

- Unity 3 includes the thorax and the vital organs and extends from the T4 to the L3. The shoulder girdle is also included.

The details of the diagnostic routine are beyond the scope of this book. For a detailed description, refer to Tom Dummer's *Textbook of Osteopathy* (see recommended reading at the end of the chapter).

The triangles of force and unities are two-dimensional interpretations. The polygons of force offer a three-dimensional interpretation.

The polygons of force

The polygons are created by combining the AP, AC and PC lines, as in Figure 3.26.

The upper polygon has a triangular base surrounding the foramen magnum of the skull, providing a base for the support of the cranium (Fig. 3.26Ai). The apex is found at the T4 and rib 3 which is the point through which the compressive and torsional forces of the head and neck act.

The lower polygon has its base in the bony pelvis (Fig. 3.26Aii). When correctly aligned this acts as a solid base for the support of the abdominal and pelvic organs and is instrumental in maintaining abdominal tension. The soft tissues are of great importance in maintaining the integrity of this polygon, as its relatively large lateral margins are formed in the abdomen and the lower two-thirds of the thorax. Loss of soft tissue tone or balance will lead to a collapse of this polygon, with a consequent

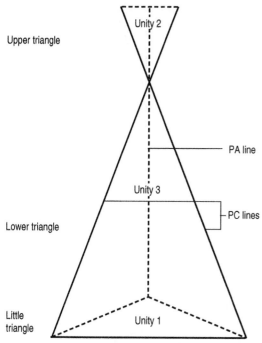

Figure 3.25 Combining the PA and PC lines gives rise to the three triangles and the three unities.

deleterious effect on the viscera within. The apex articulates with the apex of the upper polygon anterior to T4 at the point where they both cross the central gravity line. The two polygons thus pivot around this point, hence its great mechanical significance. Problems in either polygon may reflect, and thus possibly cause symptoms, at this pivot and/or its related structures.

Combined, the polygons represent the support of the spine and the viscera, and how the relative pressure differentials between thoracic, abdominal and pelvic cavities are maintained. They also represent the articular tensions (particularly spinal) as they oscillate around the central gravity line. Many of the effects of this will be addressed more fully in Chapter 5, where Littlejohn's anterior and posterior body types are analysed. In brief, the anterior and posterior weight-bearing types describe the changes that occur in the body when the centre of gravity line shifts either forwards or backwards from the neutral position, with a consequent deformation of the polygons. It is possible, by analysing the effects that it has on the lines of force, and therefore spinal integrity and cavity pressure balance, to hypothesize on the gross positional changes and possible physiological

and pathological changes that may arise as a result of this shift.

As well as modelling the changes with gross anterior and posterior shifts, the polygons offer a means of interpreting the vectors of force that may be acting on the individual in a three-dimensional manner. To illustrate this, take the example of a functional unilateral short leg (Fig. 3.27).

The pelvis will be lower on the side of the short leg; this will result in a lowering of the base of the lower triangle with a resultant increase in the vector of force represented by the ipsilateral PC line passing obliquely inferiorly and laterally from its contralateral origin at the occiput to the acetabulae (Fig. 3.27A). Generally associated with the lowering of the pelvis there will also be a movement in the anteroposterior plane. For the purpose of this discussion we will say that the acetabula has moved slightly anteriorly. This will cause the line of tension to have an additional vector of force acting anteriorly. This results in a torsional vector of force acting through the body (Fig. 3.27B). Applying this concept (where appropriate) will model the probable passage of this vector of force. Any structure lying within this vector of force will be subject to that force, be it articular, visceral, neurological, vascular, etc. Analysis of the vectors of force and an understanding of the underlying structures will enable one to anticipate the effects this will have on those structures. In the diagram an organ is positioned with its rotational axis lateral to the descending vector, thus it will be caused to rotate medially. The anterior vector of the descending force will cause it also to rotate anteriorly. When palpating this structure, its mobility will be greater on medial rotation and anterior rotation, as it will move preferentially into the direction of the lesion. If that is what is found, it would be reasonable to hypothesize that this pattern is as a result of the short leg, and as such would only resolve fully when the leg length discrepancy is resolved. However, if the findings on the organ differed from this it may indicate that it is not part of the global pattern, and therefore may itself be in dysfunction, requiring specific local treatment. The polygons can therefore help model global patterns that will be visible on observation and palpable as fascial patterns and via the tissues and organ mobility.

(Please read the conclusion with regard to the Newtonian concepts of pulleys and lever inherent with the above.)

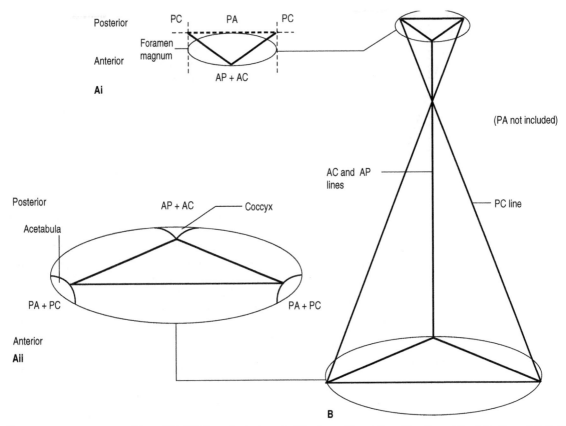

Figure 3.26 The polygons of force. **(Ai, ii)** Points of attachment of the lines of force. By uniting the points of the lines of force at the foramen magnum, and similarly at the pelvic bowl, two triangles appear: an upper one with its apex facing anteriorly, and a lower one where the apex faces posteriorly. By drawing in the lines of force passing between their points of origin on the two triangles, the polygons of force appear. **(B)** The polygons of force.

CONCLUSION

This chapter has offered numerous different interpretations of how the spine and the body may be modelled utilizing structural conceptual models. As stated in the introduction, they are all empirical. A relatively wide range of concepts has been discussed, from patterns of individual dysfunction compensation, to the planar model of patterning of the triangles or unities, to the more global view offered by the polygons. At this point in time these ideas will still appear to you as rather strange abstractions. This is partly due to the relatively wide range of approaches, which are necessary because of the infinite variety of patterns a patient can express. Also, this results from the confines of this book limiting further explanation of the diagnostic routines of the unities. An understanding of these procedures will assist in the understanding of the unities and the polygons, and you are therefore directed to Tom Dummer's own writings on the subject in the *Textbook of Osteopathy*. However, the key point of this chapter is that you start truly looking at the body. This ability to look and *actually* see is one of the most important skills, and sadly one of the ones most often neglected. The looking is not to impose any of these particular models on a patient, but to see inside the body, to see what pattern it is expressing. Michelangelo, when commissioned to create a sculpture, would go to the marble mines to look at the blocks of marble. He would look deep within them to see what sculptures the blocks themselves expressed. He did not impose the form; he revealed what was already within. This may sound flowery, but that is exactly what osteopaths aim to do.

All of the concepts above are based on a Newtonian conception of mechanics which utilizes the

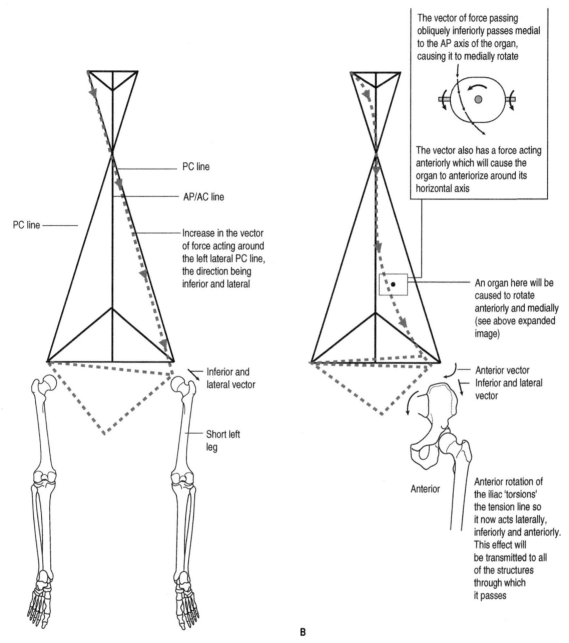

The vector of force passing obliquely inferiorly passes medial to the AP axis of the organ, causing it to medially rotate

The vector also has a force acting anteriorly which will cause the organ to anteriorize around its horizontal axis

PC line

AP/AC line

PC line

Increase in the vector of force acting around the left lateral PC line, the direction being inferior and lateral

An organ here will be caused to rotate anteriorly and medially (see above expanded image)

Inferior and lateral vector

Short left leg

Anterior vector
Inferior and lateral vector

Anterior

Anterior rotation of the iliac 'torsions' the tension line so it now acts laterally, inferiorly and anteriorly. This effect will be transmitted to all of the structures through which it passes

B

Figure 3.27   Modelling the effects on the polygons of force that will occur in the presence of a functional unilateral short leg.

compressive force of gravity to support structures that are comprised of columns, beams, levers and fulcra, such as in a conventional building. Most of our biomechanical concepts are based on these Newtonian principles. These concepts are being questioned, as there are too many features of the human form and function that cannot be explained by this model. Perhaps more impor-

tantly, over the last few decades a new model has been emerging that appears to be able to explain some of these anomalies – in fact, the more this model is tested the better the results. That model is *tensegrity*. Technically it should be discussed within this chapter, but because of the possible great importance of it, it will be 'honoured' with a chapter of its own, Chapter 4.

References

1. Weaver C. The cranial vertebrae. JAOA 1936; March.
2. Kapandji IA. The physiology of the joints, vol 3: the trunk and vertebral column. Edinburgh: Churchill Livingstone; 1974.
3. Hides JA, Stokes MJ, Saide M et al. Evidence of lumbar multifidus muscle wasting ipsilateral to symptoms in patients with acute/subacute low back pain. Spine 1994; 19(2):165–177.
4. Campbell C. A brief review of the mechanics of the spine. Maidstone: Maidstone College of Osteopathy; 22.
5. Wernham J, Hall TE. The mechanics of the spine and pelvis. Maidstone: Maidstone College of Osteopathy; 1960.
6. Dummer T. A textbook of osteopathy, vol 1. Hadlow Down: JoTom Publications; 1999: 175–200.

Recommended reading

There are few books that address the spinal lesion patterns. Most of the early part of this chapter consists of the author's own thoughts derived from the collective teachings of Tom Dummer, Harold Klug and Robert Lever, and the indirect teachings of Michelangelo, Picasso and the natural beauty of nature. Only Tom Dummer has a widely available text.

Original Littlejohn texts are rare, and those interpreted by John Wernham are somewhat opaque in nature, but are worth the effort. An excellent introductory text is that of Chris Campbell. The Maidstone College of Osteopathy prints several of the following books; however, it rarely includes the date of publication. Those dates shown are the collective opinions, but are not guaranteed.

Campbell C. A brief review of the mechanics of the spine. Maidstone: Maidstone College of Osteopathy.

Dummer T. A textbook of osteopathy, vol 1. Hadlow Down: JoTom Publications; 1999: 116–126,166–203.

Littlejohn JM. The fundamentals of osteopathic technique. Maidstone: Maidstone College of Osteopathy.

Stone C. Science in the art of osteopathy. Cheltenham: Stanley Thornes; 1999: 122–165.

Wernham J, Hall TE. The mechanics of the spine and pelvis. Maidstone: Maidstone College of Osteopathy; 1960.

Chapter 4

Tensegrity

INTRODUCTION

One of the fundamental concepts within osteopathic philosophy is the concept of *vis medicatrix naturae*, or the self-healing nature of the body. The role of a practitioner is to aid the body in this attempt. For AT Still, a devout man, this ability could be accounted for by God's perfect design of the human body, a theological vitalistic philosophy. Many subsequent osteopaths share this faith and thereby, to varying degrees, the rationale. For those that could be termed non-theological vitalists, the self-healing ability may be due to the vital force within the body, a non-physical inner force or energy that gives the body the property of life (chi, prana, ki, *élan vital* or variations on these). Another vitalistic term that is often used is 'the body's inherent wisdom'. However, for the many students and practitioners who do not have these beliefs, it is an exceptionally difficult concept to accept. Even though in practice it can be observed to be the case, a rational explanation for it is lacking. There have been attempts at creating mechanistic models (many of which are included in this book) to explain this idea, and though useful, none appear to be able to account for the truly holistic affects that osteopathy is capable of eliciting from the body.

However, more recently there has been a growing interesting concept that challenges the accepted paradigm of biomechanics. It offers a logical rationale for *vis medicatrix naturae*, as well as many other of the tenets of osteopathy such as that:

- structure and function are reciprocally related
- changes applied in one area will also have effects distally.

It may also offer routes leading to a greater understanding of the human body beyond a purely somatic level. This concept is based on principles of tensegrity. This section will explore some of the ways that tensegrity may offer novel interpretations of well observed phenomena and possibly result in a shift in the osteopathic conceptual paradigm.

TENSEGRITY

Tensegrity is, in itself, not a recent concept. The architect Richard Buckminster Fuller (1895–1983), more familiarly known as Bucky, began thinking and writing about coexistent tension and compression in the 1920s.[1] In 1948 Kenneth Snelson, a student of Fuller's, built the first tensegrity structure. Both men developed the concept of tensegrity in differing ways, with Fuller's concepts perhaps being more obviously applicable to the human body.

The word itself is a contraction of 'tensional integrity'. A simple definition of tensegrity is that it is a structural system composed of discontinuous compression elements connected by continuous tension cables, which, due to the way in which the tensional and compressive forces are distributed within the structure, is a self-stabilizing structure, i.e. stable but able to interact in a dynamic way.[2,3]

Fuller offers a more complete definition, describing it as 'a structural-relationship principle in which structural shape is guaranteed by the finitely closed, comprehensively continuous, tensional behaviours of the system and not by the discontinuous and exclusively local compressional member behaviours'.[4]

The discontinuous local compressional model referred to is that of conventional or 'classical' architecture based on Newtonian mechanics, which utilizes the compressive force of gravity to maintain structures based on columns, beams, levers and fulcrums. It is from this compressional model that our current thinking of the biomechanics of the body arises. All of the concepts discussed in the previous chapters are based on Newtonian principles.

Tensegrity structures behave very differently from structures based on the classical compressional architectural model, most notably in their ability to act as 'whole systems'. If a beam is loaded within a structure based on the classical model, the forces will be distributed locally. Within a tensegrity structure the tensegrity beam does not act independently, or locally, but acts only in concert with

'the whole building', which contracts symmetrically when the beam is loaded[4] distributing the forces throughout the structure.

Fuller considered all structures, from the atom to the solar system, to be tensegrity structures. (It is worth noting the similarities between Fuller ideas and those of Bertalanfty and General System Theory in Chapter 9). It is not always obvious why or how certain structures are tensegrities, so some examples will be briefly discussed before looking at the application of tensegrity to the human body.

A SIMPLE 'STICK AND STRING' MODEL

A simple example of a tensegrity structure is shown in Figure 4.1. It can be seen that the compression elements are acting as struts that push into the continuous cable. As the system functions as a whole, whatever occurs at one point of the structure will occur equally at all of the other points. So if you 'tighten one point in a tensegrity system, all the other parts of it tighten evenly. If you 'twang' any tension member anywhere in the structure, it will give the same resonant note as the others'.[4]

All tensegrity structures have the property that even before the application of any external load, members of the structures are already in compression or tension. This is known as 'prestress'. The stiffness of the structure depends on the degree of prestress within it; this will be determined by the position of the struts and the degree of contractility or elasticity in the tensional cable. Thus in the simple structure shown in Figure 4.1, either lengthen-

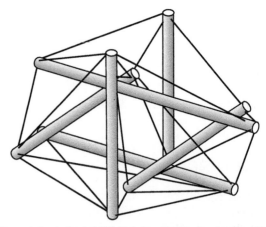

Figure 4.1 A simple 'stick and string' tensegrity structure. It consists of discontinuous compression elements maintained in their particular relationship by the continuous tension cable.

ing the struts or using a stronger elastic band will increase the degree of prestress. Increasing the degree of prestress will reduce its inherent movement (without friction) and also increase its mechanical responsiveness.[5]

The combination of tensional and compressional elements is called 'synergy'. They are mutually dependent. Synergy is defined by Fuller as 'the behaviour of integral, aggregate whole systems unpredicted by behaviours of any of their components or subassemblies of their components taken separately from the whole'.[4] Levin illustrates this clearly by stating that one would not examine the properties of the metal sodium, and the gas chlorine, and predict the properties of the combination, salt.[6]

A common example of this basic model is that of the more recent design of the dome-shaped tent, which at its simplest consists of two flexible rods that insert into the fabric of the tent.

Such a tent demonstrates many of the features of tensegrities. The structure is extremely light and though it appears to be frail, it is in fact very strong. Much of its strength is derived from the rapid omnidirectional distribution of applied forces. Thus if an external force is applied to the tent it will be dispersed throughout the fabric of the tent and poles, causing it to deform as a whole. By sharing the force throughout the whole structure it is able to withstand forces far greater than could be predicted by engineering analysis of the separate components (synergy). This is perhaps more easily envisaged with the geodesic domes and will be discussed again below.

The fact that tensegrity structures work as 'whole systems', maintaining a constant relativity between the elements of the structure, can be demonstrated in the tent by pushing or pulling on opposite sides of it: the entire tent will then expand or contract symmetrically.

Another unique and markedly significant feature of this structure is that when the external force is removed the tent will return to its original shape – it is self-stabilizing.

THE GEODESIC DOME

Geodesic is a mathematical phenomenon, being the most economical relationship between two events, i.e. a straight line between two points. A geodesic dome is a structure based on that principle. It could be considered essentially to be a more complex ver-

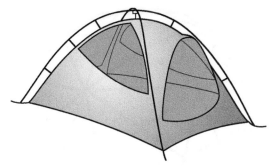

Figure 4.2 A simple tent demonstrates many of the key features of tensegrity structures. It is: light; flexible; external forces, when applied, are distributed throughout the whole structure and when that force is removed the tent returns to its original shape, thus it is self-stabilizing.

sion of the stick and string model. The tension-bearing members in these [tensegrity] structures map out the shortest paths between adjacent members (and are therefore, by definition, arranged geodesically). Tensional forces naturally transmit themselves over the shortest distance between two points, so the members of a tensegrity structure are precisely positioned to best withstand stress. For this reason, tensegrity structures offer a maximum amount of strength.[3] The name geodesic dome is somewhat misleading in that it tends to make one visualize the well-known examples such as the Geosphere at Disneyworld in Florida and the Biosphere in Montreal. However, they do not have to be symmetrically spherical, as in the examples above, but can be asymmetrically spherical, like pears, caterpillars, or elephants,[4] not to mention human beings.

By looking at Figure 4.3 it is possible to see that the geodesic dome is comprised of numerous triangles. Structures that are completely comprised of triangles are termed 'fully triangulated' structures. These are inherently stable structures and though the joints within them are flexible, they are not subject to the torque or bending movements that other structures are prone to, such as structures based on squares (imagine the torque that you can induce on a cardboard box by just compressing it obliquely).[7] The triangulation therefore contributes to the strength and rigidity of the structure. Fully geodesic structures differ from the stick and string model in that they appear to be constructed solely of rigid elements or struts; however, each strut is able to resist either tension or compression depending on the particular requirement. Thus they are able to act as either the tensile or the compressional elements required in a tensegrity. It is interesting to note that they do not require direct contact between all

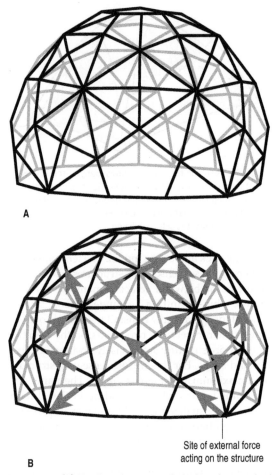

Site of external force
acting on the structure

B

Figure 4.3 **(A)** The Geosphere: a geodesic dome is comprised of numerous triangles. **(B)** Any external force will be transmitted omnidirectionally to all parts of the structure.

compressional elements for stability.[5] By observing the patterns of triangulation it is possible to conceive how an external force would be distributed from its point of contact omnidirectionally, spreading progressively to the whole structure. (See Fig. 4.3B.)

A BICYCLE WHEEL

A bicycle wheel is another commonly used example of a tensegrity structure. The spokes are the tension elements that suspend the hub, and they transmit the forces from both the ground and the frame of the bicycle to the entire rim of the wheel. Levin[8] illustrates the differences between Newtonian and tensegrity mechanics by comparing the mechanics of a wagon wheel with that of a bicycle wheel.

In a wagon wheel the load is transferred through the structure by loading of directly connected compression elements. The weight of the wagon presses on the axle which presses on the wheel hub which compresses the underlying spoke which, in turn, compresses the rim of the wheel. In bicycle wheel mechanics the weight of the frame transfers to the hub of the wheel which is hung in a tension network of wire spokes. There is continuous tension of the spokes, which are pre stressed, but the compression elements are discontinuous and do not compress one another. The hub remains suspended in its tension network. Compression loads are distributed around the rim. The compression elements behave in a counterintuitive way, not loading one another as in Newtonian construct but loaded by the tension elements. The rim of the wheel is compressed by the distributed tension of the spokes. The hub hangs from the spokes, which are always under tension, and the spoke under the hub is never compressed.

The planets of the solar system are maintained in their orbits in a similar manner. The spokes of the wheel, the constant tensional elements, are replaced by the attraction of the planets to the sun. The sun acts as the hub of the wheel. Passing from one extreme to the other, it is also possible to utilize this analogy in regard to an atom, with the electrons being maintained in their orbits by their attraction to the nucleus. It is interesting to reflect on the relatively vast distances over which this power to attract electrons occurs. If the nucleus was considered to be 1 cm across, the outer electrons would be 1 km away.

THE BALLOON

The final example for discussion is that of a balloon. To understand this it is useful to apply a slightly different terminology. Rather than using the terms 'compression' and 'tension' it is possible to replace them with 'push' and 'pull', where 'push' is synonymous with discontinuous compression and 'pull' with continuous tension. The balloon, when analysed as a tensegrity, can be seen as consisting of a continuously pulling rubber skin being discontinuously pushed by the individual air molecules contained within the balloon, thereby keeping it inflated. Any external force acting on the balloon will be dissipated by all of the enclosed air molecules to all of the skin. The same effect would be achieved by filling the balloon with water.

SUMMARY

To summarize the key features of tensegrity and tensegrities:

- Many structures, from the solar system to the atom, are tensegrity structures.
- Tensegrity is a structural system composed of discontinuous compression elements connected by continuous tension cables, with the balance between tensional and compressive (or push and pull) forces creating the stability.
- They act as 'whole systems' so that any external forces acting on them are transmitted to all elements of the structure equally, causing it to deform symmetrically rather than to collapse.
- Vibration in one part of the structure will be passed to all other parts.
- They have the property of synergy, meaning that it is not possible to deduce the function of the whole by analysis of the parts.
- The structure is efficient, requiring fewer materials than an equivalent constructed in the classical model, and though the structures may be light they are in fact very strong.
- They are self-stabilizing structures; once the external force is removed they will return to their original shape.
- They can be either symmetrically spherical or asymmetrically spherical (a dome or an elephant).
- The continuous tensional elements do not have to be visible, as in the solar system and atoms.
- Prestress and/or triangulation are essential elements in tensegrities.
- Pneumatic and hydrostatic systems can be tensegrities, e.g. a balloon or a football.

THE APPLICATION OF THE TENSEGRITY MODEL TO THE HUMAN FORM

The current model of the human body is based on classical Newtonian mechanical principles. Within this model the skeleton is perceived as being the primary support, held together by compression, with the soft tissues and viscera hanging off it or acting as local tensioners. This model has been criticized on many grounds, most notably that the mechanical laws of leverage that operate in the compressional system would create forces that far outstrip any strength of biologic materials.[6] Another criticism of the Newtonian model is that it is unidirectional, so that if the orientation of the structure

is changed it will become unstable: if a house is tilted it will fall down.

The tensegrity model shifts the emphasis, and views the bones of the skeleton as being discontinuous compression components suspended, or 'floating', within a continuous soft tissue tension network. It should be remembered that the fascial system is continuous throughout the whole body. From this it is possible to see that it complies with the definition of a tensegrity.

Caroline Stone[9] attempts to illustrate this conceptual shift in the role of the skeleton by imagining a 'rubber tent man' (see Fig. 4.4). This makes use of the example of the tent as a tensegrity structure but relates it to man! The skin acts as the tent fabric, and the bones of the skeleton as the tent poles. Without the poles it will be flat, but as the poles are inserted they push out the skin, causing it to become taut and to gradually take on the shape of a man. She later uses the concept of the balloon tensegrity model to inflate the body cavities, thereby offering greater structural support to the tent man. In drawing this analogy she is trying to illustrate the interdependence of the structures: neither the rigid structures nor the elastic structures have primacy.

As well as fulfilling the initial continuous tension and local compression definition of tensegrity, the body exhibits other features of tensegrity mechanics:

The body demonstrates prestress

The muscles of the body have a physiological resting length, meaning that they are always in slight tension. The ligaments of the spine have been shown to also be held in a degree of tension,[10,11,12] and it can be conceived that other ligaments will behave similarly. This can be interpreted as prestress.

The body cavities and their contents act as 'balloon' tensegrities

The biomechanical principles of JM Littlejohn stress the importance of the body cavities, notably the thoracic and abdominopelvic, in the maintenance of upright posture. Reflecting on this from a tensegrity perspective, they can be interpreted as functioning in the manner of the balloon tensegrity model. The cavities, being filled with viscera and fluid, exert an effect on the internal fascial compartments of the body, keeping them 'inflated' and contributing to the overall stability of the body (as used in the 'tent man').

The fact that tensegrities are self-stabilizing structures may also begin to offer the beginnings of a rationale for vis medicatrix naturae.

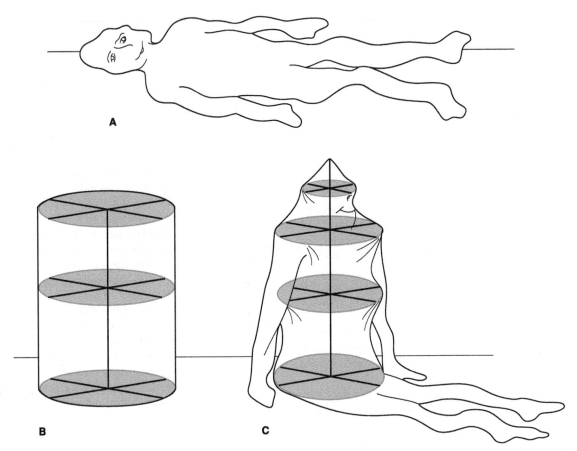

Figure 4.4 The rubber tent man. **(A)** Imagine a deflated rubber man lying flat on the ground. **(B)** Now imagine a series of rods being inserted within the rubber skin of the man. These rods push out the skin so that the man begins to stand. Instead of being filled by air, the shape of the man is formed by the rubber membrane being pushed taut by the internal rods. **(C)** Inside the trunk, limbs and head a series of horizontal membranes within the rubber skin of the man help to divide him into compartments. These are expanded by the insertion of the rods that help the man to stand upright. Further support is then offered by filling the compartments with uncompressible fluid and viscera. (Reproduced with the permission of Nelson Thornes Ltd from Science in the art of osteopathy 0 7487 3328 0, first published in 1999.)

If the evidence is beginning to become sufficient to make this hypothesis appear viable, it is interesting to reflect on the role of synergy as an important feature of tensegrities. Synergy in this context means that it is not possible to deduce the function of the whole by analysis of the parts; this concept has always been stressed within the holistic approach, in the tenet 'the whole is greater than the sum of the parts'.

THE HIERARCHICAL STRUCTURE OF TENSEGRITY

One of the principles that has not been mentioned yet is that there is a hierarchical structure to tensegrities,

the same principles applying at each level of decreasing or increasing complexity, so that the macroscopic principles just discussed should be reflected in the microscopic levels. We will now explore some of the smaller levels of organization of the body.

THE ARTICULAR LEVEL

Passing down to an articular level, Levin persuasively argues that both the sacroiliac[8] and shoulder girdle articulations[13] are clear examples of tensegrity mechanics. He utilizes the bicycle wheel analogy as the underlying model. Thus, for the pelvis, the pelvic ring would represent the rim of the wheel and the sacrum the hub. These represent the discontinuous compressive elements of the model. The sacrum is suspended between the ilia by the complex arrangement of ligaments and muscles; these represent the spokes of the wheel or the tensile elements. This offers omnidirectional stability and is independent of the position of the body, or the direction of any external forces that may be applied to it. Any forces acting on the sacrum can be dispersed around the pelvic bowl. As with the hub of the wheel, assuming that there is no structural damage to the spokes, the hub stays in the same position relative to the rim; so too will the sacrum. In order to do this, though, the movement must be in tandem with the other pelvic bones, giving rise to tension coupled movement patterns.

It is perhaps interesting to reflect on this complex pattern of supporting soft tissues and try to envisage what effects may arise in the presence of dysfunction in any one of these supporting soft tissues, particularly considering the numerous and varied functions of the pelvis.

The shoulder has been similarly envisaged with the scapula being the hub and the radiating muscles and connective tissue being the spokes.

Reciprocal tension membranes

Another example of tension coupled movements was first described by WG Sutherland in 1939.[14] He stated that the intracranial and spinal dural membranes balance and maintain the relationship between the bones of the cranium, and also synchronously maintain their relationship with the sacrum. He termed this phenomenon 'reciprocal tension', and the dura the 'reciprocal tension membrane'. This would now be described as a tensegrity arrangement, the dura being envisaged as the continuous tensional element maintaining a dynamic equilibrium between the cranial bones and the sacrum. The concepts of balanced membranous and balanced ligamentous tension (BMT and BLT) that have arisen from his work are also easily explained in tensegrity terms.

In Chapter 2 much attention was directed towards the coupled movement of the vertebrae. Perhaps in the future, tensegrity will offer a more convincing answer to this complicated problem. If so, the axial compression gravity based models that are dependent on keystones and pivots will need to be revised.

THE CELLULAR LEVEL

This, arguably, is the area in which some of the most exciting research has occurred. It also offers manual therapists the opportunity to appreciate scientifically that by addressing the gross structure it is possible to have an effect at the deepest levels of the body, including at that of the cellular physiological level. The cytologists Ingber, Wang and their team have largely been responsible for pushing this research to these new levels of understanding. (As it is only possible to discuss the findings briefly here, a list of their articles is included in Recommended reading at the end of the chapter.)

The conventional image of the cell, with which most of us are familiar, looks something like a fried egg, with the nucleus sitting in the middle, surrounded by the organelles, all floating in a viscous gel (see Fig. 4.5A). This flattened appearance is in fact an artefact due to the cell membrane adhering to the underlying plate; in vivo they take up a different shape depending on the cell type. How cells achieve and maintain their shape was poorly understood. They were known to contain a cytoskeleton comprised of microtubules, microfilaments and intermediate filaments, but an understanding of the precise roles of these elements was lacking. Ingber, having an interest in both the tensegrity sculptural work of Kenneth Snelson, and the actual concept of tensegrity, attempted to model the cell from a tensegrity perspective, and eventually succeeded in so doing. The processes that he went through to achieve this are detailed in the article 'The Architecture of Life'.[3]

To summarise Ingber described a 'hard wired' network-like structure comprised of three types of filaments: microtubules and microfilaments which act as the compression elements, and actin microfilaments which offer the continuous tension. This network occurs throughout the cell, including passing continuously into the nucleus of the cell. The structure of the cell is thus maintained by the contractile actin microfilaments creating tension, pulling towards the nucleus. This in turn is resisted by the compression elements, the microtubules and large bundles of cross-linked microfilaments. The whole network is integrated by the intermediate filaments making connections between these elements and the cell membrane. The integrins within the cell membrane connect with fibres of the extracellular matrix (ECM), anchoring it externally and further resisting the inward pull of the microfilaments. The hard wiring of the cell has been demonstrated by pulling on the cell membrane, which caused the cytoskeleton filaments and the nucleus to line up in the direction of the pull. This also demonstrates that by affecting the cell membrane it is possible to affect structures deep within the cell.[15]

Continuing on from this research, and of a most fundamental significance, was the finding that by changing the shape of a cell it was possible to cause cells to switch between different genetic programmes.[16,17] Experiments were set up that enabled the shape of the cells to be varied, from flat to spherical and even square.

By simply modifying the shape of the cell, they could switch cells between different genetic programs. Cells that spread flat became more likely to divide, whereas round cells that were prevented from spreading activated a death program known as apoptosis. When cells were neither too extended nor too retracted, they neither divided nor died. Instead they differentiated themselves in a tissue-specific manner: capillary cells formed hollow capillary tubes; liver cells secreted proteins that the liver normally supplies to the blood; and so on.

Thus, mechanical restructuring of the cell and cytoskeleton apparently tells the cell what to do. Very flat cells, with their cytoskeletons stretched, sense that more cells are needed to cover the surrounding substrate, as in wound repair, and that cell division is needed. Rounding indicates that too many cells are competing for space on the matrix and that cells are proliferating too much; some must die to prevent tumour formation. In between these two extremes, normal tissue function is established and maintained.[3]

The other key realization was that the cell membrane has globular proteins that span it, having receptor sites both internally and externally. Many of these are chemoreceptors, but some are mechanoreceptors. The mechanoreceptors are called integrins, and are connected internally to the intracellular fibrous cytoskeleton, and extracellularly to the ECM fibrous network. By these connections it is possible to convey tension and compression from the extracellular fibre matrix to the cell, and even to the nucleus: they act as mechonotransducers. The cell can now be seen as a part of a much greater structure: it is physically bound into the ECM which will then be bound to another cell and so on. The ECM and its continuity with the cell membrane and contents is the cellular expression of the fascial continuity. This entire interconnected system is variously known as the tissue-tensegrity matrix or the living matrix (see Fig. 4.5B).

The living matrix is a continuous and dynamic 'supramolecular' webwork, extending into every nook and cranny of the body: a nuclear matrix within a cellular matrix within a connective tissue matrix. In essence when you touch a human body you are touching a continuously interconnected system, composed of virtually all of the molecules of the body linked together in an intricate webwork. The living matrix has no fundamental unit or central aspect, no part that is primary or most basic. The properties of the whole net depend upon the integrated activities of all of the components. Effects of one part of the system can, and do spread to others.

The shape, form, mechanical, energetic, and functional characteristics of every cell, tissue or organ arise because of local variations in the properties of the matrix.[18]

As well as creating the structure of the body, the living matrix performs many functions, and the full impact of some of these has yet to be fully understood. It acts as a dynamic conduit for the fluid in which it is bathed and, consequently, oversees all of the humoral based communication. It can convey vibration, and tissue harmonics have been explored as possible indicators of carcinogenic tissue.[19] Chemical, mechanical and visual stimuli can all be transduced into vibration which can be conveyed throughout the matrix to the nucleus of the

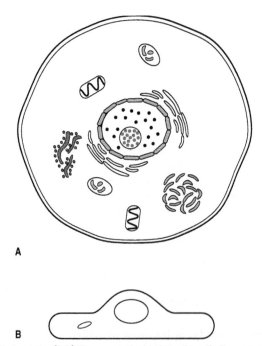

A

B

Figure 4.5   (A,B) The conventional view of a cell, demonstrating no particular organization (B = lateral view).

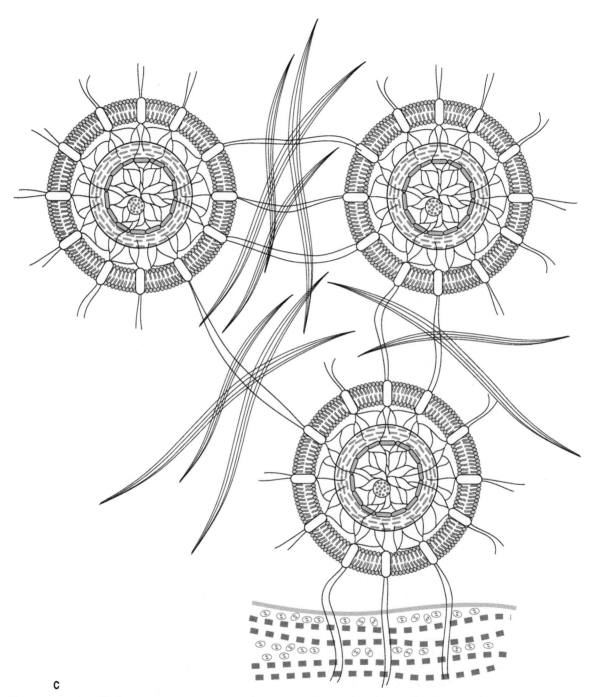

C

Figure 4.5 cont'd (C) The tensegrity view of the cell. The cell is 'hard wired'. Note that the fibres are continuous from the cell membrane to the nucleus itself, and that it is continuous via the integrins with the extracellular matrix.

cells. The matrix as a whole can be looked at as a crystalline matrix which is piezoelectric, so that when it is deformed in any way it will generate bioenergetic signals. As it is a semiconductor it is able to convey bioelectronic signals throughout the body, creating another method of communication.[18] The possibilities yet to be explored are endless.

From a manual therapist's perspective these concepts enable us to touch the body and know that we are in contact with the *entire network of the living matrix*, and that changing the relationship of one part of the body to another part will have an effect throughout the tensegrity matrix, with possible consequences at a cellular level.

It is possible to take this concept to an even smaller scale. The tensegrity hierarchy is continuous; atoms are tensegrity structures, they combine with other atoms which obey the physical laws of triangulation and close packing[11] and therefore are by definition geodesic. These then combine to form more complex molecules, e.g. proteins, which combine to form organelles, then cells, tissues, organs, systems, the whole body (known as self-assembly). The body acts as a complete system.

The synergetic concepts also apply on the ever increasing scale; we work within a family unit, within a community, in a country, being part of a species living on a planet which itself is part of the universe …

The hypothetical applications of this concept are almost limitless, but unfortunately will not be debated here. However they should provide you hours of creative debate.

CONCLUSION AND PRACTICAL APPLICATIONS

The tensegrity model of biomechanics challenges the Newtonian compressive model from which our current concepts of the biomechanics of the body arise. It is a system composed of discontinuous compression elements connected by a continuous tension cable that are arranged in such a way as to distribute forces omnidirectionally throughout the structure. It focuses on the structure's ability to work as an integrated whole unit.

All structures can potentially be viewed as tensegrities. To help understand the way the body might achieve support from these structures it is possible to utilize some basic examples: A simple stick and string model, the geodesic dome, a bicycle wheel and a balloon.

The bones of the skeleton may be considered as discontinuous compression components suspended within a continuous soft tissue tension network. The muscles and ligaments exhibit pre-stress, and the body cavities and their contents act on the fascial compartments keeping them 'inflated', contributing to the overall stability of the body.

On a cellular level, the cells are hard wired intracellularly, but also connected, via the transmembranous integrins, to the ECM, the whole forming the massive living matrix that permeates every part of the body.

This chapter started with the premise that tensegrity may offer some explanation of vis medicatrix naturae. As the whole of the body is permeated by the living matrix, which is in essence a human-shaped geodesic dome, it should theoretically have the ability to self-stabilize. This is similar to stating that if one can correct the primary lesion of the body it will resolve all the other problems therein. There is truth in both statements, but the reality is a lot more complex. Tensegrity structures will transmit forces throughout their structure when they are functioning well. When one element is dysfunctioning it will distort the whole structure, but by adding a focus (i.e. the dysfunctional or rigid element) in a system that should by rights not have any, it is as if a Newtonian lever has been introduced into the body, destabilizing the tensegrity. Where many of these occur it may be possible for tensegrity and Newtonian biomechanical patterns to be present simultaneously.

This model offers excellent examples of structure functional reciprocity and reveals a coherent rationale for how changes applied in one area will also have effects distally. Perhaps most significantly it enables us to realize changes in the gross structures will have an effect, via the living matrix, on the most fundamental levels of organization (molecular, cellular structure and physiology).

From a more practical osteopathic perspective it removes the primacy from the bony structures and highlights the very great importance of the soft tissues. This does not make the bony concepts redundant, but will cause one to analyse how these models achieve their results (as they certainly have for over 100 years) from a slightly different perspective. It should be remembered that continuous tension and local compression are interdependent.

It also reveals the true genius of WG Sutherland (and the many others who have promulgated similar theories) with regard to his concepts of 'reciprocal tension', and the treatment models that have arisen from it BLT and BMT (see Section 3).

The full expression of all components of the body is manifest in the living matrix, both in function and in dysfunction. Careful assessment of the matrix will inform the practitioner of where they should direct their efforts. The choice of treatment approach is not important from a tensegrity perspective – it may be structural, fascial or cra-nial – as long as normal function is reinstated the self-stabilizing effects of the human geodesic dome will restore the structural, physiological and possibly psychological homeostasis.

References

1. Fuller RB. 4D time lock. Online. http://www.cjfearnley.com/fuller-faq-5.html.
2. Lee P. Tensegrity. The Cranial Letter 2000; 53(3):10–13.
3. Ingber DE. The architecture of life. Scientific American 1998; 278(1):48–57.
4. Fuller RB, Applewhite EJ. Synergetics: explorations in the geometry of thinking. New York: Macmillan; 1975. Online. http://www.bfi.org/synergetics/index.html.
5. Chen CS, Ingber DE. Tensegrity and mechanoregulation: from skeleton to cytoskeleton. Osteoarthritis and Cartilage 1999; 7(1):81–94.
6. Levin SM. Continuous tension, discontinuous compression: a model for biomechanical support of the body. The Bulletin of Structural Integration 1982; 8 (1): 31–33.
7. Levin SM. A different approach to the mechanics of the human pelvis: tensegrity. In: Vleeming A, Mooney V, Snijders C et al, eds. Movement, stability and low back pain: the essential role of the pelvis. Edinburgh: Churchill Livingstone; 1997: 162.
8. Levin SM. The tensegrity system and pelvic pain syndrome. Online. Available: http://www.biotensegrity.com/.
9. Stone C. Science in the art of osteopathy. Cheltenham: Stanley Thornes; 1999: 102.
10. Nachemson A, Evans J. Some mechanical properties of the third lumbar inter-laminar ligaments. J Biomechanics 1968; 1:211.
11. Tzaczuk H. Tensile properties of the human lumbar longitudinal ligaments. Acta Orthop Scand; 1968; Suppl. 115.
12. Kazarian LE. Creep characteristics of the human spinal column. Orthop Clinics of North America; 1975; Jan:6.
13. Levin SM. Putting the shoulder to the wheel: a new biomechanical model for the shoulder girdle. Online. Available: http://www.biotensegrity.com/.
14. Sutherland WG. The cranial bowl. Mankato: Free Press Company; 1939.
15. Maniotis A, Chen C, Ingber DE. Demonstration of mechanical connections between integrins, cytoskeletal filaments and nucleoplasm that stabilize nuclear structure. Proc Natl Acad Sci USA 1997; 94:849–854.
16. Chen CS, Mrksich M, Huang S et al. Geometric control of cell life and death. Science 1997; 276:1425–1428.
17. Singhvi R, Kumar A, Lopez G et al. Engineering cell shape and function. Science 1994; 264:696–698.
18. Oschman JL. Energy medicine. Edinburgh: Churchill Livingstone; 2000: 48.
19. Pienta KJ, Coffey DS. Cellular harmonic information transfer through a tissue tensegrity matrix system. Med Hypotheses 1991; 34:88–95.

Recommended reading

The best introduction is Ingber's 'Architecture of Life'; it is easily read and is inspirational. Fuller's Synergetics *is heavy on the mathematics side. Levin has an excellent website where he posts all of his articles. But for sheer beauty, visit Snellson's website.*

Fuller RB, Applewhite EJ. Synergetics: explorations in the geometry of thinking. New York: Macmillan; 1975. Online. http://www.bfi.org/synergetics/index.html (if that fails, try: http://www.rwgrayprojects.com/synergetics/synergetics.html).
Ingber DE. The architecture of life. Scientific American 1998; 278(1):48–57.

Levin SM. A different approach to the mechanics of the human pelvis: tensegrity. In: Vleeming A, Mooney V, Snijders C et al, eds. Movement, stability and low back pain: the essential role of the pelvis. Edinburgh: Churchill Livingstone; 1997.
Levin SM. Online at: http://www.biotensegrity.com/.
Oschman JL. Energy medicine. Edinburgh: Churchill Livingstone; 2000: 48.
Snelson K. Online. http://www.kennethsnelson.net/.

Chapter 5

Biotypology

INTRODUCTION

Biotypology is the study and classification of the human race with regard to elements of people's physical appearance or morphology. From this it is possible to make generalizations about their anatomical structure, physiological processes and psychological attitudes. It also aids in predicting potential pathological problems to which each biotype may be prone.

This attempt at introducing some order to the infinite variation within the human race has its formal roots in the Orient, notably in Ayurvedic and Traditional Chinese Medicine. The Western world was thought to be introduced to this concept via the writings of Empedocles and Hippocrates. Every subsequent generation has then added its own interpretations.

In fact, if one reflects, we, as individuals, perform a similar process of classification every day. In our dealings with people we consciously or unconsciously assess them from their appearance and demeanour. We may be able to know instantly whether we could get on with someone or not, often even before they have spoken; or understand how to engage someone and what topics of conversation may interest them. Of course, this initial opinion may subsequently change, but more often than not we are quite astute at assessing people's interests and attitudes from their physical appearance. We can utilize these same observations in a more formalized, objective and clinical way to enable us to make hypotheses concerning health from similar observations.

Perhaps not thought by all osteopaths to be truly 'osteopathic', it is largely through the work of Tom

Dummer that biotyping has been incorporated into the body of osteopathic study. He integrated the work of several of the foremost exponents of biotyping to develop a model of osteopathic significance. It is not difficult to see why he became interested in this field when you consider that WH Sheldon, creator of one of the most widely used biotypical models stated that 'physique and temperament are clearly two aspects of the same thing ... it is the old notion that structure must somehow determine function' – a reiteration of Still's famous principle.

There are numerous models of classification or biotypology. For this discussion we will principally be discussing those of WH Sheldon, JE Goldthwait, E Kretschmer, L Vannier and T Dummer. These have been chosen as they are generally well known, utilize terminology that is easily understood, and their application to osteopathy, or in fact to any holistic therapy, is very apparent. Most other models could be applied equally well, and those of you who have grounding in Eastern philosophy or medicine will find much to interest them by exploring the Oriental 'biotypes'.

Goldthwait, an orthopaedic surgeon as would be expected, considers the overall structure of the body, how this may differ from one biotype to the next and the effects that will arise from disturbance of the overall posture. There is a large overlap with the latter element and the anterior and posterior biotypes derived from Littlejohn and described by TE Hall and later by J Wernham (this will be discussed within this chapter). Kretschmer's work is principally based on the psychological tendencies relating to certain types. Sheldon's classification is perhaps one of the models most commonly utilized in all forms of therapeutic intervention. It is a thorough and integrated analysis of biotype from both a structural and a psychological perspective. It does suffer somewhat in that the research was done purely on males, and though many believe it can be applied equally well to women, this cannot be supported by the original research. Vannier's model is based on a homeopathic interpretation of the three calcareous constitutions. This results in a somewhat complicated analysis, enabling predictions to be made on morphology, intellect, character, possible diseases to which they may be prone, and what their constitutional remedies may be. Both Sheldon's and Vannier's models use a two-level classification addressing the 'structural' consequences and the psychological effects. Put another way, 'that which is', the immutable elements that are genetic or atavistic, termed 'physical traits'

by Sheldon, or 'constitution' by Vannier; and 'that which can be', which is mutable and dependent on all of the environmental and psychosocial elements, defined by both as 'temperament'. Dummer extracted elements from all of these models and compiled an osteopathic interpretation, enabling these useful concepts to be applied clinically.

Each of these interpretations is a complete and thorough entity, and it is not possible, within the confines of this book, to do them justice. Rather, an attempt is made to introduce some of the key concepts of each, especially those that have the most obvious application osteopathically. Examples are discussed in an attempt to explore the underlying concepts. These concepts should then be applicable in other areas of the body, or across the body types. For a more complete understanding of these models it will be necessary to refer to the original texts (listed in the Recommended reading at the end of the chapter).

It is interesting to note that although Goldthwait (orthopaedic surgeon), Sheldon (psychologist), Kretschmer (clinical psychologist) and Vannier (doctor and homeopath) had different conceptual backgrounds, and pursued their observations from different perspectives, there is a notable concordance between their biotype definitions. The criteria utilized by the above authors for including individuals in a particular group, though not identical, have sufficient similarities to make useful comparisons between the classifications; this is shown in Table 5.1.

This area of study is often criticized. The two major concerns are:

- The types stated never appear in reality and are just hypothetical concepts.
- These are stereotypical models that, at best, are prescriptive and, at worst, lead to judgemental behaviour and, in extremis, fascism or racism.

In response to the first criticism, each of the researchers take great pains to state that they have utilized the extreme, or 'perfect' example, as the

Table 5.1 A comparison between the biotypical classifications

Author	Biotype classification		
Sheldon	Ectomorph	Mesomorph	Endomorph
Kretschmer	Asthenic	Athletic	Pyknic
Goldthwait	Slender	Intermediate	Stocky
Vannier	Phosphoric	Carbonic	Fluoric
Dummer	Functional	Structural	Functional

defining descriptor for each group (Fig. 5.1).

They also state that these extreme types will occur very infrequently in reality. More usually, an individual will have a mixture of characteristics from two or more of the classifications within their model, and the traits expressed will reflect the relative proportions of these characteristics. The pure examples are often explained as being points on a continuum, with a gradual shift in dominance from one type to the next as the cycle progresses. This is shown figuratively in Figure 5.2.

The second criticism has some validity, in that individuals *have* utilized these models inappropriately, most notably in eugenics. Kretschmer's work was subverted and used to justify the Nazi logic about racial differences. This is not a fault of the model, but rather the fault of those people applying it. This material is not intended to be prescriptive, but rather indicative of a potential relationship between structure, function/dysfunction and psychological attitudes. It is there to help us towards a first level of hypothesis about an individual, which will then be 'tested' throughout the rest of the clinical interaction, from case history to treatment.

Another point sometimes raised is that the relationship between body type and personality are not direct, as is implied, but possibly indirect. People with different body types do differ in personality, but they may do so because of the different treatment to which they are exposed. Currently in

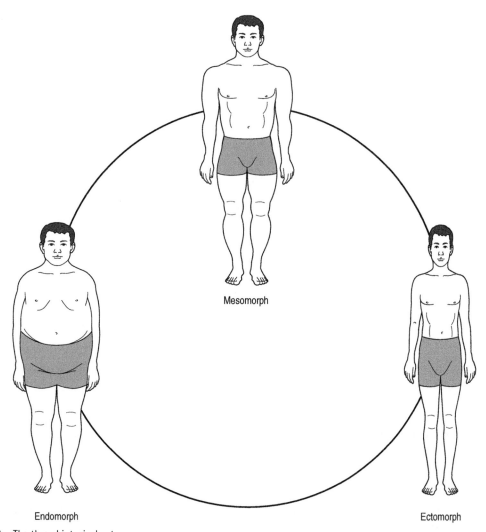

Mesomorph

Endomorph

Ectomorph

Figure 5.1   The three biotypical extremes.

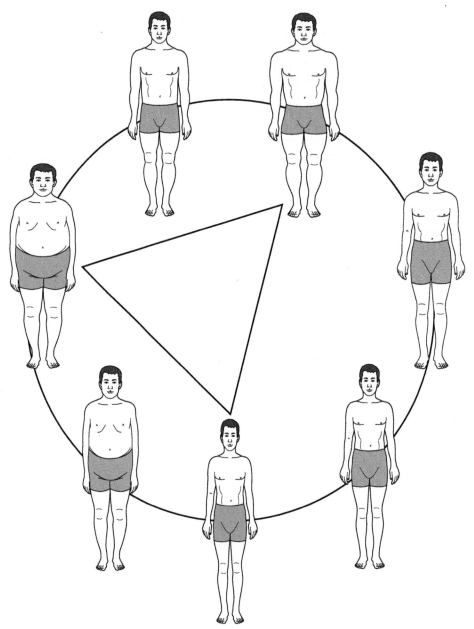

Figure 5.2 Biotypical extremes can be seen as points on the continuum, with a gradual shift from one type to the next. The individual will demonstrate characteristics from both, dependent on their relative proportions.

the Western world the slender (ectomorph) type is considered to be the most desirable, the stocky (endomorph) type less so. Is it the difference in treatment between the types that contributes to the development of their personalities? This is a more complicated point, and in all probability there are elements that are direct and some that are indirect.

An awareness of this possibility should help to distance the practitioner from the possible stereotypical 'labelling' application of these models.

A list of recommended reading is to be found at the end of this chapter. The original texts will give a much more complete understanding of the concepts.

Before exploring these models we will briefly consider the early history of biotypical models which has influenced subsequent models.

HISTORICAL PERSPECTIVE

From ancient times, the principal medical cultures tried to classify individuals according to their morpho-functional characteristics in order to study and understand their tendencies in terms of health and sickness. Ayurveda, India's traditional medicine, is thought to have been in existence for 5000 years and is considered the world's oldest and most complete medical system. Ayurveda regards the human being as consisting of body, mind and spirit. These respond to the vital forces known as doshas, classified as Vata, Pitta and Kapha, which together control all bodily functions. The full range of physiological, psychological and behavioural characteristics is based on the balance between these forces.

Chinese medicine is nearly as old as Ayurveda, and has similar holistic roots. Two principal concepts are that of the duality Yin and Yang, and the Five Elements Theory, which proposes that all things, including the human body, are comprised of five basic elements: fire, earth, metal, water and wood. Our physical tendencies and personality type are dependent on the relevant proportions of Yin and Yang and the Five Elements.

It seems probable that these Oriental philosophies will have significantly influenced Western medicine. In Ancient Greece, Empedocles (495–435 BC), a Pythagorean philosopher, scientist and healer, stated that all matter is comprised of four 'root elements': earth, air, fire and water. These could be combined in an indefinite number of variations and proportions to create all matter. He supported this rather bold statement by drawing an analogy to the great variety that painters can produce with only four pigments.

Hippocrates (c 460–c 377 BC) based his system of constitution and temperament on the Pythagorean system and the teachings of Empedocles. Hippocrates based his system on four bodily fluids or humors. Fire is akin to blood, earth to phlegm (lymph), air to yellow bile, and water to black bile. According to his humoral theory, just as with the Oriental models, the general health or constitution of man entirely depends on an appropriate balance among the four bodily humors. Though there is a balance of the humors, in most individuals one will predominate, and that will

therefore define the constitution of that individual. Inherent with this concept is that each constitution will demonstrate particular characteristics in the sense of anatomy, i.e. body shape, dominance of body systems and physiology, with each type having a greater susceptibility or inclination to particular diseases. This relationship between certain characteristics and the tendency to certain disease is referred to as diathesis.

Similarly, an individual's temperament will depend on the relative predominance of the humors in the individual:

- Sanguine (*sanguis* – Latin – blood): warm, pleasant, active and enthusiastic.
- Phlegmatic (*phlegma* – Latin – lymph): slow moving, apathetic and sluggish.
- Choleric (*khole* – Greek – bile): changeable, quick to react and irritable.
- Melancholic (*melas khole* – Greek – black bile): depressed, sad and brooding.

Other relationships within the humoral concept are summarized in Table 5.2.

These terms have passed into general usage – a few phrases that have their origins in the humoral concept are:

- humourless
- in good/bad humour
- melancholic
- jaundiced
- sanguine
- bitter or sour attitudes
- seeing red when angry
- feeling black when depressed.

This was further developed by Galen and was used as recently as 1764 by Kant in his typology of temperament in *Observations on the Feeling of the Beautiful and Sublime*.

Temperament and constitution together form the so-called biotype.

RECENT MODELS OF BIOTYPOLOGY

JOEL E GOLDTHWAIT: SLENDER, INTERMEDIATE AND STOCKY TYPES

Goldthwait (1866–1961), an American orthopaedic surgeon, observed the variation within anatomical structures and their positions. He attempted to describe two aspects of this, firstly the differences that will be found in the three classifications:

Table 5.2   A summary of certain key features of the humors

Humor	Temperament	Nature	Taste	Temperament in action
Red blood	Sanguine	Hot and moist	Salty	Active, enthusiastic and pleasant in nature
Phlegm	Phlegmatic	Cold and moist	Sweet	Sluggish, dull, or apathetic coldness or indifference
Yellow bile	Choleric	Hot and dry	Bitter	Easily moved to unreasonable or excessive anger
Black bile	Melancholic	Cold and dry	Sour	Marked by depression of mind and spirit

- the slender type
- the intermediate (or normal)
- the stocky type.

The intermediate type is seen as being the ideal or normal, and variations from this are classified within the other two types.

Secondly, he described the anatomical and physiological changes that will occur as a result of poor posture.

By analysing the gross changes in the anatomy that occur as a result of these differences from the norm, he and his fellow researchers proposed that it is possible to predict the likely problems, both functional and pathological, that may arise as a consequence. In his own words:

> not all human beings are made alike, and a study of these anatomical differences is helpful in the understanding and treatment of disease. The recognition of structural differences is also of great value in the maintenance of health and physical well being, for differences within the organs accompany those changes seen externally. This leads to a somewhat different normal function and a different reaction to the environment. Individuals of different body types show different susceptibility to various diseases. The pattern of the body is inherited and depends upon the body type of ancestors. However while the body type cannot be changed, the manner in which it is used can be modified greatly. The health of the individual depends largely on this, as well as whether he will succumb to one of the diseases of which he is a potential victim.[1]

This is based on the premise that structure governs function, and its relevance to osteopathy can immediately be understood.

The findings of Goldthwait and his colleagues were published in 1945 in *The Essentials of Body Mechanics in Health and Disease*. Unfortunately at that time the medical paradigm was shifting to a more specific, 'invading pathogen'-led approach and so the work was largely overlooked by his allopath colleagues.

In discussing the biotypes, the features mentioned are variations from the intermediate type; the intermediate type can be conceived as 'ideal' (to use Goldthwait's preferred term) and will not therefore be discussed. The descriptions below are taken from Goldthwait[1] and Spring.[2] Please note that all of the descriptions are of the 'classical' example of each type, and though the terms 'usually' and 'normally' are used sporadically throughout, every statement could be qualified by these and similar words: nothing is 'written in stone'.

The slender type

This type is generally small and delicate, or tall and slender, with a narrow face, soft, thin skin and abundant hair. The limbs vary greatly, but are often proportionately long, with the hands and feet being small, with long and tapering toes and fingers. The muscles are delicate, lacking bulk and rather straplike in nature, further exaggerating the slender appearance. Similarly, the ligaments (and connective tissue generally) are delicate and therefore lax, leading to a relative articular hypermobility.

The stocky type

This is essentially the opposite of the slender type. They are generally much more heavily built, with a proportionately much greater width in relation to the height. The head is rounded, sitting on a short and thick neck. The face is broad with a square jaw and closely set eyes. The skin is relatively thick and the hair sparse. The limbs are stocky and short, as are the hands, feet and digits. The muscles are large and rounded with coarse fibres; they may be well delineated but are often covered with a layer of fatty tissue, softening their appearance. The ligaments are tight and strong, leading to a relative hypomobility.

An overview of some of the key defining features of the types is shown in Table 5.3.

By extrapolating from these basic observations, one can begin to be able to understand why and

Table 5.3 Some of the key features of Goldthwait's three types. (With permission from Spring L. Body morphology. Unpublished dissertation. Maidstone: European School of Osteopathy; 1998.)

	Intermediate	Slender	Stocky
Torso	Moderate length and breadth	Tall and slender	Short torso and neck
Subcostal angle	70–90°	Less than 70°	Greater than 90°
Ligaments	'Ideal'	Lax with an average 15–30° increased ROM from norm	Tight and strong with an average 10–20° decreased ROM from norm
Visceral	Optimal	Ptosed	Tightly bound
Spinal curves	'Ideal'	Increased lumbar lordosis and thoracic kyphosis	Normal

how many of the changes in the body may occur, and the consequences that arise as a result of these.

For example, Goldthwait describes the slender type as having weak or lax ligaments. This will apply to all of the connective tissues, including the muscles. Static support of the spine and body generally is achieved in the ideal situation by the person 'leaning' on his ligaments, notably the iliofemoral ligament (the "Y" ligament of Bigelow), the anterior longitudinal ligament, and the posterior knee ligaments. The ankle cannot be "locked", but by leaning forward only a few degrees the gastrocnemius must contract to support the entire body. Relaxed erect posture is principally ligamentous with only the gastrocsoleus muscle group active'.[3]

The Y ligament prevents hyperextension of the hip; it also limits the anterior movement of the pelvis and body, as the person leans into it. It is supported in this role by the anterior longitudinal ligament. In the slender type these ligaments are lax and therefore allow the body to glide further anteriorly, causing the lumbopelvic angle to increase and a consequent increase in the lumbar lordosis. As the body attempts to maintain its centre of gravity there also will be an increase in the thoracic and cervical curves, hence the finding stated above for the slender individual of increased lumbar and thoracic spinal curves. As there is such a great overlap between this model and the posterior type of Littlejohn the global and physiological effects will be discussed with the posterior biotype later in this section.

Another example that can be extrapolated is related to the viscera. Goldthwait states that the skeletal muscle of the slender type is much finer and less bulky than that of the stocky type. This also holds true for the smooth muscle found in the walls of many of the viscera. As such the viscera in the slender type are much less well defined, and hold their shape

less obviously. As well as the intrinsic soft tissues maintaining the shape of the organs they are also supported externally by connective tissue, which holds them in the 'correct' position and is partly responsible for maintaining the shape of the organ.

The position of an organ and the effects of lax connective tissue of a slender individual are well illustrated by the large intestine. The transverse colon is essentially supported by its connective tissue attachments at the hepatic and splenic flexures. Laxity of these will result in the large intestine dropping into the lower abdominal and even pelvic cavity; see Figure 5.3. This will affect its ability to function effectively on a physiological level as well as possibly causing pain.

Another example of this is the stomach in the slender type. Having a fine muscular wall it is unable to maintain its inherent shape easily, and lacking any firm connective tissue support, the stomach changes from its 'normal shape' into that described as a 'fish hook' stomach, as seen in Figure 5.4. In the stocky individual the stomach is 'normal'. The structure is appropriate to its function. The curve of the stomach is designed to allow some pooling of the contents, permitting the process of digestion to occur. Contraction of the strong muscular walls then causes the partially digested food to pass over the slight incline of the pylorus of the stomach, through the pyloric sphincter and into the duodenum. In the slender individual's stomach, as can be seen in Figure 5.4, there is a large curve in the lower part of the stomach. This acts rather like the 'U' bend of a toilet, pooling the contents of the stomach in the deep curve. The muscle wall is thin and relatively weak and the incline that needs to be overcome before the contents can be conveyed to the small intestines is great. The combination of these two factors means that the contents remain in the stomach

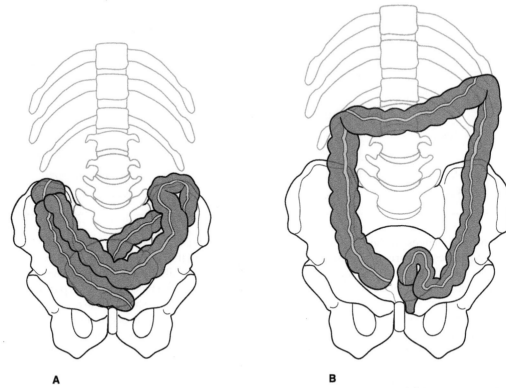

A   **B**

Figure 5.3   A comparison of the position of the large intestine in a stocky and a slender individual. **(A)** Slender individual's colon. **(B)** Stocky individual's colon.

for too long, resulting in poor digestion, flatus and possible ulceration from the prolonged presence of the gastric secretions. This may appear to be a somewhat naïve rationale, but, empirically, slender types are prone to gastrointestinal problems, and stocky types, due to the efficiency of their gastrointestinal system, tend to put on excessive weight.

Tables 5.4, 5.5 and 5.6 summarize Goldthwait's findings within the viscera, the physiological function and the susceptibility to disease.

The postural changes that predominate in Goldthwait's *The Essentials of Body Mechanics in Health and Disease* relate largely to those of a postural slump. The findings are very similar to those of Littlejohn's posterior type.

JM LITTLEJOHN'S ANTERIOR AND POSTERIOR WEIGHT-BEARING TYPES

The anterior or posterior types relate to the shifting, either forward or backward, of the central gravity line from its ideal position, forward leading to the anterior type, and backward the posterior type. The central gravity line is found by resolution of the anteroposterior (AP) and the posteroanterior (PA) lines, and the anterocentral (AC) and posterocentral (PC) lines (see Ch. 3). For Littlejohn, the 'ideal' position of the central gravity line has it passing between the occipital condyles, then inferiorly to pass through the centre of the body of the L3, through the anterior promontory of the sacrum, and medial to the centre of the hip, knee and ankle, where it bifurcates and passes anteriorly to the metatarsal heads and posteriorly to the calcaneum. When the gravity line shifts from this position a series of changes in the structure of the body and therefore its function will occur. Littlejohn modelled these changes, and they are conveyed via J Wernham and TE Hall in *The Mechanics of the Spine and Pelvis*.[4]

As already mentioned, the types that will be discussed represent perfect examples or the extremes of their type, although this in fact rarely exists. However, once the underlying principles are understood, it is an easy task to moderate them or apply them to individuals with a mixed presentation.

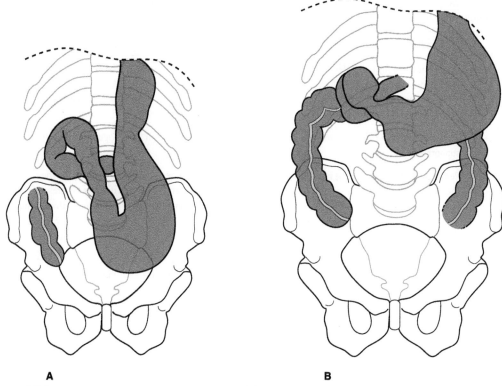

Figure 5.4 **(A)** The 'fish hook' stomach of a slender individual. **(B)** The more 'usual' shape of the stomach in a stocky individual.

When attempting to analyse these models the author has found it useful to attempt to put his own body into a similar position to that being analysed: it is then possible to work a large part of the findings by assessing the information coming from one's own body. This is useful in clinical practice with any complicated postural patterns, but do beware of mirrors!

The anterior type generally appears more easy to envisage, making it easier to interpret the possible anatomical and physiological consequences. For this reason, the discussion will start with the anterior type and then draw conclusions from that to the posterior type.

The anterior type

In this type, the central gravity line has shifted forward. Their posture is similar to that of a ski jumper in flight, though obviously less marked.

The key features can be seen in Figure 5.5. The following text explores a selection of these key features. The head is held forward and the chest is held in a position of relative inspiration. To achieve

this, the thoracic spine will extend, 'flattening' the spine to the upper lumbar spine. This is compounded by the whole extensor apparatus of the posterior thorax contracting, as if trying to prevent the person from falling anteriorly. This will also cause the scapulae to retract, resulting in external rotation of the upper extremities (try getting into the posture!). The suboccipital muscles also contract to extend the upper cervical spine to keep the eye line horizontal.

As a consequence of this, the thorax is in a position of relatively full inspiration, causing the diaphragm to be similarly in inspiration, its position being lower than its 'normal' resting position. The lower diaphragmatic position will compress the abdominal viscera inferiorly into the abdominopelvic cavity.

The anterior position causes the pelvis as a whole to rotate anteriorly and the hip extensors contract in an attempt to limit this. The abdominal muscles, the rectus abdominis and the internal and external obliques take origin from the ribs and insert at the inguinal ligament and the pubic

Table 5.4   Viscera. (With permission from Spring L. Body morphology. Unpublished dissertation. Maidstone: European School of Osteopathy, 1998.)

	Intermediate	Slender	Stocky
Abdomen	Upper abdomen firm, rounded and of equal circumference at the mammary line; no marked depression below subcostal margin	Peculiarities in shape and attachments of viscera	Cavities and internal organs larger than that of the Intermediate type
Fat	Plenty of firm perivisceral fat for support and protection	Less, especially retroperitoneal of fat for the kidneys	Plenty excess retroperitoneal, perivisceral and abdominal fat
Stomach	Pear-shaped, easily emptying into the duodenum	Long and tubular with longer attachments; the downward displacement increases on standing	Roughly oval. The transverse diameter is greater. It is firmly attached with consequent decreased downward displacement
Liver	Lower edge level with subcostal border, it should not be felt inferior to that	Small, often sags down and to the right. The right lobe can even rest on right iliac crest	Firmly attached beneath diaphragm
Kidney	At lower margin, reaches the upper edge of L3	Reaches lower than Intermediate, very mobile	
Small intestine	About 20 ft long	10–15 ft long, thin walled and small lumen; long mesentery leads to sag into pelvic cavity on standing	25–35 ft, thick walls and relatively large lumen
Large intestine	5/6 ft long; adheres to posterior abdominal wall on right; only slight downward and forward sagging as it crosses to the splenic flexure; it then reattaches posteriorly down to sigmoid colon	3–5 ft long; the attachments are long leading to increased mobility. The whole colon may be below the iliac crests. The transverse colon may have an entirely free mesentery	5–8.5 ft long, with short, firm retroperitoneal attachments, reducing the sag
Appendix		Long and well developed	
Pelvic organs		Differences (unspecified)	

ramus. As the thorax is lifted superiorly and anteriorly, and the pelvis is rotated anteriorly and inferiorly, there will be a distancing of origin and insertion of the abdominal muscles, putting them under tension. This will cause the viscera to be compressed posteriorly into the abdominopelvic cavity.

The knees will be hyperextended and the gastrocnemii under tension.

One of the principal roles of the polygons of force and the PA and PC lines is to maintain the pressure differentials in the cavities. Looking at the above it is clear to see that an imbalance between the pressures must occur in the anterior type. The thorax is essentially a flexible box that can be opened and closed; the viscera are constant. Opening the box reduces the pressure exerted on them, and closing it increases it. In this case, the thorax is in relative inspiration and the diaphragm descended, thus there is 'greater space' within the thoracic cavity and, therefore, a relative decrease in pressure within the thorax. Conversely, below the diaphragm the abdominopelvic cavity is being compressed from above by the diaphragm, anteriorly by the abdominal muscles, and possibly posteriorly with the extension of the thoracic and upper lumbar spine taking the vertebral bodies anterior to their norm. Thus there is a relative increase in pressure below the diaphragm.

Table 5.5   The physiological function. (With permission from Spring L. Body morphology. Unpublished dissertation. Maidstone: European School of Osteopathy, 1998.)

	Intermediate	Slender	Stocky
Physiological function	Because this type is the norm with optimum gut length, easy emptying of stomach and little sag of the transverse colon, it is most efficient and least susceptible to disturbance	Generally *everything is rapid*. However, stomach empties with difficulty against gravity. Due to GIT shortness, this type needs a more concentrated diet, to prevent problems of poor assimilation. Increased length of attachments can lead to visceral ptosis and constipation	Stomach empties easily and long GIT leads to good nutrition and tendency to fat. Because increased function, process slightly slower
Circulation	Good venous and pulmonary function	Is more rapid (BP is lower) but poorly adapted to long sustained effort. Slowing/partial stagnation of the pulmonary and venous systems due to postural sag; with cold, clammy extremities and venous varicosities; also a tendency to 'eye-strain' with increased AP eye diameter	Usually adequate; a tendency to high BP. Face 'ruddy and plethoric'. There is greater development of left side of heart
Puberty	No comment	Comes early for both sexes; the female tends to dysmenorrhoea	Tends to be later; basal metabolism often less than the norm
Psychological tendencies	No comment	Tendency to learn fast and impatience with slower heavier types. Often dogmatic and fanatical, quick to anger, limited endurance, but quick recovery from fatigue. Adjusts rapidly to changes in environment	Easy-going socially and in temper; good sense of humour; tolerant. Make poor reformers. Slow but greater endurance; slow recovery from fatigue. Extrovert, not self-conscious. Does not adjust easily to changes in the environment

Table 5.6   The susceptibility to disease. (With permission from Spring L. Body morphology. Unpublished dissertation. Maidstone: European School of Osteopathy, 1998.)

	Intermediate	Slender	Stocky
Susceptibility to disease	This type is least susceptible to disease. (Beyond that, Goldthwait makes no comment)	Rapidity of response in this type can lead to problems of reaction in the immune system. Greater tendency to contract influenza, bronchitis, TB and acute infectious diseases. Fevers are common, as is hypotension. Inadequate gastric secretion, gastric and duodenal ulcer and spastic colon common. Also common: hyperglandular disturbances and rheumatoid arthritis	Less susceptible to acute infections but chronic disease common: chronic bronchitis, emphysema, hypertension and arteriosclerosis, myocardial degeneration, chronic nephritis, gallstones and gallbladder disease. Gout and osteoarthritis. Hypertrophy of prostate more common. Also hyposecretion of endocrine glands, early hair loss and baldness
Cephalic and psychiatric		Melancholia, depression and acute nervous and mental disorders	Cerebral haemorrhage. Degenerative and chronic nervous and mental disorders

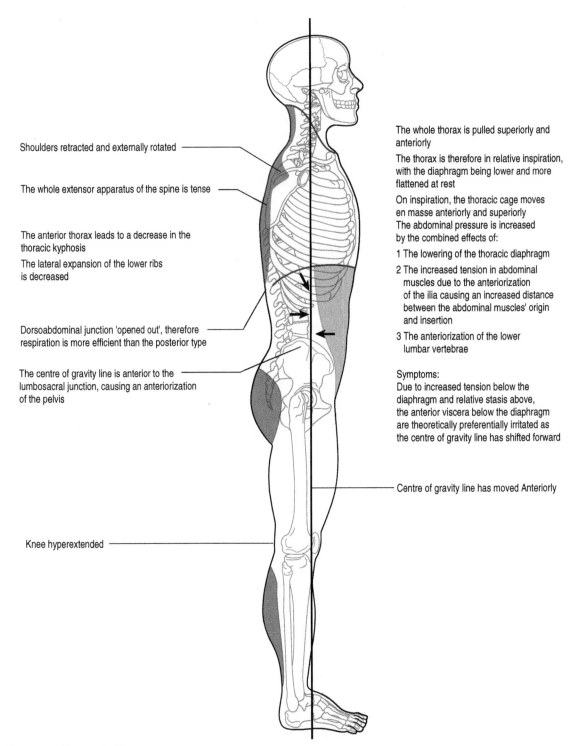

Shoulders retracted and externally rotated

The whole extensor apparatus of the spine is tense

The anterior thorax leads to a decrease in the thoracic kyphosis
The lateral expansion of the lower ribs is decreased

Dorsoabdominal junction 'opened out', therefore respiration is more efficient than the posterior type

The centre of gravity line is anterior to the lumbosacral junction, causing an anteriorization of the pelvis

Knee hyperextended

The whole thorax is pulled superiorly and anteriorly

The thorax is therefore in relative inspiration, with the diaphragm being lower and more flattened at rest

On inspiration, the thoracic cage moves en masse anteriorly and superiorly
The abdominal pressure is increased by the combined effects of:

1 The lowering of the thoracic diaphragm

2 The increased tension in abdominal muscles due to the anteriorization of the ilia causing an increased distance between the abdominal muscles' origin and insertion

3 The anteriorization of the lower lumbar vertebrae

Symptoms:
Due to increased tension below the diaphragm and relative stasis above, the anterior viscera below the diaphragm are theoretically preferentially irritated as the centre of gravity line has shifted forward

Centre of gravity line has moved Anteriorly

Figure 5.5   The anterior biotype.

Global fluid exchange will be disturbed as the pressure gradients that are present in the ideal state are modified. Thus in the anterior type there is an increase in pressure in the abdomen and pelvis. Blood returning from the lower extremities now has to overcome a greater pressure to enter the cavity as the pressure gradient has increased. Clinically the result is that there will be congestion in the lower extremities. The suboccipital muscle tension will have a similar effect at the cranium, possibly affecting the supply via the vertebral arteries and/or the drainage via the internal jugular vein, resulting in headaches of differing nature – more of a migrainous, hemicranial type headache with arterial compression, and more congestive, whole head type headache with venous congestion.

Compression tends to cause an irritative state in the tissues subject to it, whereas a decrease in pressure tends to lead to a hypofunctioning state and stasis.

All of the viscera below the diaphragm are subject to an increase in pressure. As the gravity line has shifted anteriorly, the body and the structures within are tractioned forward. The clinical changes are noticed more in the anterior structures than in the posterior ones. To illustrate the changes that can occur below the diaphragm we will look at the relationship between the bladder and uterus. In the ideal position they are both supported in place by their fascial attachments supporting them over the pelvic diaphragm. As the person walks, the foot plant will cause a downward movement of the viscera, which, as they are supported above, will cause them to fractionally elongate and will cause a relative increase in pressure within the viscera. As the viscera returns to its normal position and normal shape the pressure will drop again: this has the effect of acting as a local pump promoting fluid exchange. This movement is limited and softened by the pelvic floor.

In the anterior type, the pelvis rotates anteriorly, so that the bladder, rather than resting on the pelvic floor, is now resting on the posterior aspect of the pubic ramus. The uterus will tend to antevert, compressing the bladder more firmly against the ramus. When walking occurs in this situation, the bladder is unable to stretch freely as before, but is squashed against the pubic ramus. The stretching effect will be reduced, impairing local perfusion and, therefore, its physiological function, and the compressive element will, with time, make it painful and tender. This could be a rationale for the presence of cystitis of a non-infective nature. The anteversion and relative compression of the uterus will possibly lead to dysmenorrhoea, and could possibly be a contributing factor to difficulty conceiving.

Above the diaphragm, the relative decrease in pressure leads to a tendency for stasis and hypofunction. Respiration is slightly impaired as the relative fixity of the thorax in inspiration limits the full range of thoracic movement.

The posterior type

The posterior type, as with the majority of these models, is the converse of the above, see Figure 5.6.

The thorax is held in relative expiration, causing the ribs to be more sharply inclined inferiorly, thereby reducing the anteroposterior diameter of the thoracic cavity and the intercostal spaces, but also slightly increasing the lateral expansion of the ribs. The diaphragm will be held high in the expiration position, approximating its origin and insertion on the central tendon, thereby reducing its ability to contract efficiently. The heart is attached firmly to the central tendon of the diaphragm, and relies partly on the traction and relaxing effects of the diaphragmatic excursion to aid its own perfusion. As the diaphragm passes inferiorly it tractions the heart, creating a relative increase in pressure within the coronary arteries and the myocardium itself, and the reverse as it passes superiorly. This positive effect will be reduced as the diaphragmatic excursion is also reduced in this type. It is possible that this action aids cardiac contraction and therefore disturbance of this movement may even affect the body's perfusion generally.

Additionally, as the potential space within the thoracic cavity is effectively reduced by the position of the ribs and diaphragm, there will be a relative increase in intrathoracic pressure, further compromising perfusion of any intrathoracic structures. There will be a tendency to cardiac hypertrophy, as the heart is having to contract against a greater resistance. Venous return from other areas of the body will be diminished as the pressure gradient entering the thorax has been increased. The changes in the abdominopelvic cavity are essentially the reverse of those in the thorax. Thus there is a relative decrease in pressure within these cavities. Stasis occurs due to the increased pressure in the thorax. Symptomatically, the posterior weight-bearing type is characterized by irritability in the structures in the thorax and congestion of the abdominopelvic cavity contents being most prevalent in the posterior structures, e.g. haemorrhoids, constipation, retroversion of the uterus, menorrhagia.

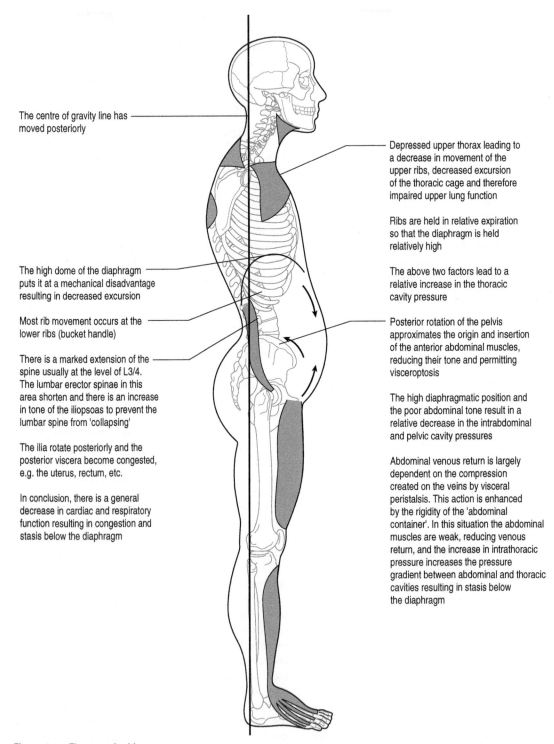

The centre of gravity line has moved posteriorly

The high dome of the diaphragm puts it at a mechanical disadvantage resulting in decreased excursion

Most rib movement occurs at the lower ribs (bucket handle)

There is a marked extension of the spine usually at the level of L3/4. The lumbar erector spinae in this area shorten and there is an increase in tone of the iliopsoas to prevent the lumbar spine from 'collapsing'

The ilia rotate posteriorly and the posterior viscera become congested, e.g. the uterus, rectum, etc.

In conclusion, there is a general decrease in cardiac and respiratory function resulting in congestion and stasis below the diaphragm

Depressed upper thorax leading to a decrease in movement of the upper ribs, decreased excursion of the thoracic cage and therefore impaired upper lung function

Ribs are held in relative expiration so that the diaphragm is held relatively high

The above two factors lead to a relative increase in the thoracic cavity pressure

Posterior rotation of the pelvis approximates the origin and insertion of the anterior abdominal muscles, reducing their tone and permitting visceroptosis

The high diaphragmatic position and the poor abdominal tone result in a relative decrease in the intrabdominal and pelvic cavity pressures

Abdominal venous return is largely dependent on the compression created on the veins by visceral peristalsis. This action is enhanced by the rigidity of the 'abdominal container'. In this situation the abdominal muscles are weak, reducing venous return, and the increase in intrathoracic pressure increases the pressure gradient between abdominal and thoracic cavities resulting in stasis below the diaphragm

Figure 5.6 The posterior biotype.

WH SHELDON: ENDOMORPH, ECTOMORPH AND MESOMORPH

Sheldon's classification is perhaps one of the most thoroughly researched and perhaps one of the most widely used. It is a simple model, easily applicable in the clinical situation, offering an interesting insight into the relationship between the body structure and an individual's psychological predispositions. His studies are divisible into two distinct but interrelating areas. Those relating to the morphology of man are published in the book *The Varieties of Human Physique: An Introduction to Constitutional Psychology* (1940),[5] and those relating to the psychological correlates are published in *The Varieties of Temperament: A Psychology of Constitutional Differences* (1942).[6]

Sheldon's interest was that of a psychologist attempting to find morphological and psychological correlates. He was critical of the difficulty of clinical application of the earlier biotypological classifications based solely on anthropometric criteria. He and his team wanted to produce an easily applicable useful morphological taxonomy. In order to do this they carefully examined thousands of photographs of young men, and experimented in organizing them in several different ways. Initially they were aware that there were no specific types, but that there were obvious variations. By selecting the most extreme of these variations they eventually arrived at three main components of morphological variation, termed endomorphy, mesomorphy and ectomorphy. They then selected a small number of anthropometric criteria to enable objective assessment of these features, and subsequent classification utilizing these components. Sheldon's research has received criticism from certain quarters in that it did not include any women. The reason Sheldon gave for this omission was that he could find no true female ectomorphs. It is the authors' experience that though no women were included within the research, the findings are equally applicable in the clinical situation to both men and women.

The physical correlates or somatotype

Sheldon arrived at the threefold classification based on the predominant embryological tissue, the endoderm giving rise to the viscera; the mesoderm the musculoskeletal system; and the ectoderm the neural tissue and skin. The physical correlates derive from this.[5]

Sheldon called the pattern of the morphological components the 'somatotype'. This was expressed by three numerals. The first digit relates to the degree of endomorphy, the second to mesomorphy and the third to ectomorphy. Subjects were rated on a on a 1–7 scale. Thus a 117 would be an extreme ectomorph, whereas 711 would be an extreme endomorph and an extreme mesomorph would score 171. Very rarely, though, does any individual belong to a single, extreme somatotype. People often have the features of two or even three of the types. An average person who has some ectomorphic tendencies would score 446, whereas 444 is a mixture of all three types. Sheldon referred to the analysis of the physical traits as the 'statics' of psychology (remember, he was trying to classify psychological predispositions via morphology). He believed that these characteristics define the individual and that they are immutable.

However, the classical definitions are:

Endomorphy: this means a relative predominance of soft roundness throughout the various regions of the body. When endomorphy is dominant the digestive viscera are massive and tend relatively to dominate the body economy. The digestive viscera are derived principally from the endodermal embryonic layer.

Mesomorphy: this means a relative predominance of muscle, bone and connective tissue. The mesomorph physique is normally heavy, hard and rectangular in outline. Bone and muscle are prominent and the skin is made thick by heavy underlying connective tissue. The entire body economy is dominated, relatively, by tissues derived from the mesodermal embryonic layer.

Ectomorphy: this means a relative predominance of linearity and fragility. In proportion to his mass, the ectomorph has the greatest surface area and hence relatively the greatest sensory exposure to the outside world. Relative to his mass he also has the largest brain and central nervous system. In a sense, therefore, his bodily economy is relatively dominated by tissues derived from the ectodermal embryonic layer. See Figure 5.7.

There is sufficient overlap between the physical characteristics expressed by Sheldon and Goldthwait that this will be only briefly discussed here. Sheldon assessed the physical performance of each body type in five categories: strength, power, endurance, body support and agility. The endomorphic type is low in all categories, the mesomorphic type is high in all categories, and the ectomorphic type is high in endurance, bodily support and agility but low in strength and power.

Figure 5.7 The endomorph, mesomorph and ectomorph.

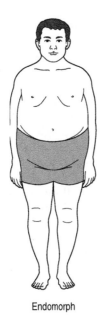
Endomorph

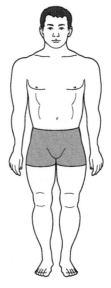
Mesomorph

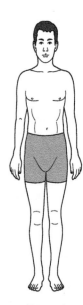
Ectomorph

The psychological correlates or temperament

The second element of his classification was to assess the psychological correlates of the somato-type. This he termed 'temperament'. Unlike the physical traits, which are immutable, the temperament is influenced by the environment. He tried to explain this by using the term 'statics of psychology', and 'the balance among the components comprising the morphology of man at rest' as descriptors of the immutable physical traits. To complement this he utilized the term 'dynamics' for the mutable temperament or psychological component. He described this as 'the science of man in motion. When man gets up and moves around, expressing his desires and motivations and interacting with his fellows'.

Sheldon used 60 traits to devise three categories of temperament:[6]

- Viscerotonia
- Somatotonia, and
- Cerebrotonia.

Sheldon's full definitions are included here, as their language is well suited to the description of these types. Table 5.7 also presents the typical characteristics of each type.

[Viscerotonia] in its extreme manifestation is characterised by general relaxation, love of comfort, sociability, conviviality, gluttony for food, for people

and for affection. The Viscerotonic extremes are people who 'suck hard at the breast of mother earth' and love physical proximity with others. The motivational organization is dominated by the gut and by the function of anabolism. The personality seems to centre around the viscera. The digestive tract is king and its welfare appears to define the primary purpose of life

[Somatotonia is] roughly predominance of muscular activity and of vigorous bodily assertiveness. The motivational organization seems dominated by the soma. These people have vigour and push. The executive department of their internal economy is strongly vested in their somatic muscular systems. Action and power define life's primary purpose.

[Cerebrotonia is] roughly a predominance of the element of restraint, inhibition, and of the desire for concealment. Cerebrotonic people shrink away from sociality as from too strong a light. They 'repress' somatic and visceral expression, are hyperattentional, and sedulously avoid attracting attention to themselves. Their behaviour seems dominated by the inhibitory and attentional functions of the cerebrum, and their motivational hierarchy appears to define an antithesis to both of the other extremes.

The genius of Sheldon's classification lies in his use of the primitive germ layers of the embryo as the foundation of his system.

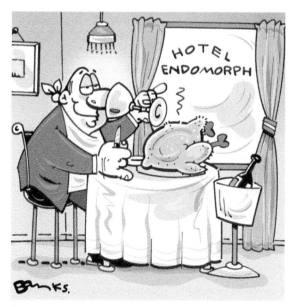

Figure 5.8　The viscerotonic individual.

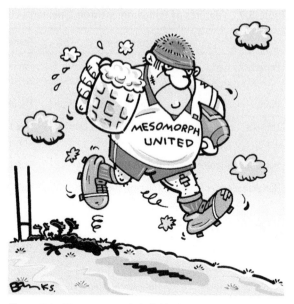

Figure 5.9　The somatotonic individual.

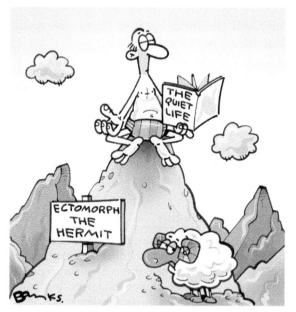

Figure 5.10　The cerebrotonic individual.

Thus the endodermal layer gives rise to the viscera, particularly the gastrointestinal system and liver, pancreas, thymus, thyroid and parathyroids. In the endomorph these tissues predominate and they therefore seek to express themselves via this system – hence viscerotonia. Endomorphs have a tendency to enjoy food, and as they have perhaps the most efficient digestive systems of the somatotypes they have a tendency to easily put weight on. However, it is not just food they like; they take pleasure in elegant and sumptuous surroundings, good friends to dine with, and the presentation and smells of the food. This is an expression of the sensual and sensitive side of the viscera (see also Table 5.7).

The mesodermal layer gives rise, essentially, to the musculoskeletal system. As these tissues predominate in the mesomorph they achieve expression through activity of the somatic muscular system, somatotonia. Somatotonic individuals enjoy physical activity and perform well at it. They have a tendency to be aggressive, not in a physically violent way (though that is possible) but working hard at what they do; they are competitive and can be dominating. Their pursuits similarly reflect these attitudes – they enjoy physical team sports.

The ectodermal layer gives rise to the nervous system and the skin, the ectomorph therefore expressing itself through the central nervous system, cerebrotonia. These are sensitive individuals, some would say hypersensitive. They have a tendency to intellectual over-stimulation and introspection. All senses are acute; they dislike noise, and (with

Table 5.7   Features of temperament from Sheldon's classification

	Viscerotonia	Somatotonia	Cerebrotonia
Personality type	Sociable, loving, secure	Physical, assertive, adventurous, a risk taker	Intellectual, restrained, self-conscious, artistic
Wants	Have a want of affection	Desire power and dominance	Need of privacy, peace and quiet
Lifestyle	Love of food and comfort	Need of enjoyment and physical activity	Mentally and emotionally over intense
Relations with others	Relaxed, easy-going	Competitive, active and noisy	Inhibited, quiet, introverted
Social tendencies	Tolerant, sociophilic, indiscriminate amiability	Indifference to what others think or want	Socially anxious, sociophobic
When troubled seek out	People	Action	Solitude
Orientation towards	Childhood and family relationships	Goals and activities of youth	Later periods of life
Sporting pursuits	Not greatly interested	Team sports, aggressive, i.e. rugby, fast burst activities such as sprinting	Solitary pursuits often including endurance, cycling, long-distance running, mountaineering

regard to the skin as a sense organ) tend to be 'thin skinned' and therefore to avoid social interaction.

Thus Sheldon's classification unites the mind and the body.

MARTINY'S ENDOBLASTIC, MESOBLASTIC AND ECTOBLASTIC TYPES

M Martiny created a system of biotypology utilizing the same concept of embryological tissues as the basis for the classification. There follows a very brief review of his biotypological classifications, primarily for the sake of comparison and interest. It is not certain whether Sheldon and Martiny communicated with each other, but the similarities between the two classifications are great. Martiny utilized the terms endoblastic, mesoblastic, ectoblastic and chordoblastic constitutions to distinguish his types.[7,8]

Endoblastic constitution

These people are generally short in height, fat, pale and flaccid with a round and relaxed face. The parasympathetic system prevails, with the individual being a slow, passive, not very emotional or strong person. They are easily fatigued and need regular sleep.

Mesoblastic constitution

These people are stocky to fat, with good musculoskeletal development and muscle tone. Their faces are generally oval with a ruddy complexion. Being both active and powerful, this results in a strong and self-confident person, who needs to expand and communicate. It is because of this that they do not consider sleep very important.

Ectoblastic constitution

These people are tall, thin, pale, and look weak, but have a good muscular tone. Their temperament is nervous because of the dominance of the sympathetic system. A poor vitality, but high nervousness explains their tendency to catch everything going, but also to a remarkable sensitivity. Ectoblastics are complicated people, closed in their own inner world, and consider the environment to be an external reality which contrasts with their own somewhat idealized perception of it. This results in the individual displaying an apparently strong personality, generally indifferent to popular opinions.

Chordoblastic constitution

This person is an equal combination of the three other types, and is therefore perfect!

ERNST KRETSCHMER: PYKNIC ATHLETIC AND ASTHENIC TYPES

Ernst Kretschmer (1888–1964) is only discussed briefly here, due to the strong similarities between his and Sheldon's findings. A German psychiatrist, he proposed the classification of three basic constitutional types: pyknic, athletic and asthenic. Also sometimes included within this classification is 'dysplastic', a combination of the three types. He suggested that asthenics and, to a lesser degree, the athletic types were more prone to schizophrenia, while the pyknic types were more likely to develop manic-depressive disorders. He has received much criticism as his work was used by the Nazis for eugenics purposes; however, the classifications are still valid. He modified his terminology throughout his research; the terms in parenthesis are the earlier terms.[9]

Pyknic (cyclothyme)

This derives from the Greek word puknos meaning 'thick'. These are plump, rotund, macrosplanchnic types. Kretschmer proposed that these people were more likely than others to develop manic-depressive disorders.

Asthenic (leptosomic or schizothyme)

These are the tall, thin, microsplanchnic types, who were said to be more prone to schizophrenia.

Athletic

These are the more muscular, athletic types. This type is less inclined to any psychological disturbance. When present it is more likely to be schizophrenic than manic-depressive.

Dysplastic

This is a combination of the first three basic types. This is not always used within the general classification.

Table 5.8 compares Kretschmer's classification with that proposed by Sheldon.

LEON VANNIER

Leon Vannier (1880–1963), during his practice as a homeopath, observed that there was a correlation between the constitution of individuals and the characteristics of three homeopathic remedies: Calcera Carbonica, Calcera Phosphorica and Calcera Fluorica. He felt he could roughly divide the human species into three distinct types which he described as Carbonic, Phosphoric and Fluoric.

Like Sheldon, he stated that the biotype was comprised of two levels, and termed these 'constitution' and 'temperament'.

'Constitution' is 'the unchangeable structure out of which the body develops'[10] arising from heredity, being observable in the structure of the musculoskeletal system and its relations.

'Temperament' is a mutable element, described as 'that which becomes'. It is affected by the environment and may also be influenced, to good or ill effect, by the individual.

Vannier's is an exceptionally rich and highly complex interpretation of biotypes. By reducing it to the elements shown in Table 5.9, we are doing it some injustice. See Recommended reading at the end of the chapter for the original texts.

TOM DUMMER'S CONTRIBUTION

Tom Dummer was an eclectic individual with an avid interest in people and philosophy. In his *Textbook of Osteopathy* (1999) he commented on a broad range of biotypology approaches from the East and the West, psychological, physiological and structural. He created an empirical bipolar

Table 5.8 A brief comparison between the key temperament findings of Kretschmer and Sheldon

Kretschmer	Athletic	Asthenic	Pyknic
	Competitive	Serious	Social
		Quiet	Friendly
		Solitary	Lively
		Introvert	Extrovert
Sheldon	Mesomorph	Ectomorph	Endomorph
	Vigorous	Introverted	Jovial
	Aggressive	Inhibited	Pleasure-loving

Table 5.9   A summary of key elements of Vannier's classification of constitution and temperament. (With permission from Spring L. Body morphology. Unpublished dissertation. Maidstone: European School of Osteopathy; 1998)

	Carbonic	Phosphoric	Fluoric
Structure	Rigid and straight	Elegant and shapely, expressive and variable in appearance	Unstable and flexible
U/E limb angle	When standing, forearm projects slightly forward, and in forced hyperextension still forms small angle with upper arm	Hyperextension shows forearm forms straight line with humerus	Forearm forms reflex angle with humerus, more so when in forced hyperextension
L/E limb angle	Thigh and leg not precisely aligned, but show no angular deformities	Thigh and leg in perfect alignment	Thigh and leg show an angular deformity, a forward-facing obtuse angle
Orthodontic	Lower and upper rows of teeth are in perfect occlusion. Teeth very white, central incisors almost square	Upper and lower rows of teeth in perfect contact at all points. Palatine arch ogival (gothic arch). Teeth long and yellow, central incisors' transverse diameter less than vertical	Undershot jaw is normal. Upper and lower rows of teeth do not meet correctly
Function	No comment	Fragile with low resistance	Irregular
Psychological/ social	Basic and fundamental: is resistant and stubborn. Directing principle is order, reasons logically. Likes to establish, to organize, to construct and in whatever situation, has strong sense of responsibility	Aesthetic considerations rule his spirit and dictate his smallest actions. He loves beauty and seeks to express it	Unstable in attitude. Uncertain and irresolute, takes decisions on spur of moment; his plans are often contradictory, always sudden and unpremeditated. Gifted with extraordinary mimicry, variety of brilliant performances
Heredity	No comment	Tubercular	Syphilitic

model of typology based on a synthesis of these many sources, modified specifically to help the osteopath in the clinical situation. He included a third classification, which was a mixture of the two.

He based this classification on Still's concept of structure and function, classifying the types as either 'Structural' or 'Functional' or a mixture of the two types which he called 'Mixed'. Table 5.10 draws on some of the key elements of this model, but yet again you are referred to the original texts for a more complete understanding.[11,12]

Dummer's basic premise was that structure governs function. Spring succinctly states the concept underpinning this:

If Structure was to refer to the musculoskeletal body, the body's literal structures and Function was to refer to the physiological processes within the body, the Structural approach in treatment would be a direct appeal to the musculoskeletal structures leading to an effect of the local tissues upon the physiology via circulation and nervous tissues; a Functional approach in treatment would be a direct appeal to the physiology, via intracellular behaviour, leading to effects upon the musculoskeletal structures.[2]

Both structural and functional approaches achieve similar results; it is just the methods of application that differ. This statement does not perhaps emphasize the more psychological aspects, but these would be considered within the approach to the patient.

Dummer makes clear that there are numerous factors, other than just biotype, that will play a part in dictating the mode of treatment most suitable for

Table 5.10   The structural functional classification of Tom Dummer, including features of level of dysfunction and preferred treatment approach. (Modified after Dummer T. Specific adjusting technique. Hove: JoTom Publications; 1995, and Spring L. Body morphology. Maidstone: Unpublished dissertation. European School of Osteopathy; 1998)

Structural	Functional	Mixed
Solid frame, big muscles with strong tonus, hypomobile joints, tendency to put on fat	Either: 1. Short with decreased muscle tonus and hypermobile joints, under-reactive. Or: 2. Tall with slightly more muscle tonus , mediate joints, mobility, over-reactive	Combination of aspects of both structural and functional
Any activity that allows them to utilize their physical abilities, or express their competitiveness and aggression, such as a 'hard-headed businessman'	1. Tending to the caring professions 2. Activity that allows them to express their artistic tendencies	Dependent on the proportions of the structural or functional components
Level: physical level, i.e. anatomical, physiological, biochemical	Level: vital energy. The energy matrix	Dependent on the proportions of the structural or functional components
Depth: superficial, involving structure more than function. Often at the musculoskeletal level, or structure of organs and vessels	Depth: profound on a bioenergetic level; involving the dysfunction of all tissues with emphasis on the viscera, and also the psyche and particularly the emotional level and subconscious mind	Dependent on the proportions of the structural or functional components
Treatment approach: most open to appeal in the musculoskeletal field. Structural mechanical: General osteopathic treatment (GOT), general articulatory treatment (GAT)	Treatment approach: most open to change in fascial or fluid fields. Cranial and indirect (functional*)	Treatment approach: care required to assess the relative balance of mix of structure/function

*It should be noted that the term 'functional' is used by Dummer to mean both the treatment approach developed by Bowles and Hoover, and as a term for a group of approaches more widely termed indirect. In this incidence it is intended to mean indirect approaches.

a patient. He also states that the *intention or mode of application* of any treatment can make it structural or functional. However, this classification does give some indicators that will assist in making the final treatment plan.

SUMMARY AND APPLICATIONS

This chapter has covered what is perhaps one of the more 'difficult' concepts in the book. As mentioned previously, there is an inherent disquiet amongst many individuals about the application of labels or stereotypes to people, and this is right, to an extent. However, there are differences between people, and these differences are not so great that people cannot be grouped together in some manageable and useful form.

The other relatively difficult aspect of this chapter is that the models are radically summarised and those features listed are numerous and are presented in tabular form. You are not expected to memorize all of the traits specific to each classification; in fact, I would actively encourage you *not* to do that. Rather, it is the intention that you read the words and from them build a picture in your head of each of the three major types. This will be a condensation of the work of some of the foremost biotypologists, each coming from differing scientific and philosophical backgrounds. As you observe more people and think about them as whole and unique individuals, you will develop your own interpretation of these models and will be able to place each patient somewhere on the continuum of typology. (This is not a situation of 'once placed, never moved'; this is a dynamic process, to be reviewed at each consultation. As you learn more about the person, their position on the continuum will subtly change.)

Most importantly, do not forget that you are a human being too, with an ability to empathize and understand fellow human beings. You can see when an individual is sad or happy. It is written in the body, gestures, face, eyes and voice. So often in teaching clinics the authors have observed students who have these abilities to 'read people', but the moment they put on their white coat and shut the treatment room door, fail to recognize or utilize these inherent skills, becoming a practitioner rather than a person. This is obviously partly due to the stress and relative novelty of the situation, but a practitioner must be a person too.

The benefit of applying these models is enormous. The moment you see your patients you can start the process of getting to understand them as a whole. Firstly, the gender and estimated age of patients will immediately narrow down the differential diagnostic possibilities. (These, too, are another form of biotype; male/female, child, youth, middle-aged, elderly.) Then, a rough assessment of biotype will begin to permit you to create hypotheses on their body structure, organ position, problems that they may be predisposed to, as well as the way they may think and communicate.

These early hypotheses are then progressively tested. While taking a history, it will be possible to explore patients' mental approach and attitudes to life, and their views of themselves and of the problem that they have consulted you about.

With regard to communication, and utilizing the extreme examples of their type, ectomorphs will be detailed in the explanation of their problem, and will expect a similarly detailed reply. They will want to know the intricate details of what the problem is, how it could have been caused, whether it is likely to occur again, what can be done to prevent this, and what the long-term consequences may be … be prepared to explain all.

Mesomorphs, in comparison, generally will not want to know much about the process. They are more pragmatic, and if you were to start explaining the underlying causes and what you intend to do, you would probably be interrupted and told that they are not interested in what you do, and that they simply want you to do what is necessary to permit them to continue their sport or life free of pain as quickly as possible.

Endomorphs will be more interested in engaging you in conversation about life in general.

Obviously these are the extremes of the types, but they often appear to be reasonably accurate and give an indication to the practitioner on what level,

initially, to engage the patient. Later the subtleties of the mixed biotypes can be explored.

Functional and pathophysiological changes are varied, depending on the biotype. This is due to a combination of the differing structure and support of the organs, and the nature of their overriding motivations (visceral, musculoskeletal or cerebral). The examination can confirm or refute the constitutional elements. It is equally important for the hypothesis to be proven right or wrong. If it is wrong, this gives you the opportunity to re-examine why you thought it was so in the first place, to reassess, rethink and create a new hypothesis. This serves two purposes: firstly, it prevents you from going down investigative cul-de-sacs, and secondly, it is by reflecting on such aspects of your practice that you will continue to develop your skills as an osteopath.

Analysis of all of the above leads you to the point of deciding what treatment to apply. Dummer's classification of the structural and functional will assist in this, but as stressed in his writings, the model should not be followed blindly. There are numerous other factors that need to be considered such as patients' vitality, and the environmental moulding to which their temperaments have been subjected, which may override those qualities you would have expected, based on their biotypes.

Within this modelling, those individuals that are paradoxical are perhaps of greatest interest to the practitioner. That is, those people who have, for whatever reason, attempted to achieve something to which their biotype is not particularly suited. An example would be an ectomorph attempting to compete at a high level in sprinting, the normal domain of mesomorphs. Such a person will be aware that they have to work harder than others that they come across. Being naturally introspective they will question why. This will range from a logical analysis to the extreme of self doubt. Discussion around the particular strengths of a biotype may lead to either an acceptance of the problem from an informed perspective, leading to the person adopting realistic coping strategies, both mental and physical; or to the realization this may not be their particular area of expertise – perhaps this person should attempt a different form of running more appropriate to their biotype.

Patients may find it reassuring if it is explained that what they are feeling or experiencing is within the normal realms of their biotype. More often than not we feel that we are the only ones that are experiencing such problems, and it can be a great relief to know that it is nothing unusual and that the feelings or problems have been experienced by many before, allowing a degree of connecting with one's fellows. Often 'problems' do not need to be resolved, but just understood for what they are; this in itself can lighten the 'load'. The real problem may be fear of the unknown.

This is a vast area of study, and the above discussion has just skimmed the surface of it. It is a matter of concern that, in so doing, the depth of thought underlying these bare statements may have been sacrificed, despite constant reiterations of the continuum of the classifications, and warnings about not dogmatically following the models. The most important point to take away from this subject is that a natural curiosity and interest in people will enable you to more effectively communicate with your patient and help you find the most effective approach to enable your patient to achieve better health. The models are there just to provide some structure for your thoughts.

References

1. Goldthwait JE, Lloyd T, Loring T et al. Essentials of body mechanics in health and disease, 5th edn. Philadelphia: JB Lippincott; 1952.
2. Spring L. Body morphology. Maidstone: Unpublished dissertation. European School of Osteopathy; 1998.
3. Caillet R. Low back pain syndrome, 3rd edn. Philadelphia: F.A. Davis Company; 1986: 34.
4. Wernham J, Hall TE. The mechanics of the spine and pelvis. Maidstone: Maidstone College of Osteopathy; 1960.
5. Sheldon WH, Stevens SS, Tucker MD. The varieties of human physique: an introduction to constitutional psychology. New York: Harper; 1940.
6. Sheldon WH, Stevens SS. The varieties of temperament: a psychology of constitutional differences. New York: Harper; 1942.
7. Martiny M. Essai de biotypologie humaine. Paris: J Peyronnet; 1948.
8. Notes on Martiny. Online. http://www.giuseppeparisi.com/framesetipiumanx.htm.
9. Kretschmer E. Physique and character: an investigation of the nature of constitution and of the theory of temperament. New York: Harcourt Brace; 1925.
10. Vannier L. La doctrine de l'homeopathie Francaise. Paris: G Doin; 1931.
11. Dummer T. A textbook of osteopathy, vol 1. Hadlow Down: JoTom Publications; 1999: 133–154.
12. Dummer T. Specific adjusting technique. Hove: JoTom Publications; 1995: 36–43.

Recommended reading

Unfortunately nearly all of these books are out of print, and devilishly difficult to get hold of. The British Library can get them for you, but be prepared for a long wait. If you are going to use them for a final project, ordering them should be your first priority. It is only by reading these original texts that you will get a true feel for each particular model. Lizzie Spring's excellent (unpublished) undergraduate project, from which most of the tables came, is available at the ESO library in Maidstone.

Dummer T. A textbook of osteopathy, vol 1. Hadlow Down: JoTom Publications; 1999: 133–154.
Goldthwait JE, Lloyd T, Loring T et al. Essentials of body mechanics in health and disease, 5th edn. Philadelphia: JB Lippincott; 1952.
Keuls K. Osteopathic medicine: Part 1 osteopathic principles. Brighton: Keuls; 1988.

Kretschmer, E. Physique and character: an investigation of the nature of constitution and of the theory of temperament. New York: Harcourt Brace; 1925.
Martiny M. Essai de biotypologie humaine. Paris: J Peyronnet; 1948.
Sheldon WH, Stevens SS, Tucker MD. The varieties of human physique: an introduction to constitutional psychology. New York: Harper; 1940.
Sheldon WH, Stevens SS. The varieties of temperament: a psychology of constitutional differences. New York: Harper; 1942.
Spring L. Body morphology. Maidstone: Unpublished dissertation. European School of Osteopathy; 1998: 53.
Vannier L. Typology in homoeopathy. Beaconsfield: Beaconsfield Publishers; 1992, or
Vannier L. La typologie et ses applications thèrapeutiques: les temperaments, prototypes et mètatypes. Paris: Doin Editeurs; 1976.

Chapter 6

The nervous system

CHAPTER CONTENTS

INTRODUCTION

The nervous system has always been perceived as having a fundamental role in the coordination of the body. Classically the somatic nervous system was thought to be responsible for the musculoskeletal system, and the autonomic nervous system (ANS) regulates the visceral function. The understanding of the nervous system has advanced dramatically over the last few decades; the old concept of it being an independent and discrete 'hard wired' system has now been replaced by the concept of it as a complex integrated system, communicating bidirectionally with the endocrine and immune system (neuroendocrine immune system) and being affected by changes in the psyche as well as the soma (giving rise to the new area of study psychoneuroimmunology [PNI]). Information is conveyed by a multiplicity of possible pathways which are neuroplastic in nature, i.e. capable of being conditioned or learning in response to particular requirements or environmental factors.

The nervous system has always been understood to be involved in the causation and maintenance of the osteopathic lesion. The understanding of its actual role has been modified in relation to the prevalent knowledge of neuroanatomy and neurophysiology. Much of the early work in this area was performed by Professor Irvin Korr and his co-workers, notably Dr JS Denslow. The results of this research have given several decades of osteopaths a scientific rationale for the practice of osteopathy. This research is now slowly beginning to show signs of age and new models are appearing that, in light of the advancing knowledge, offer slightly differing interpretations. This reevaluation will continue as long as these sciences continue to advance. This chapter will review the key concepts, offering a historical perspective and examining the current proposed models of the neural basis of osteopathic medicine.

THE BASIC ORGANIZATION OF THE NERVOUS SYSTEM

The function of the nervous system is to control and regulate various activities of the body and to enable the body to react to the continuous changes of its internal and external environments. It is the nervous system that mediates most of the inputs made during an osteopathic treatment, and thus a sound knowledge of neuroanatomy and neurophysiology is essential. Anatomy texts will often divide the nervous system structurally into the central and peripheral nervous systems, and functionally into the somatic and autonomic nervous systems. It is the interaction of these divisions that underpins osteopathic medicine and hence treatment.

The central nervous system (CNS) consists of the brain and spinal cord and it receives, interprets and creates responses to all of the information passed to it. The information is passed to it via the peripheral nervous system (PNS) which is comprised of the peripheral nerves and ganglia. The PNS is divided into afferent (sensory) and efferent (motor) systems, the afferent system gathering the sensory information and the efferent system transmitting the responses to the effector muscles or organs. Broadly, the somatic system organizes information related to the musculoskeletal system and the ANS coordinates the visceral system (cardiac muscle, smooth muscle and glands). The ANS is divided into a sympathetic branch (sympathetic nervous system, SNS) or thoracolumbar outflow, and a parasympathetic branch (parasympathetic nervous system, PSNS) or craniosacral outflow. The SNS essentially prepares the body systems for action whereas the PSNS has a more vegetative calming role.

The nervous system does not work in isolation but via a complex interaction with other body systems, perhaps most significantly in an osteopathic context with the endocrine and immune systems, the whole generally being known as the neuro-endocrine-immune system. This system is largely responsible for maintaining homeostasis and will be addressed later in this chapter. There are many

excellent texts that contain more specific information regarding the nervous system and its function; elements that have a specific relevance osteopathically will be discussed in this text.

We will begin by looking at the basic level of neurological organization, the neural reflex, and what role this has in creating and maintaining somatic dysfunction in the musculoskeletal and other systems. The concept of the facilitated segment will also be addressed.

NEURAL REFLEXES

The neural reflex is an involuntary response of an effector to a stimulus from a receptor. This simple statement belies the complexity of even the simplest of reflexes. Much of the early research in this area was done by Sir Charles Scott Sherrington (1857–1952) and published in 1906 in his classic text, *The Integrative Action of the Nervous System*.[1]

By working with decerebrate animals, he explored the spinal reflexes and demonstrated that they did not function as a series of isolated processes, as was then currently accepted, but rather that they work as an integrated part of the total organism's activities. The truth of this integration was supported by his discovery in the late 1890s of the 'reciprocal innervation' of muscles, also known as Sherrington's second law: when a muscle receives a nerve impulse causing it to contract, its antagonist receives, simultaneously, an impulse causing it to relax.[2] His significance in the early genesis of neurophysiology is revealed by the fact that he was responsible for coining such terms as neurone, synapse, interoceptor, exteroceptor and proprioceptor.

The research in this area has advanced rapidly, with the phenomenal complexity of the nervous system being progressively revealed. Even so, there are still innumerable questions yet to answer. In order to appreciate how reflexes work we will begin by looking at one of the so-called simple reflexes, the spinal reflex.

THE SPINAL REFLEX

Figure 6.1 shows the simple monosynaptic spinal reflex consisting of an afferent limb comprised of a peripheral receptor, that when stimulated, passes an action potential via the afferent fibres to enter the spinal cord at the posterior horn. The spinal

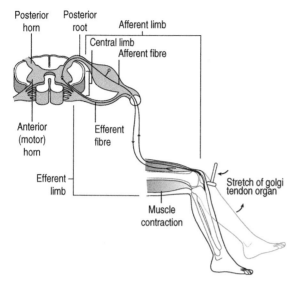

Figure 6.1   The monosynaptic stretch reflex.

cord is part of the central nervous system, so is sometimes referred to as the 'central limb' of the reflex. The fibres, having entered the posterior horn of the cord, pass via the grey matter to the anterior horn where they synapse with the nuclei of the motor neurones. Passing out of the cord by the anterior root, the motor fibres form the efferent limb of the reflex arc, conducting the impulses to the effector muscle, causing it to contract. In fact this type of reflex exists only in the myotatic (stretch) reflex – in reality reflexes are far more complex, but this simple example serves well to give a basic understanding on which to build.

THE MONOSYNAPTIC MYOTATIC OR STRETCH REFLEX

The monosynaptic stretch reflex contains two neurones with one synapse linking them together. Stretching a muscle will stimulate sensory endings of the receptor, the muscle spindle, to pass an action potential to the spinal cord by way of a primary afferent fibre. This will then synapse with an alpha motor neurone at spinal cord level, the impulse then passing along the axon and subsequently causing contraction of the effector muscle. It is this reflex that forms the basis of the deep tendon reflexes that are used as part of the clinical testing of the nervous system. Its role in the body is that of an important postural reflex.

The receptor in this stretch reflex is the muscle spindle (Fig. 6.2). Muscle spindles are small structures (3–12 mm) lying within and attached by fibrous connections to the muscle itself. They lie parallel to the fibres of the overlying muscle. As they are an integral part of the whole muscle, the spindle's length is directly related to the muscle length of the muscle that they are within, i.e. when the muscle shortens or lengthens, so does the spindle.

The spindle consists of a fibrous outer sheath encapsulating several small muscle fibres which are referred to as intrafusal fibres ('intra' is Latin for 'inside', 'fusus' is Latin for 'spindle') to differentiate them from the larger extrafusal fibres of the surrounding muscle. There are two types of intrafusal fibres and each has different stretch characteristics. Attached to these are the sensory receptors of which there are also two types. One reports on the static length of the intrafusal fibre, increasing the output proportionate to the increase in length, and both report on the change in length of the fibres. This combination permits the spindle to have both a static and a dynamic response. Impulses are constantly passing to the cord from these endings.

The sensory fibres from the receptors connect, some monosynaptically, with the same alpha motor neurones that supply the surrounding extrafusal fibres. The afferent input from these receptors is excitatory to the alpha neurones with which they synapse. Thus when the muscle is stretched the spindle via the reflex causes the muscle to contract, thus opposing the stretch. Conversely when the muscle shortens there is a diminution of spindle output leading to less stimulation of the alpha neurone, resulting in relaxation or lengthening of the muscle. Thus they oppose change of length in both directions.

THE GAMMA EFFERENT SYSTEM

The motor supply to the spindles consists of gamma efferent fibres. Their full function appears to be relatively poorly understood, but their significance is evidenced by the fact that they appear to make up almost a third of the efferent ventral root fibres. Collectively this is termed the gamma efferent system. Of those aspects of its role that are understood it appears that its principal action is to cause contraction of the intrafusal fibres. When the motor cortex initiates a movement, a barrage of impulses are passed to the alpha motor system to cause the appropriate muscles to contract. At the same time

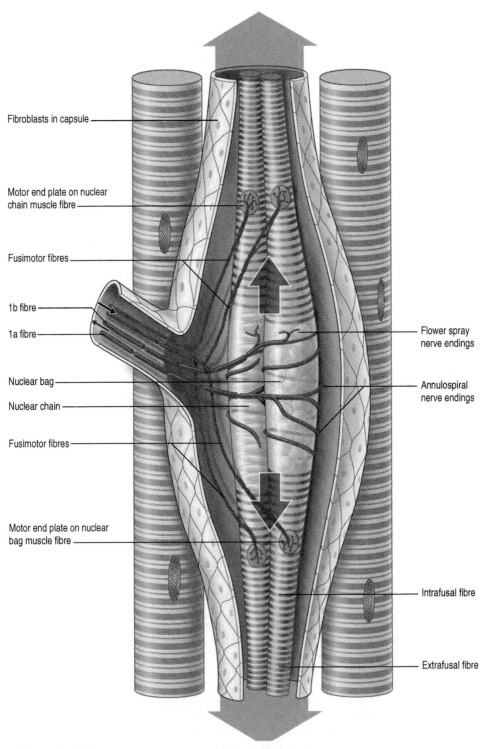

Figure 6.2   The muscle spindle.

there is a similar barrage passing to the gamma system with the intention of causing the intrafusal fibres to contract in a similar proportion to that of the alpha fibres, thus maintaining the same length and tension relationship between the two sets of fibres. Thus the same degree of tension is maintained within the extrafusal fibres, permitting a 'damping' of the movement and a constant responsiveness of the muscle. If the intrafusal fibres were to lag, they would be stretched, causing tensioning of the extrafusal fibres. It is thought that the registering and balancing of the length of the spindle with regard to the surrounding muscle fibres, and hence the ultimate length of the muscle, is controlled via a system termed the gamma loop (the reflex spinal loop between the spindle afferents and the gamma efferents).

As well as this role, it is thought to have a function in preparing the body for anticipated work. For example, when one is about to lift a box, the higher centres make an assessment as to how heavy it is and what will be required of the muscles. This information is passed to the spindles via the gamma efferents, 'warming up' the relevant muscles via the spindle afferents and the alpha motor neurones loop.

Another proposed role is almost that of an amplifier. When a muscle is contracted and static the extrafusal fibres are notably shorter than their normal resting lengths; similarly, as the intrafusal fibres are in parallel with the extrafusal fibres, they too will be shortened. This will result in a decreased sensory afferent output from the intrafusal fibres, and so there will be a lack of information as to the mechanical state of the muscle. If the muscle has shortened to balance the stretching of its antagonist there will be reciprocal inhibition from the stretched muscle to the shortened muscle, further reducing its afferent output. The body is dependent on the gamma afferent output to 'know' where that part of the body is. So it is thought that the gamma efferent system fine-tunes the spindle to amplify any feedback that exists. As an analogy it is rather like turning up the volume control of a hi-fi to full, in order to listen to a quiet passage of music.

THE GOLGI TENDON ORGAN

The muscle spindle works in tandem, but almost antagonistically, with the Golgi tendon organ, a sensory receptor in the muscle tendons. This works in a similar manner to the spindle but responds to levels of tension in the tendon. Once a particular level of tension is exceeded the receptor inhibits the related muscle. As with the spindle it has both a dynamic and static response, but whereas the spindle detects length and rate of change of length, the Golgi tendon organ detects degree and rate of change of tension. Both are constantly feeding information into the spinal cord and to the higher centres and have significant roles in maintaining posture and in controlling movement. These are just two of a large range of proprioceptors present in the muscles, tendons, skin and labyrinth apparatus that are responsible for this control.

POLYSYNAPTIC REFLEXES

The myotatic or monosynaptic reflex as described above is suitable for producing a simple response, such as a withdrawal response from a painful stimulus. However, to obtain coordinated movements necessitates the uniting of the contraction or relaxation of numerous independent muscles simultaneously and this requires much more complicated processes. To this end the primary afferents that project to the spinal cord not only synapse with the motor neurones of the stretched muscle but also to muscles having a synergistic function to complement the action of the prime mover.

In addition, as demonstrated by Sherrington, stretching a particular muscle or group of muscles will cause a relaxation response in the antagonist muscles; this is termed reciprocal inhibition. The mechanism for this was found to be that the primary afferents, in addition to synapsing with the alpha motor neurones of the prime mover and its synergists, also synapse with inhibitory interneurones that pass to the alpha motor neurones of the antagonist muscles.

By using a simple example it is possible to demonstrate how these reflexes work and to introduce another, the crossed extensor reflex. If we step onto a nail, free nerve endings, acting as pain receptors in the skin, will send impulses to the spinal cord which will synapse with the alpha motor neurones passing to the flexor muscle of the leg, causing a reflex withdrawal of the limb from the painful stimulus. In fact, the afferent fibres will also synapse with interneurones in the dorsal horn of the spinal cord, which then in turn act upon the motor neurones of several spinal cord segments in order to activate a number of muscle groups. In addition to activating the flexor response, the interneurones will inhibit the actions of the extensor muscles in the same limb, permitting the flexion to take place. Furthermore, there will be commissural interneurones that cross to the contralateral side of the spinal cord that create an extensor contraction and flexor relaxation in the opposite limb. This so-called crossed extensor reflex serves to prepare the opposite limb to support the change in weight-bearing due to the raising of the flexed limb. Once again, this whole process is a spinal cord reflex, but has now become a polysynaptic reflex. It is by employing these simple spinal cord reflex circuits that the higher centres of the nervous system are able to control the more complex coordinated movements with relatively simple input.

The higher centres can modify these reflex arcs. An example of this has already been mentioned, whereby there is an increased output of the gamma efferent system causing the spindles to shorten slightly and therefore increase the tone of the extrafusal fibres of the muscles in anticipation of lifting a heavy load. Overall, the higher centres have an inhibitory effect on the reflex arcs. This is demonstrated by upper motor neurone problems in which the central control is lost and the deep tendon reflexes become brisk; however, it appears to have a limitless overriding role responding to circumstances as they arise.

From the above it is possible to see that there is a constant feedback from the muscles to the spinal cord as to their state of mechanical tension. This allows the body to regulate the state of contraction and relaxation within individual muscles and within muscle groups and therefore the position of the underlying articulation. This mechanism is equally true for the limb muscle groups and for the axial muscles; the complex interplay between these permits postural control and coordinated movement.

THE REFLEX IN A SIMPLE MODEL OF SOMATIC DYSFUNCTION

By simplifying the model of somatic dysfunction and analysing it from the perspective of a single muscle or group of muscles at a spinal segmental level, it is possible to examine what processes occur in normal postural functioning, and, from that, to extrapolate to what would occur under abnormal conditions, such as a somatic dysfunction of the articulation. See Figure 6.3.

It is possible to see from the diagram that an intersegmental muscle is part of the erector spinae group of the paravertebral muscles and joins the

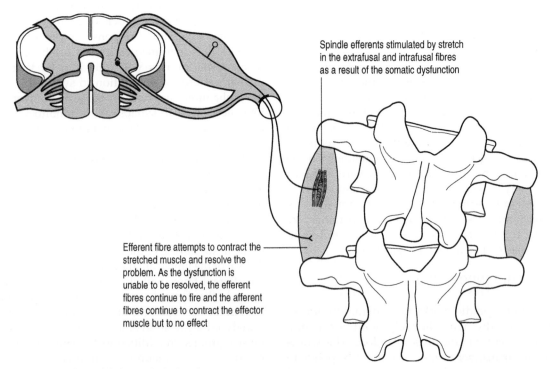

Spindle efferents stimulated by stretch in the extrafusal and intrafusal fibres as a result of the somatic dysfunction

Efferent fibre attempts to contract the stretched muscle and resolve the problem. As the dysfunction is unable to be resolved, the efferent fibres continue to fire and the afferent fibres continue to contract the effector muscle but to no effect

Figure 6.3   A simple model of somatic dysfunction.

two vertebrae. The structure of this muscle is similar to any other skeletal muscle; it comprises a belly and two tendons of attachment. Within the muscle itself are the muscle spindles and within the tendons are the Golgi tendon organs, i.e. the structures that are responsible for monitoring the muscle length and tone. These structures, as we have seen, are linked to the respective spinal cord segments by afferent fibres and the responses are mediated back to the muscle by way of the efferent motor neurones.

If an excessive tension is applied to a muscle, by, for example, making a side-bending movement to the opposite side, there will be an increase in the rate of firing in the muscle spindles of the muscle on the lengthened side. This will then be relayed to the spinal cord to produce a contraction of the muscle in an attempt to restore its normal length and tension, and hence the position of the vertebra. In effect a simple spinal reflex is being used to restore the segment to the normal position and tension. If for some reason the position cannot be restored, it will then set up a constant barrage of impulses into the spinal cord at this level and the segment will become, in Irvin Korr's terms 'facilitated' (the 'facilitated segment' will be further explored below). This abnormal positioning of the vertebra and the increased neural activity would be termed a somatic dysfunction. It may be the result of a trauma, or repetitive strain, which in the case of postural muscles could be as a result of a compensatory pattern (as we have seen earlier when we looked at the biomechanics of the spine) or many other sources, visceral, psychic, etc. This explains some of the 'local', purely mechanical features of dysfunction (muscle hypertonicity, asymmetry of position and movement). However, there are many more aspects, both local and distant, that are involved within somatic dysfunction. These are not dependent on just the nervous system, but on the complex bidirectional interplay between the nervous, endocrine and immune systems. These aspects will be discussed more fully later in this chapter.

SOMATIC AND VISCERAL REFLEXES

Thus far, in the reflexes discussed, both the sensory receptor and the motor effector have been within the somatic or musculoskeletal system. Osteopathically, this reflex would be termed a 'somaticosomatic reflex', the first word indicating where the sensory part has arisen from and the second word where its efferent effect will be felt. It is the body's way of controlling the musculoskeletal system unconsciously. The nervous system is such an inherent part of this process that most people refer to the neuromusculoskeletal system.

The visceral systems, logically, have a similar feedback system, e.g. the presence of food in the stomach will be noted by receptors on the stomach lining which will then feed this information via the afferent limb of the reflex arc to the appropriate spinal segment, which will cause the effector glands to increase secretion. Thus it is the same process and would be termed a viscerovisceral reflex. There is one major difference, in that the part of the nervous system mediating the visceral reflex is the autonomic nervous system rather than the somatic nervous system of the somatic reflex.

A BRIEF REVIEW OF THE ANATOMY OF THE AUTONOMIC NERVOUS SYSTEM

The autonomic nervous system (ANS) is primarily involved with the day-to-day automatic functions of the visceral processes of the body. It is ultimately controlled by the brain and brain stem structures, but as with the somatic nervous system, it has a peripheral system that functions at a spinal level. In fact, much of the time the peripheral autonomic fibres 'hitch a lift' in the somatic nerves. This discussion will concentrate on the peripheral aspects of the ANS. See Figure 6.4.

The sympathetic part of the ANS is also known as the thoracolumbar outflow, as the nuclei of the sympathetic outflow arise from an extra horn of the grey matter of the spinal cord section termed the lateral horn or intermediolateral cell column. This is present only from the first thoracic segment to the second or third lumbar segments. The axons of the sympathetic neurones pass from the spinal cord to the sympathetic ganglionic chain and hence are termed preganglionic nerves. They pass from the spinal cord to the ganglionic chain by way of the white rami communicantes, so called because the axons are group B myelinated fibres and appear whiter due to the presence of the myelin. Within the ganglionic chain, there are four options open to them:

- They may synapse at that level with a postganglionic fibre that will then pass on to its target viscus.
- They may pass through the ganglion without synapsing and pass to a sympathetic ganglion

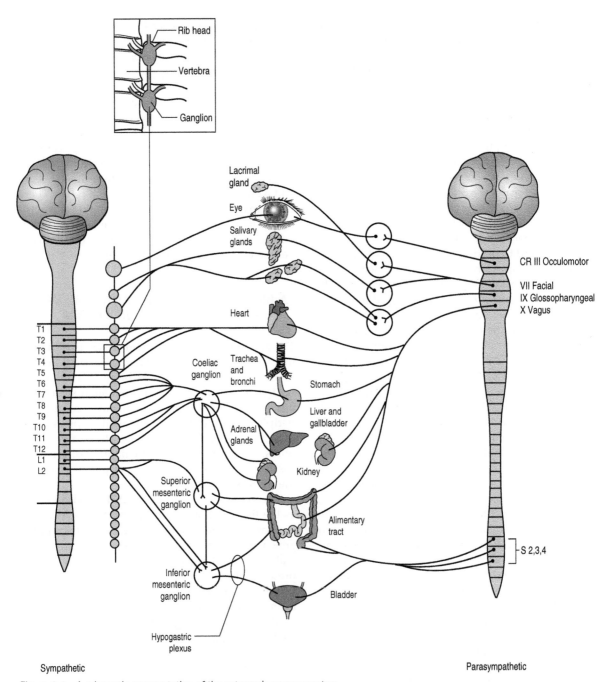

Figure 6.4   A schematic representation of the autonomic nervous system.

closer to their target viscus where they will synapse.
- They may ascend or descend within the ganglionic chain and synapse at a level different to their exit level.
- They may ascend or descend within the ganglionic chain without synapsing and then exit to

pass to a sympathetic ganglion closer to their target viscus where they will synapse.

It is by ascending and descending that the preganglionic fibres reach the ganglia to which there are no white rami communicantes, i.e. those areas where there are no sympathetic nuclei in the lateral horn – the cervical, lower lumbar and sacral regions. Axons leaving the ganglia pass in the grey rami communicantes that is made up almost exclusively of unmyelinated group C postganglionic fibres then pass into the spinal nerve to be carried to their ultimate destination.

The sympathetic ganglionic chain extends from the upper cervical region down to the coccyx. At most levels there exists a pair of ganglia, one either side of the vertebral column. In the cervical region the ganglia lie on the anterior aspect of the transverse processes just posterior to the carotid sheath. In the thoracic region the ganglia lie on the anterior aspects of the costovertebral joints, whilst in the lumbar region they lie on the lateral aspect of the bodies of the lumbar vertebrae. In the pelvis, they are to be found on the anterior aspect of the sacrum just medial to the anterior sacral foramina. Finally, the sympathetic chains from either side join together to form a single ganglion at the coccyx, known as the ganglion impar. In the upper cervical region the ganglia are normally coalesced to form a series of three ganglia, the superior, middle and inferior cervical ganglia. In addition, the inferior cervical ganglion may be joined to the first thoracic ganglion to form the so-called stellate ganglion. Above the cervical region, the sympathetic nerves pass into the interior of the skull with the internal carotid artery. There may be a single ganglion which arises from the joining of the two sides that is known as the ganglion of Ribes. In this manner, although there are 31 paired spinal nerves, the number of paired ganglia will normally be fewer.

Many of the preganglionic fibres that pass out of the ganglionic chain continue into the body where they form ganglia. This is most pronounced in the abdomen and the pelvis where they form the paraaortic ganglia, the coeliac, mesenteric and hypogastric ganglia.

The parasympathetic part of the ANS is also known as the craniosacral outflow as the nuclei of the outflow arise in the cranial nuclei of cranial nerves III the occulomotor nerve, VII the fascial nerve, IX the glossopharyngeal and X the vagus, and the lateral horn of the sacral segments S2, 3 and 4. They pass as preganglionic fibres in their respective nerves to ganglia either in or very near to the target organ where they synapse and the short postganglionic fibres pass to the organ. The fibres are also found in the sympathetic ganglia.

It can be appreciated that though the nuclei arise in only parts of the CNS, all visceral structures receive an autonomic supply.

An awareness of the position of the various elements of the ANS will help in understanding why dysfunction in a certain area may result in more complex effects than anticipated. For example, somatic dysfunction at the cervicothoracic region will possibly affect the motor and sensory supply to the upper extremity via the somatic nervous system, leading to any combination of weakness, pain and paraesthesia; but it could also have an effect on the blood supply to the cranium via disturbance of the sympathetic fibres ascending from their T1 lateral horn nuclei, possibly resulting in migrainous or vascular type headaches.

Much osteopathic treatment is directed at affecting the peripheral, and thereby the central, aspects of the ANS. There are numerous examples of how this can be achieved. Simple rib raising/articulation techniques will have a major effect on the sympathetic chain; how this can occur can be understood by observing the close proximity of the rib heads and the ganglionic chain. Releasing tension in the cervical muscles and fascia will affect the autonomic supply to the head, as a sacral toggle will affect the parasympathetic supply to the pelvis. These are obvious examples, but by understanding the organization of the ANS, and where it may be disturbed, you will be able to treat systemic complaints much more effectively.

VISCEROSOMATIC AND SOMATICOVISCERAL REFLEXES

From the earliest days of osteopathy, the osteopathic lesion has been known to have both local effects and distal effects. The relationship between visceral dysfunction and spinal tenderness and the mechanism through which this was mediated had been proposed well before the founding of osteopathy. As early as 1836, Professor Jean Cruveilhier (1791–1874) observed points of tenderness on the spine related to certain pathological problems, and these occurred at specific levels of the thoracic spine dependent on the site of the pathology. He termed these points 'dorsal points'. Moreover, if treatment was applied at these sites rather than to the tissue overlying the affected organ, the effect was greater and longer lasting.

The mechanisms mediating this were established by numerous researchers, though perhaps the most significant were Sir Charles Sherrington and Sir Henry Head (1861, 1940). Both were pioneers in the area of spinal reflexes and they were in regular communication, pooling their respective findings.

In 1893, Head coined the term 'referred pain' to describe visceral pain that is felt in regions of the body other than in the organ that has the pathology.[3] He discovered reproducible zones of tenderness and hyperalgesia of skin, associated with visceral disease; these became known as Head's zones. For example, a patient with hepatic disorders may feel pain or dysthesia in the skin on the right side of the thoracic cage and the right shoulder. As well as the sensation changes, there were also trophic changes noted in the somatic area of referral. The trophic changes include changes in the blood flow, in the texture and structure of the skin, thickening of the subcutaneous connective tissue structures and muscle atrophy. The reflex zones do not form as soon as a clinical picture of original disorder is established: certain elements such as blood supply changes and sudomotor changes may be present very soon, but the more chronic tissue changes such as skin texture change can take 2–3 months after the onset of the visceral disturbance to manifest in the somatic zones.

Head also demonstrated the mechanism responsible for this phenomena, revealing that a sympathetic nerve supplying an internal organ has a corresponding nerve which supplies particular areas of skin, and perhaps most importantly, that these two nerves are linked by a reflex in a spinal cord segment. He also realized that the viscera were poor at registering pain and that in the case of a noxious stimulus affecting a viscera there may be diffuse poorly localized minor pain felt in the viscera, while the pain was generally felt more strongly at its associated referral area of the skin, or Head's zone. Many early osteopathic texts quote an interpretation of this as Head's law: 'When a painful stimulus is applied to a part of low sensibility in close central connection with a part of much greater sensibility, the pain produced is felt in the part of higher sensibility rather than in the part of lower sensibility to which the stimulus was actually applied'.[4] This law will appear particularly pertinent with regard to the neurological lens concept within the discussion on segmental facilitation below.

The reflex mediating the production of changes in the somatic structures, the skin and its associated connective tissue, as a consequence of a primary visceral problem, is termed the viscerosomatic reflex. (Early osteopathic texts refer to it as a secondary reflex lesion.) If the viscera can have an effect on the somatic structures it is logical that the reverse can occur. This is described as a somaticovisceral reflex or, in the early osteopathic texts, as a primary reflex lesion.

A simple representation of these reflexes is shown in Figure 6.5.

It has now been shown that there are numerous synaptic connections between the somatic and autonomic systems. The earlier representations of clear, well-divided somatic and autonomic reflex arcs dramatically oversimplify the reality. In fact there appears to be a marked overlap between these two systems. This is well demonstrated by looking at the organization of the grey matter of the spinal cord. This has been divided into 10 zones termed Rexed layers. Nociceptive afferents from both visceral and somatic structures enter the spinal cord and pass into Lissauer's tract, passing superiorly and inferiorly in this tract and sending branches to synapse in Rexed layers I, II, V and X.[5] There they synapse with interneurones, many of which are wide dynamic range (WDR) neurones. These interneurones are multireceptive, receiving inputs from both visceral and somatic afferents, thus they are common to both. The interneurones then stimulate both the visceral efferents and motor efferents, including both alpha and gamma motor neurones. To date there do not appear to be any ascending tracts that are solely for the transmission of visceral sensation, so all transmission of sensory information to the higher centres is via shared tracts.[6] Thus the systems act in an integrated and mutually dependent manner.

THE RELATIONSHIP BETWEEN SOMATIC AND VISCERAL STRUCTURES

The patterns of the relationships between the somatic structures and the viscera have been studied by numerous individuals and there have been many charts drawn of these relationships. They can be divided broadly into two general classifications, those related to the spinal segmental supply, and those concerned with viscerosomatic tender points.

The segmental supply model

The distribution of nerve fibres is more or less segmental throughout the body. This is the result of the preservation by the sensory levels of the nervous system of the original embryologic division of the body into metameres. A metamere consists of the spinal segment that provides sensory and motor

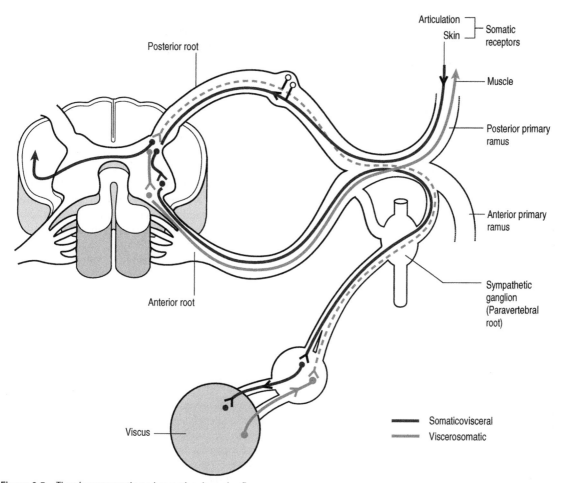

Figure 6.5   The viscerosomatic and somaticovisceral reflexes.

innervation to one embryologic division.[7] It is composed of:

- A dermatome, which is the cutaneous area supplied by a single pair of posterior (sensory) roots and their ganglia.
- A sclerotome, which is the area of bones supplied by the unit.
- A myotome, which is the area of skeletal muscle supplied by the anterior (motor) roots of the segment.
- A viscerotome, which is the area of viscera supplied by the same unit.
- It also includes all the vessels, arteries, veins and lymphatics at each level.

Thus it is probable that when a particular spinal segment is disturbed, changes will occur in any or all of those structures supplied by that spinal segment.

The autonomic spinal segmental supply of each viscera is known. For the heart it is from T1 to T6. As there is a direct relationship between the autonomic and somatic nervous systems, the skin changes would be expected to be found in the dermatomal areas of T1 to T6. There may also be referral to the relevant myotomal or sclerotomal levels, causing muscle or bone pain predominantly in the upper left thorax.

The converse is obviously the case where areas of spinal dysfunction will have an effect on the viscera. It is possible to predict what viscera are going to be affected by the same means as above, but in reverse. Littlejohn attempted to model these relationships in his work on the 'osteopathic centres'; these generally mirror the autonomic supply though there are notable exceptions. For example, the uterus has an osteopathic centre at C2/3, which is far away from its autonomic supply.

Viscerosomatic tender points model

In this model, there are points that are reproducible but not obviously related to the segmental spinal supply. Head's zones are an example of this type of referral, as are the dorsal points described by Cruveilhier. Other examples are Chapman's reflexes, Jones' tender points, myofascial trigger points and Jarricot's Dermalgies reflexes. These are discussed in more detail in Section 3.

Awareness of these models has great advantages clinically. They offer an objective means, other than assessing the viscera locally, of confirming diagnostically the presence of an underlying visceral dysfunction, and, after treatment, a means of assessing whether there has been full resolution. By observing the autonomic changes present at the skin it is possible to relate those to the associated viscera; thus if the skin has chronic changes with atrophy, hypoperfusion and coarsening, it would be possible to hypothesize that the related viscera will similarly have undergone chronic changes. The converse will be the case for an acute presentation with oedema, heat sweat and tenderness at the skin and a related recent problem at the viscera.

Conceptually they enable one to hypothesize where a particular problem, in the somatic or visceral systems, may have a related dysfunction via these reflex links. This is particularly important in that they are branches of a reflex arc. If only one aspect of the arc is corrected it is possible for the untreated aspect to reinstate the one previously resolved. With regard to treatment they offer an additional 'way in' to a problem: either end of the reflex can be treated to give some relief. This is particularly useful in the case of an especially acute problem where it is too tender to address the problem locally, or where there is some underlying condition that precludes a direct approach; treatment applied distally at the tender points may have a palliative effect.

It is important to be aware of the individual differences present in people; we are not anatomically identical, and the relationships are not always exactly as they are stated in the charts or texts. These are only conceptual models – they serve to create hypotheses that need to be tested against the case history and other examination findings before one can act on them.

There is another very important reflex that needs to be mentioned – the psychosomatic, and its reverse, the somaticopsychic.

PSYCHOSOMATIC AND SOMATICO-PSYCHIC REFLEXES

In our hectic and stressful society the psychosomatic reflex and its effects are now well known, for example, the effects of stress in the pathogenesis of cardiovascular disease. Similarly there is now a much greater awareness of the psychological effects of somatic dysfunction. Reflecting on the integration of the nervous system it is possible to extend this reflex to psychovisceral and visceropsychic. The mechanism of this is essentially similar to the reflexes already discussed, but will be addressed in greater depth in the next chapter, on psychology.

Much of the work of relating these reflexes to osteopathy and researching their validity has fallen to Professor Irvin Korr, an American physiologist who has dedicated his life to these studies.

PROFESSOR KORR'S CONTRIBUTION

In his work entitled 'The Neural Basis of the Osteopathic Lesion', Korr stated:

> Within the nervous system, in the phenomena of excitation and inhibition of nerve cells, and in synaptic and myoneural transmission, lie the answers to some of the most important theoretical and practical osteopathic problems. The existence of a neural basis for the lesion has been known, of course, for a long time. The segmental relation of the osteopathic lesion to its somatic and visceral effects is explicable in no other way.

> The activity and condition of the tissues and organs are directly influenced, through excitation and inhibition, by the efferent nerves which emerge from the central nervous system and which conduct impulses to these tissues and organs.[8]

His aim was to explain how various effects of the osteopathic lesion, both local and distant, were produced. The effects included hyperaesthesia, hyperirritability, tissue texture changes of the skin, muscle and connective tissue, local circulatory changes and altered visceral and other autonomic functions. (See Qualitative considerations in articular somatic dysfunction on p.22.)

EARLY STUDIES

Professor Korr worked with Dr JS Denslow to investigate the relationship between the osteopathic lesion and the control of efferent activity. One study involved the application of a certain amount of pressure via a calibrated pressure meter to the spinous processes of the thoracic spine and measurement of the resulting muscular activity electromyographically at the corresponding levels. Essentially this was measuring the activity in a simple spinal reflex arc. The pressure at each segment was gradually increased in order to initiate muscular activity at each particular level, thus the researchers determined the 'reflex threshold' that needed to be exceeded to cause a motor response. By comparing 'lesioned segments', which they determined by palpation, with the non-lesioned reflex thresholds, it was found that thresholds were lower in lesioned segments. In addition, it was found that the more severe the lesion, the lower the threshold.

The spread of excitation

Next, they explored the manner in which neural activity may spread from its original site throughout the spine, and the possible consequences of this. Four vertebral levels in the thoracic spine (T4, 6, 8 and 10) were selected, and using the above methods the reflex thresholds for each level ascertained. The muscle activity was monitored at every level in response to pressure applied to each of the separate spinous processes, i.e. 16 readings were taken.

Their principal findings were that there was a far greater spread of excitation towards a lesioned segment than away from it. So that if, for example, T6 was a severely lesioned segment (i.e. it had a low reflex threshold), only very slight pressure at T6 was required to elicit an EMG response at T6. But even a very high pressure at T6 did not evoke responses in T4, 8 or 10. Whereas, at T4, 8 or 10 application of a low pressure would produce no response at the level where the stimulus was applied, but elicit a response at T6. See Figure 6.6. Korr expressed this in a simple analogy:

The anterior horn cell of a lesioned segment represents a bell easily rung from a number of push buttons, while the spinous process or push button of the lesioned segment does not easily ring bells other than its own.[8]

The hyperexcitable segment they termed a 'facilitated segment' from the Latin word 'facilis' meaning 'easy' – it is more easy to elicit a response at that particular segment. This reflects Head's law: 'When a painful stimulus is applied to a part of low sensibility in close central connection with a part of

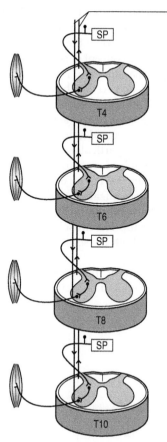

Figure 6.6 The reflex spread of excitation. See the section on spread of excitation for an explanation. (After Korr IM. The neural basis of the osteopathic lesion. In: Peterson B ed., The collected papers of Irvin M Korr. Colorado: American Academy of Osteopathy; 1979.)

much greater sensibility, the pain produced is felt in the part of higher sensibility rather than in the part of lower sensibility to which the stimulus was actually applied.'

The facilitated segment: a simple explanation

Many students find this concept difficult to grasp. The author has found that a simple analogy sometimes helps. The premise is based on the true concept that for a nerve to pass an action potential it has to receive a stimulus that exceeds the threshold potential of that nerve – anything below that will fail to illicit a response. This is termed the threshold stimulus, being the difference between the resting potential and the threshold potential. See Figures 6.7A and B.

Where there is somatic dysfunction there will be a barrage of afferent information from the receptors, relaying information about the aberrant position of the lesioned structures to the cord, in an attempt to get the efferent system to contract the effector muscles and to resolve the problem as in Figure 6.3. Inherent in the concept of somatic dysfunction is the principle that the body is not able to resolve the problem itself, and so the above process continues unabated. This will cause the affected segment to have a higher level of neural activity than before. Thus this could be perceived as having raised the resting potential of that particular segment, so that a lesser threshold stimulus is required to elicit a response from that segment. See Figure 6.7C.

Due to the metameric organization of the spinal cord this means that the resulting facilitation will affect the segmentally supplied muscles, viscera and associated tissues via both the somatic and visceral efferents.

Figure 6.7D is a schematic representation of Korr's experiment on the spread of excitation. This aims to pictorially represent how the facilitated segment can act as a 'neurological lens'.

The neurological lens

Korr's team used this term to describe the effects that a facilitated segment will have (see Fig. 6.7D). The term is an analogy based on the action of a magnifying glass. A magnifying glass will focus a wide range of light rays to one point, concentrating them sufficiently to be able to burn paper, as all children know. The facilitated segment acts like the magnifying glass, taking any neural inputs passing up or down the spinal cord and focusing them on that segment and its associated structures, hence the neurological lens.

Tissue texture changes

In the discussions above, mention has been made of the possible autonomically mediated visceral

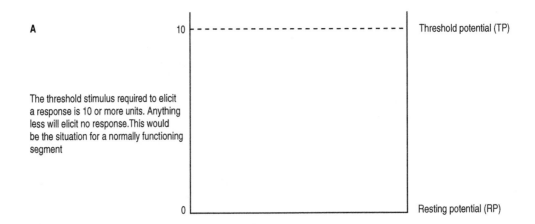

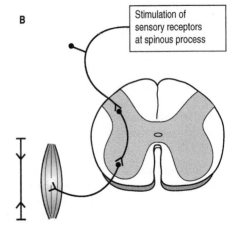

Figure 6.7 A schematic view of the facilitated segment. **(A)** Basic premise: the all or nothing principle. Stimulation of the spinous process of the vertebra, if able to overcome the threshold potential of the segment, will cause the anonciated paraspinal muscles to contract. **(B)** No segmental lesion. This concept will be applied to the spinal segments and for the purpose of this exercise the actual figures are not going to be used, but rather it is proposed that the resting potential of the segment is 0 units and the threshold is 10 units, thus the threshold stimulus has to exceed 10 units.

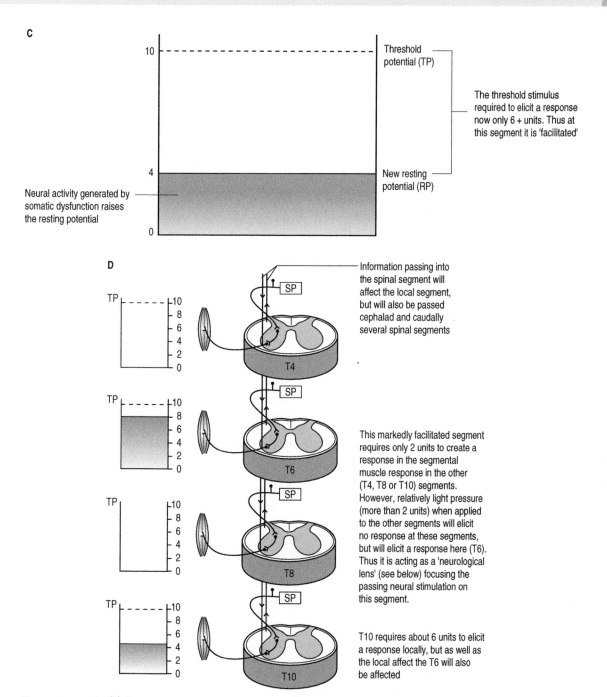

C

Neural activity generated by somatic dysfunction raises the resting potential

Threshold potential (TP)

The threshold stimulus required to elicit a response now only 6 + units. Thus at this segment it is 'facilitated'

New resting potential (RP)

D

Information passing into the spinal segment will affect the local segment, but will also be passed cephalad and caudally several spinal segments

SP

T4

SP

T6

This markedly facilitated segment requires only 2 units to create a response in the segmental muscle response in the other (T4, T8 or T10) segments. However, relatively light pressure (more than 2 units) when applied to the other segments will elicit no response at these segments, but will elicit a response here (T6). Thus it is acting as a 'neurological lens' (see below) focusing the passing neural stimulation on this segment.

SP

T8

SP

T10

T10 requires about 6 units to elicit a response locally, but as well as the local affect the T6 will also be affected

Figure 6.7 cont'd **(C)** Segmental dysfunction. Pressure on T8 (unlesioned and resting potential of zero). No local response will be elicited until a large force equivalent to 10 units is applied. However, before this occurs there will be a spread of the neural stimulus to distal segments. If the stimulus transmitted exceeds 2 units a response will be elicited at T6, and if it exceeds 6 units then T10 will also have a motor response. Thus neural stimuli are passed superiorly and inferiorly through the spinal cord, eliciting responses preferentially in areas of increased neural activity (such as that associated with somatic dysfunction). The dysfunctioning segment is thought of as being facilitated and acting as a neural lens, preferentially focusing neural activity at the facilitated and lesioned segments. **(D)** Where lesioned segments occur, they may act as foci to neural activity within the spinal cord.

or systemic effects that may accompany the musculoskeletal consequences of somatic dysfunction. However, the above experiments only demonstrate the musculoskeletal effects. So Korr and his coworkers formulated a series of experiments to attempt to demonstrate the relationships between the osteopathic lesion and sympathetic activity.

They focused their attention on the tissue texture changes that occur in the region of an osteopathic lesion: localized oedema, temperature changes and fibrous alterations of the muscles, which appear to be mediated by the sympathetic nervous system causing altered vasomotor activity, fluid balance, capillary permeability and trophic factors. They monitored the tissue changes that occurred with changes in autonomic supply.

Initially they utilized electrical skin resistance as a possible index of changes in vasomotor and sweat gland activity. They found that reducing the flow of impulses over a sympathetic pathway to a given area of skin caused marked elevation of resistance in that area (due to a decrease in vasomotor and sweat gland activity), and the converse, that stimulation of sympathetic pathways either locally or systemically lowered the skin resistance.[9] They utilized the electrical skin resistance (ESR) and skin temperature as an indication of the degree of local sympathetic activity. The backs of numerous subjects were assessed, and each individual exhibited a unique pattern of resistance, and, by implication, facilitation. Interestingly, these individual patterns remained relatively constant in some subjects for time spans that ran into years.

The researchers then attempted to see the effects that could be induced by introducing a factor that would cause a change in the mechanical balance of the individual, thus reflecting the changes that might arise consequent to the presence of a somatic dysfunction. One way that this was done was by using a heel lift under one foot only. Changing the postural mechanics of patients caused an exaggeration of the existing sudomotor patterns, and additional regions of sudomotor activity appeared which related to the new areas of postural adaptation and consequent dysfunction and discomfort.[10] This was interpreted as a direct correlation to areas of dysfunction and changes in superficial segmental sympathetic activity.

The segmental relationship of soft tissue changes and segmental facilitation was reinforced when later the researchers demonstrated that there was often lowered skin resistance in the areas of referred pain and in the dermatomes related to the musculoskeletal disturbances.[11]

In their summary, they state:

These studies suggest that the patterns of aberrant areas of sudomotor and vasomotor activity, which we have previously described in apparently normal subjects, may reflect subclinical and asymptomatic sources of afferent bombardment, over selected dorsal roots, or of direct irritation of nerve fibres or ganglion cells. That is, the altered patterns of sympathetic activity appear to be either reflex manifestation of changes in sensory input arising in nerve endings and receptors in the musculoskeletal tissue or the effects of direct insults to nerve fibres (or ganglion cells) or a combination of both.

Observation of the organization of the peripheral nervous system allows one to take this hypothesis one step further. The anterior and posterior rami arise from the same spinal segment and therefore will be subject to the same influences with regard to the degree of facilitation. The posterior ramus carries the sympathetic fibres to the posterior blood vessels and sweat glands, the action of which was assessed in the previous experiment. The anterior ramus, as already stated, is subject to the same degree of facilitation as the posterior; therefore the sympathetic changes occurring in the skin should be the same as those occurring in the structures supplied by the sympathetic fibres carried in the anterior ramus. Thus it is possible to theorize on the state of the deep visceral function of the body by just observing the tissue changes overlying the dermatomal region of the relevant spinal segments.

By observing these changes it is possible to correlate them to actual or possible disease states. It also has a preventive function in that subclinical and asymptomatic disease states will have this superficial representation before the patient shows any outward symptoms of frank disease. They are on the first stage of the continuum from the normal physiological state, about to pass to the pathophysiological change. This stage is still reversible with treatment, but if it were to continue further it would pass into possibly irreversible pathology.

A SUMMARY OF KORR'S CONCEPTS

Korr demonstrated that a spinal osteopathic lesion, as well as having the musculoskeletal component of aberrant position and muscle tone, has a neurophysiological component. The prime coordinator of this is the muscle spindle and its gamma loop. The spindle is disturbed by the change in position, and bombards the cord via the afferent branch of the reflex, in an attempt to stimulate the efferent branch and its effector muscle to normalize the position of the vertebrae. As it is unable to do this, the increase in neural activity continues. This activity 'warms up' the segment, making it easier for it to respond, thus it becomes a facilitated segment. The facilitation causes that segment to respond to passing neural activity which may otherwise fail to illicit a response in less facilitated segments. Thus it acts as a neurological lens.

By assessing the sympathetic activity at the skin surface, Korr and his colleagues demonstrated that somatic dysfunction does have an effect on it, resulting in the palpable tissue texture changes noted around somatic dysfunction. The distribution of nerve fibres is more or less segmental throughout the body, therefore the dermatomal area of skin that is affected will be related to a myotome, viscerotome, sclerotome and all the vessels, arteries, veins and lymphatics at that level. Korr's work poses the hypothesis that all of these structures will be similarly affected, so if the skin is demonstrating features that would indicate hypersympatheticotonia then all of those elements supplied by that segment will be subject to the same degree of sympathetic activity. If this disturbance is sustained it will be deleterious to the target tissues, possibly leading to clinical rather than subclinical conditions, the nature of which will be determined by the particular response of the tissue or organs to the atypical stimulation.[12]

THE NOCICEPTIVE MODEL OF SOMATIC DYSFUNCTION

The work of Korr and Denslow focused on the muscle spindle as the mediating factor of somatic dysfunction. Van Buskirk offers another model for somatic dysfunction, based on the concept of the nociceptive input. The following discussion is based on his paper, 'The Nociceptive Reflex and the Somatic Dysfunction: A Model'.[13]

Nociceptors belong to the myelinated type III and unmyelinated type IV peripheral neurones. They have sensory receptors that respond to pain in all its forms. The receptors are free nerve endings that originate in great numbers in most tissues, including the 'dermis, sub dermis, joint capsules, ligaments, tendons, muscle fascia, periosteum, all blood vessel stroma except that of the capillaries, in the meninges, and in the stroma of all internal organs'.[13]

Typically, they have many peripheral branches that innervate adjacent areas of the same structure. When one branch of the neurone is stimulated sufficiently to pass an action potential, it passes both centrally to the spine and the CNS (referred to as the centripetal action) and peripherally to its other branches (the centrifugal action). To transmit the action potential there will be a release both centrally and peripherally of neurotransmitters including substance P and somatostatin.

The centrifugal actions

Neurotransmitters will be released from the nerve endings of the neurone branches directly affected by the noxious stimulus. It will also cause its peripheral branches (that have not been directly affected) to similarly release neurotransmitters from their nerve endings into the surrounding tissues. The effect of these neurotransmitters in the periphery is to act as vasodilators and chemical attractors for tissue macrophages and lymphocytes. They also have an action which will both stimulate the release of, and act as synergists to, the inflammatory chemicals (cytokinins) such as histamine from mast cells and interleukin-1 (IL-1), and tumour necrosis factor (TNF) from leucocytes and complement activators whose role is to stimulate vasodilatation, phagocytosis and inflammatory chemotaxis. In doing this the nervous system is having a direct influence on the immune system, something that only a few years ago was not understood.

The local effect of this response is to irritate the surrounding nociceptors so that the threshold is decreased, leading to a greater sensitivity locally, and to create local oedema. Both of these are signs of acute somatic dysfunction. What also is now known to occur is that the locally produced cytokinins, IL-1 and TNF, are able to cross the blood brain barrier to have a wide variety of effects on CNS functions, one of which is activating the hypothalamic pituitary axis. They also lead to behavioural changes designed to limit activity and therefore aid healing, such as fatigue, fever, malaise, and reduced interest in feeding, drinking and socializing.[14]

Having looked at the effects of peripheral branches of the fibres it is now necessary to follow them as they pass to the spinal cord.

The centripetal action

The afferent nociceptive fibres from both visceral (nociautonomic) and somatic (nocifensive) structures travel with the somatic and autonomic fibres in the peripheral nerves. The nociceptive afferents enter the spinal cord at the dorsal horn and pass into Lissauer's tract. The majority of these fibres pass straight to their relevant spinal segment, while a portion remain in Lissauer's tract to pass either cephalad or caudad for approximately five segments before sending branches into the grey matter to synapse. The synapses occur in relaxed layers I, II, V and X. There they connect with WDR interneurones that receive inputs from both visceral and somatic afferents, thus they are common to both. The interneurones then stimulate both the visceral efferents and motor efferents, the alpha and gamma motor neurones. As mentioned earlier this complex and convergent arrangement of fibres from mixed origins synapsing with non-specific neurones is the probable explanation of the observed reflex relationships (somaticovisceral, viscerosomatic, viscerovisceral and somaticosomatic). An example of this convergence is that when there is visceral dysfunction, there will be contraction of the abdominal muscles that are related segmentally to the affected viscus.

Some of the axons pass into the spinothalamic and spinocervicalthalamic tracts, to pass to the higher centres, to give an appreciation of pain, while the others remain at a segmental level.

Those that remain at the segmental level are responsible for such nocifensive reflexes as the withdrawal reflex, whereby if a painful or noxious stimulus is touched, the reflex causes the hand to be withdrawn. This is a simple example, equivalent to the myotatic stretch reflex discussed earlier. The withdrawal and myotatic reflexes are the most simple examples present in the body. The majority of the other reflexes are phenomenally more complex than those examples, with the nocifensive and noci-autonomic reflexes creating complex and wide-ranging connections throughout the somatic and autonomic systems.

If there is sufficient nociceptive input this may lead to facilitation within the relevant spinal segment(s). If sustained, this may lead to a shift from physiological pain, which is the normal response to injury, to clinical pain, where there may be hyperalgesia or allodynia, and perpetuation of the somatic dysfunction causing the original problem. If sustained, this may be accompanied by metabolic and anatomical changes and possibly central sensitization (see p. 130) and chronic pain.

The rationale for the maintenance of somatic dysfunction is essentially no different from that proposed by Korr. The prime difference between the nociceptive model proposed by Van Buskirk and that proposed by Korr is the receptor that provokes the response, the nociceptors in Van Buskirk's model and the muscle spindle in Korr's. The centrifugal effects of the nociceptive impulse and the local release of substance P does also offer a slightly better explanation for the local tissue changes that occur at the site of dysfunction. While the circulating cytokinins and the central action on the HPA (see below) explain some of the systemic effects, in all probability both processes (those described by Korr and Van Buskirk) occur simultaneously in most somatic dysfunction. See Figure 6.8.

In summary, Van Buskirk proposed a hypothetical model of somatic dysfunction based on these observations:

- A somatic insult of any type will lead to the stimulation of the local nociceptors. They will pass the action potential centrifugally to its peripheral branches where release of substance P leads to the local irritation of the nerve endings and local inflammation aided by its synergistic action on the local humoral/inflammatory response.
- The action will be sent simultaneously centripetally to its central connections. There it will either pass to the higher centres to be recognized as pain; or remain at a spinal reflex level where it will potentially create changes in the visceral system via the autonomic nervous system or changes in the somatic system via the somatic motor system.
- The combination of these effects could account for the local tissue changes associated with somatic dysfunction, including all of those features typified by the mnemonic TART, and possible segmentally related changes in both the somatic and visceral systems.

Van Buskirk also briefly mentions the effects, direct and indirect, that the nervous system may have on the immune system as a result of the dysfunction. The relation to the nervous system and the immune system will be explored below.

THE NEUROENDOCRINE–IMMUNE SYSTEM

It was demonstrated in the earlier discussion on the peripheral effects of the centrifugal action potential of the nociceptors, that secretion of the neurotransmitters substance P and somatostatin could have a

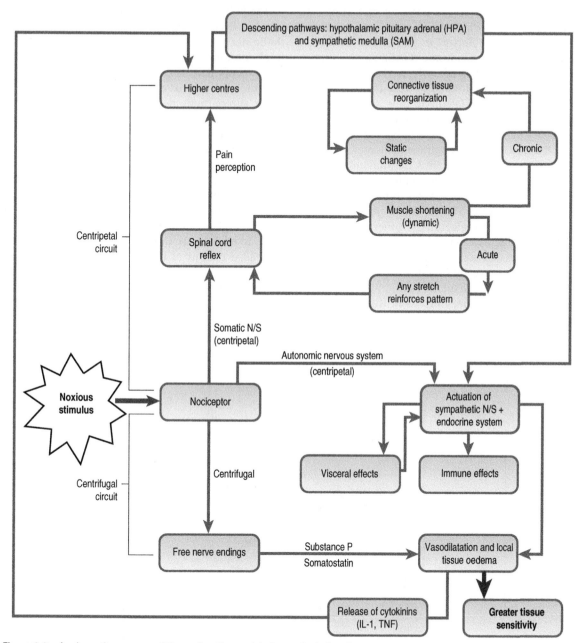

Figure 6.8   A schematic summary of the nociceptive model of somatic dysfunction.

direct influence on the immune system. Thus, the nervous system is directly affecting the immune system. Similar interactions also occur centrally. The complex interplay between these systems offers a rationale for the systemic effects that have been noted in the presence of chronic somatic dysfunction, but until now have not been adequately explained.

Recent research has revealed that the centripetal action potentials have a major effect on the immune response. The ascending fibres pass into the spino-reticular and spinothalamic pathways. The spino-reticular tract is of particular importance as it blends with the reticular network in the brain stem. This area plays a major role in the control of the general adaptive response (GAR). The GAR is the response that occurs in the presence of a stressful stimulus of any origin. (This concept was first discussed by Hans Selye[15] in what he termed the general adaptation syndrome (GAS). Selye's work and the GAS are explored in the next section; however, the material about to be discussed and the GAS are intimately related and thus would benefit from being studied at the same time.)

To date there do not appear to be any ascending tracts that are solely for the transmission of any discrete source of sensation, thus the transmission of sensory information, regardless of its origin, somatic, nociceptive or autonomic passes to the higher centres in shared tracts.[6] Thus it can be perceived that the systems act in an integrated manner.

The ascending nociceptive information passes to the brain stem where it synapses, most notably with two nuclei that are involved with the GAR, the nucleus paragigantocellularis (PGi) in the medulla, and the paraventricular nucleus of the hypothalamus (PVN).

The PGi receives sensory information from many sources. It is responsible for activating the sympathetic nervous system and can be considered the final common pathway for initiating the sympathetic component of the GAR.[16] The PGi is also able to stimulate the locus ceruleus (LC) in the midbrain, a key sympathetic nervous system control centre responsible for vigilance and arousal. The LC itself communicates with the PVN causing it to release corticotropin-releasing hormone (CRH). The PVN receives input from many sources including the limbic system. The PVN modulates both the autonomic system via descending neural pathways, and the endocrine system via its relationship with the pituitary gland. Stimulation of the LC–PVN axis leads to an increase in sympathetic activity and an increased output of the hypothalamic–pituitary–adrenal (HPA) axis.

Before this becomes too confusing, let us break it down into its major constituent parts: the hypothalamus, the HPA, the sympathetic neural axis

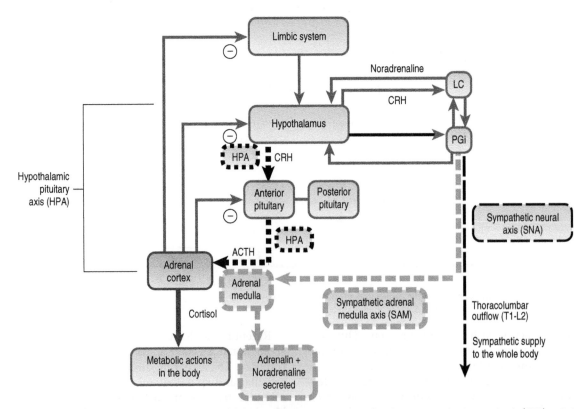

Figure 6.9   A schematic representation of the hypothalamic–pituitary–adrenal axis (HPA), the sympathetic neural axis (SNA) and the sympathetic adrenal axis (SAM). ACTH – adrenocorticotropin hormone; CRH – corticotropin-releasing hormone; LC – locus ceruleus; PGi – paragigantocellularis nucleus.

(SNA) and the sympathetic adrenal axis (SAM) (Fig. 6.9).

The body's response to a stressor or noxious stimulus has two components: the rapid acting 'fight or flight' response mediated by the SAM and SNA and the slower onset cortisol response, mediated by the HPA, which creates favourable conditions for wound healing and makes extensive metabolic adjustments designed to enable the body to face the stressor.

The key point of this discussion is that somatic dysfunction could be the origin of the noxious stimulus resulting in activation of these processes. Fundamental to all of these responses is the hypothalamus.

THE HYPOTHALAMUS

The hypothalamus is the major link between the nervous and endocrine systems. The hypothalamus is also the centre of all vegetative function in the body. It controls the function of the autonomic nervous system, and has a role in sleep, sexual behaviour and temperature regulation. To perform this, the hypothalamus has extensive connections with other areas of the nervous system. These are bidirectional, meaning that any of these connections can have an effect on its action. It also has direct effects on the autonomic nervous system via its descending projections (SNA and SAM). It coordinates the endocrine system via its vascular relationship with the anterior pituitary gland. This secretes numerous hormones that control the body's metabolism; of particular interest to this discussion is the release of adrenocorticotropin hormone (ACTH).

THE SYMPATHETIC NEURAL AXIS AND THE SYMPATHETIC ADRENAL AXIS

It has already been mentioned that the LC, PGi and the hypothalamus are key coordinators of the autonomic nervous system. It has also been stated that there is a close relationship between the LC, the PGi and the PVN, and that they are susceptible to any nociceptive input. The response to this input is mediated largely via the SNA and SAM.

The SNA is the direct neural link from the hypothalamus to the ANS. Fibres project from the hypothalamus to the medulla where they synapse with a group of cells that descend to the sympathetic system in the spinal cord. Predominant within these are the cells within the PGi. Via this system the hypothala-

mus can directly control many functions such as the heart rate, digestive function, and vasoconstriction.

To support this action, the SAM is also activated simultaneously. The adrenal medulla receives a direct sympathetic preganglionic innervation from the spinal cord, and when stimulated will cause the adrenal medulla to secrete adrenaline and noradrenaline directly into the bloodstream, which further support those changes listed above.

Therefore activation of the SAM and SNA in response to a noxious stimulus or stressor will result in:

- increased heart rate and force of beat
- constriction of blood vessels to viscera and the skin
- dilation of the blood vessels to the heart and the skeletal muscle
- contraction of the spleen
- conversion of glycogen to glucose in the liver
- sweating
- dilation of bronchial tubes
- decrease in enzyme production by digestive organs
- decreased urine output.

These responses are rapid and short-lived, and are designed to counteract an immediate danger by mobilizing the body's resources for immediate physical activity (fight or flight).

These descending autonomic pathways also have a direct immunomodulatory action. The production sites of immune cells, the bone marrow and thymus are richly supplied with autonomic fibres; these fibres also supply all of the lymphoid organs and lymphoid tissues of the respiratory tract and gastrointestinal system. Their exact function is not yet fully understood, but they appear to have a role in the maturation and activation of the immune cells and therefore the immune response, and would appear to be able to regulate all of the cells involved with inflammation.[14]

THE HYPOTHALAMUS AND THE HYPOTHALAMIC PITUITARY ADRENAL (HPA) AXIS

The HPA is the communication link between the nervous system and the immune system. In response to a stressor, the PVN of the hypothalamus produces CRH which passes via the hypophyseal portal system to the anterior pituitary. This stimulates the pituitary to secrete ACTH into the bloodstream. The ACTH passes to the adrenal glands where it causes the adrenal cortex to release cortisol.

The cortisol levels are controlled by two negative feedback loops that function to stop further production of CRH by the hypothalamus: one that passes to both the hypothalamus and limbic system (this is a long-term loop taking minutes to hours); and another short-term quick-acting loop passing to the anterior pituitary, where it is directly inhibited by the cortisol.

Thus, activation of the PVN by a stressor from any source will lead to an increase in the activity of the HPA axis and therefore a consequent increase in cortisol levels. It should be remembered that the hypothalamus can be affected by any of its numerous relations. Within this discussion we will be particularly interested in the excitation of the PVN via the numerous ascending nociceptive fibres; via stimulation from the PGi–LC (which is itself stimulated by the ascending nociceptive fibres); and through its links with the limbic system which mediates emotion.

Cortisol, a glucocorticoid, readies the body to face the stressor. It aims to ensure that energy is available, by breakdown of proteins and amino acids in the liver, leading to gluconeogenesis. The increase in glucose makes the body more alert, and assures sufficient energy availability should rapid activity be required. Cortisol causes vasoconstriction and therefore leads to an increase in blood pressure. It also attempts to moderate the inflammatory response by decreasing the production and release of proinflammatory regulators, such as the interleukins (IL), interferon and tumour necrosis factor; decreases capillary permeability; and decreases phagocytosis by monocytes.

As it is an immunoregulator, long-term high levels of cortisol will decrease antibody formation and lead to atrophy of the thymus gland, spleen and lymph nodes leading to a decrease in immune response. It also retards connective tissue regeneration.

From this, it should be possible to deduce the effects that this would have if a dysfunction, either physical or psychological, were to chronically facilitate the HPA axis. The effects in extremis are demonstrated by someone suffering from Cushing's syndrome. Excessive action of the HPA has also been implicated in melancholic depression, atypical depression, rheumatoid arthritis and chronic fatigue syndrome.[17] Excessive and long-term stimulation of the LC (and by implication the LC–PVN axis) has been shown to be associated with depression and chronic maladaptive physiological states.

It was also demonstrated that the LC can be sensitized by nociceptive input, possibly indicating that the nociceptive input from a somatic dysfunction may provoke the GAR.[16]

The HPA and immunoregulation

As briefly mentioned earlier in this chapter, the cytokinins released locally at the site of dysfunction, such as IL-1 and TNF, can pass via the humoral system across the blood–brain barrier to have numerous effects on CNS function, including activation of the HPA.

Several hormones released by the pituitary gland in response to the hypothalamus also appear to have an immunoregulatory effect, including growth hormone, thyrotropin-releasing hormone, thyroid-stimulating hormone, human chorionic gonadotropin, arginine vasopressin, gonadotropin-releasing hormone, androgens and prolactin.[14]

DISCUSSION

The above pathways are present to combat potentially harmful situations, mobilizing the body for immediate (SAM and SNA) and short-term (HPA) responses to these situations. This represents a coordinated effort on the part of the nervous, endocrine and immune systems. Recent research has modified the interactions of these systems. Perhaps one of the most important revelations is with regard to the 'messenger' molecules of the three systems. In the past they were thought to be system specific: neuroregulators, hormones and immunoregulators. It is now understood that they communicate freely between the systems via a receptor-mediated mechanism. Thus the communication is bidirectional, uniting the neuroendocrine and immune systems into one incredibly complex network responsible for controlling and maintaining homeostasis. Figure 6.10 is an attempt to represent the various levels of integration within the neuroendocrine-immune system.

Reactions discussed are thus a short-term coordinated response of the neuroendocrine-immune system to a noxious stimulus. However, there are situations in which the noxious stimulus persists, causing the short-term responses to continue longer than intended. This results in pathophysiological changes and possibly pathology.

It is of great interest to osteopaths, and to any other body workers, that it is possible to demonstrate that nociceptive information from somatic dysfunction will have an effect on this system. The range of possible disease states that may be

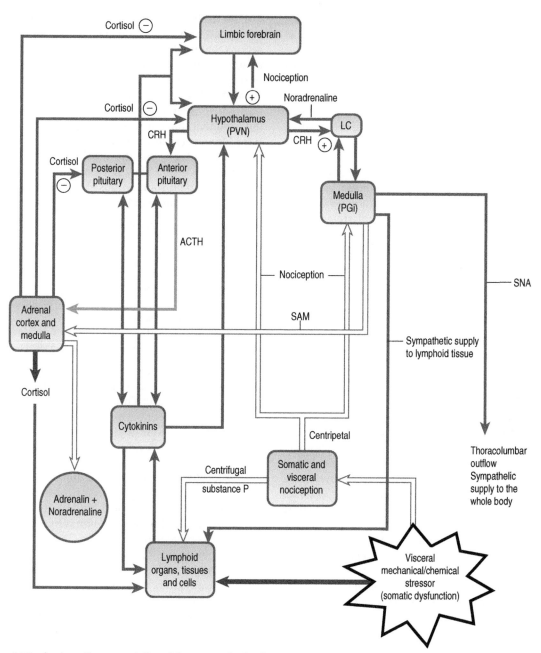

Figure 6.10   A schematic representation of the neuroendocrine-immune system.

involved with a shift in this homeostatic system is potentially great, including chronic fatigue, depression, feelings of malaise, fibromyalgia and RA.

Knowing that this is the case, we have a conceptual model of possible aetiological, contributing and maintaining factors that will form the basis of a rational management plan for individuals suffering from such conditions. Also, from a practical perspective, it is of interest to reflect on the anatomical position of the hypothalamus and the pituitary gland. The pituitary is suspended by the infundibulum in the sella turcica of the sphenoid. The hypothalamus forms the floor of the third ventricle, overlying the clivus, being the posterior part of the sphenoid, the sphenobasilar symphysis (SBS), and the basilar part of the occipital bone. The SBS is very often prone to somatic dysfunction. The possible consequences of this can be imagined, such as torsioning the infundibulum, or loss of the regular 'pumping' action resulting from the flexion extension movements of the cranial rhythmic impulse that occur at the SBS. These would affect the communication between the hypothalamus and the pituitary. It is also possible to imagine the positive benefits of techniques, such as the CV4, that aim to affect the ventricular systems.

The hypothalamus has numerous connections with the limbic forebrain and its 'emotional' nuclei such as the hippocampus and the amygdala. It is possible to conceive that emotional states could have an effect on the hypothalamus and activate the above systems. However, this discussion will be saved for the next chapter.

CENTRAL SENSITIZATION

In clinical practice you will always find a minority of patients who do not present with clinically consistent signs and symptoms: patients who complain of pain wherever you touch them on their body, even with a very light touch, but physical findings do not match the reported symptoms; and others who will not respond as expected with their pain perhaps lasting longer than expected, or who may become worse, with the pain spreading to other areas. Also, there will be numerous individuals with chronic pain syndromes often diagnosed as fibromyalgia, postwhiplash syndrome, chronic fatigue syndrome or similar, or perhaps they have been written off as 'fat file syndrome' or malingerers. All of these individuals are very difficult to treat, and attempting to find a clinical rationale for their management is almost impossible.

It is possible to explain these problems in terms of central sensitization. Stated simply, this is an increased excitability and responsiveness in the central nociceptive pathways. It is the situation that arises in states of chronic pain. An important part of the pain manifestation (e.g. tenderness and referred pain) related to chronic musculoskeletal disorders may result from peripheral and central sensitization.[18] As with any concept it is almost certainly only part of the answer; however, an understanding of central sensitization will enable you to develop a management plan based on rational theory, and through more effective treatment, give some relief to these long-suffering individuals.

Pain itself has an important function in alerting us to possible damage, and encouraging us to avoid actions that might increase the damage. This 'physiological pain' resolves over a period of time, under normal conditions and with appropriate management. Most conditions or complaints, allowing for individual differences such as age, health state and environment, have a reasonably predictable duration. However, with certain individuals the pain does not resolve within the anticipated time, and in fact it may worsen. They have made the transition to a chronic pain state. In this state they may present with one or more of the following:

- pain in the absence of a noxious stimulus (spontaneous pain)
- increased duration of response to brief stimulation (ongoing pain or hyperpathia)
- reduced pain threshold (allodynia)
- increased responsiveness to suprathreshold stimulation (hyperalgesia)
- spread of pain and hyperalgesia to uninjured tissue (referred pain and secondary hyperalgesia).[19]

This situation has long been recognized, but the underlying mechanisms have been debated for more than a century. The principal argument has been over the role of peripheral and central neural mechanisms in the initiation and maintenance of these pathological conditions. It is now generally accepted that both have a role.[20]

The peripheral and central nervous systems become sensitized, peripheral sensitization being an increase of sensitivity of nociceptive primary afferent neurones. Central sensitization is hyperexcitability of nociceptive neurones in the CNS.

Peripheral sensitization is thought to be produced by the action of inflammatory mediators such as bradykinin, prostaglandins, neuropeptides and cytokines which activate corresponding receptors of nerve fibres.[21] This works synergistically with the action of the neurotransmitters such as substance P and somatostatin secreted from the nerve endings, which will stimulate the release of cytokinins.[13]

The mechanism behind central sensitization is not so clearly understood. Some of the currently accepted theories are briefly discussed below.

PROLONGED OPENING OF NMDA RECEPTORS

The significant role of N-methyl-d-aspartate (NMDA) receptors and the production of nitric oxide (NO) in central sensitization, hyperalgesia and chronic pain has often been demonstrated.[22] Blockade of the NMDA receptors prevents and reduces central sensitization.[21] It is thought that an abnormally high transmission of C fibre inputs leads to high levels of glutamate in the synaptic cleft. These eventually cause the postsynaptic NMDA receptors to open, permitting an influx of calcium into the neurone. This is further exacerbated by NO stimulating more transmitter release. This will have a progressive effect on other neurones in the dorsal horn locally and via the numerous synaptic interconnections, and sensitization has begun.[23]

CYTOKINE ACTION ON THE CNS

The action of the cytokines, particularly the interleukins and tumour necrosis factor, on the CNS is another possibility. As mentioned earlier, they are produced at the site of tissue damage, and appear, in certain situations, to be able to cross the blood–brain barrier where they have a part to play in centralized sensitization. They are also responsible for producing the 'malaise' type symptoms associated with disease and injury that are often part of the chronic pain pattern. A review of recent research in this area is to be found in LR Watkins and SF Maier's article 'The pain of being sick: implications of immune-to-brain communication for understanding pain'.[24]

NEURAL PLASTICITY

Another area possibly involved in centralized sensitization is the concept of neural plasticity. The nervous system has an ability to change in response to its environment; without this we would not be able to learn. Pain perception has traditionally been perceived as a 'hard wired' system in which a receptor is stimulated by a noxious trigger, causing an impulse to pass into the CNS where it may elicit a spinal response (reflex arc), or be passed via specific ascending tracts to the relevant area of the cortex for interpretation. It is now being realized that this is not the case, and that the structures of these pain pathways are very diffuse and changeable. It has also been demonstrated that the receptive field (i.e. those areas of the brain that are the receiving areas for the afferent information) will change in response to even relatively small changes in the afferent input.[25] This will lead to new ways of the CNS perceiving pain, resulting in patterns of pain presentation that differ from those expected from the standard dermatomal or myotomal distributions. The potential for such neural plasticity is demonstrated at both the peripheral and central elements of the nervous system.[23]

CORTICAL MODULATION

Nociceptive input into the CNS is not simply passively received but rather is subject to modulation through spinal cord neuroplasticity and descending influences from supraspinal sites activated by a variety of environmental signals, including the acute or persistent nociceptive input itself and behavioural and emotional stimuli.[22]

Cortical modulation has a significant effect on the way that pain is perceived, and it is known that the effects created by this modulation can lead to the same type of changes as those found in centralized sensitization. Often called 'gating', the cortical control has both facilitatory and inhibitory influences from supraspinal sites. The descending facilitatory influences possibly account for secondary hyperalgesia, the hyperalgesia observed in uninjured tissue, distant from the site of insult. The inhibitory effect may be used to block certain areas of receptivity, thus making those not blocked proportionately more reactive – thus, in effect, having an excitatory effect on those not blocked. An extreme example of a purely inhibitory effect on the ascending information is illustrated by stories of farmers having cut their arm off, calmly heaving it onto their shoulders and walking to the hospital to have it sewn back on. This type of inhibitory pain gating can also be provoked consciously in methods such as biofeedback techniques of pain control.

Research is rapidly progressing and will 'firm up' our understanding of the underlying processes of sensitization. Perhaps most importantly, from an osteopathic viewpoint, it is necessary to be able to observe the signs in your patients that will lead you to suspect that this process is happening, i.e. that the patient is passing from acute to chronic pain presentation. It goes without saying that it is better to prevent this occurring, than to attempt to treat the chronic problem. David Butler[23] details some of the key features that would make a practitioner suspect that this process may be occurring; as it is difficult to improve on his descriptions, these will be quoted at length:

Area and description

The following pain areas, descriptions and clinical scenarios may relate to central sensitivity:

- *Symptoms are often not within neat anatomical or dermatomal boundaries.*
- *Any original pain may have spread.*
- *In the case of multiple area symptoms, pains may be linked, in that they either occur together, or the patient has one pain or the other pain.*
- *The contralateral side to the initial pain may be painful, though rarely as much as the initially injured side. There can be mirror pains, which are hard to explain in terms of primary hyperalgesia.*
- *Clinicians may 'chase the pain'. This is a common practice in manual therapy. For example, back pains may ease but then the patient complains of thoracic pains. It is almost as though the pain processing networks need to include a somatic component.*
- *There could be unexpected sudden stabs of pain.*
- *Patients may say 'it has a mind of its own'. The pain is called 'it', suggesting that it has lost the neat stimulus–response relationships of familiar, and to the patient, understandable tissue-based pains.*

Behaviour

The behaviour of the pain state may provide clues to a central mechanism. For example:

- *The perception of pain is ongoing. If pain persists past known healing times of tissues and a comprehensive subjective evaluation reveals no occupational provocation, disease or other reason for pain maintenance, then a central mechanism could be suspected.*
- *Summation. A number of repeated similar activities evoke pain, for example, using a computer, an exercise bike, or interpreters using sign language.*
- *The stimulus/response relationship is distorted. The pain state worsens or is evoked at variable times after the input. This could be after 10 seconds or even after a day or so. Most clinicians are familiar with the often uncomfortable situation where they examine a patient and then pain starts a short time after the examination.*
- *Responses to treatment and input are unpredictable. What may appear a successful treatment technique one day may not be successful the next. There is a pattern though, where traditional manual therapy may help for a day or two, but then symptoms invariably return.*

- *It could be that every movement hurts, yet there may be no great range of movement loss. These patients are often labelled as 'irritable' or 'unstable'. I believe that it is more likely that patients present with instability of symptoms rather than instability of structure. In routine physical examination, such as a straight leg raise, a patient may complain of pain, yet you, the therapist, may feel no resistance. It is as though the movement has touched a memory rather than a damaged tissue.*
- *Patients may say 'it hurts when I think about it'.*

Other features

There are other features which could be a part of a central sensitivity pattern:

- *These pains can be cyclical, with perhaps more in winter, and perhaps at anniversaries or reminders of traumatic times in life.*
- *With the CNS dysregulation, changes in response and background homeostatic systems such as the autonomic, endocrine, motor and immune systems are likely. Sometimes these responses may be overt in some systems, for example, focal dystonias of the hand in musicians, central contributions to complex regional pain syndromes (CRPS), or sickness responses in the case of the immune system.*
- *There may be links to traumatic and multiple traumatic events in life. These events could be during childhood or around the injury time.*
- *This state may be associated with anxiety and depression.*
- *'Miracle cures' are possible. Every clinician has hopefully had a 'miracle' in the clinic. If there is sudden, dramatic and apparently miraculous relief of severe and long-lasting symptoms from little input, then the pathobiological mechanisms are unlikely to be from local tissues. Miracles are great, but they are even better if you have some idea of why they happened. It is more likely a central change involving some alteration in cognitions and emotions.*
- *Central sensitivity is likely to be involved in syndromes such as fibromyalgia, myofascial syndrome, reflex sympathetic dystrophy, chronic low back pain and post-whiplash pain syndromes, in fact anywhere pain persists or the word 'syndrome' is paired with a part of the anatomy.*
- *The cortical modulation, or put another way, psycho-emotional and psychosocial factors, have been shown to have a correlation with the development of chronic pain patterns. The New Zealand*

government have published a list of psychosocial factors that have been shown to be involved in this process. They termed these factors 'yellow flags' (to contrast with the pathological 'red flags'). Put simply, the more yellow flags present, the greater the chance of that individual developing chronic pain.

These 'yellow flags' are covered in the next chapter.

From this it is possible to see that the clinical presentation can be varied, complex and above all confusing. In the past these patients may have been termed malingerers, or worse. It is also clear that individuals suffering from this condition will require an holistic approach, possibly involving appropriate referral to other practitioners. From a patient's perspective, just the reassurance that they are not going mad and that there is a scientific rationale for the problems that they are experiencing can go a long way towards resolving them.

SUMMARY AND CONCLUSION

This chapter has attempted to explore some of the more fundamental neurological concepts that underpin our understanding of osteopathy. The discussion started by looking at the most simple of the reflex arcs, and attempted to model somatic dysfunction on a monosynaptic reflex. It is clear that no dysfunction is really that simple; however, the principle of this simple model does hold true, and it almost acts as a foundation upon which can be loaded the progressively more sophisticated models. The polysynaptic models, that involve complex harmonious function, requiring simultaneous inhibition of certain areas and excitation of others, are in effect just more complicated versions of the basic model. An awareness of how they function will enable you to manipulate them to achieve the desired effect. For example, if an individual had a very contracted and acutely painful biceps, which was in fact too painful to address directly, it would be possible to address its antagonist, the triceps, and by stimulating it to contract, cause an inhibitory reflex to pass to the biceps and cause some degree of relaxation.

The visceral and somatic systems were shown to work in a coordinated manner, with the afferent information from both sources synapsing with multireceptive WDR neurones, with problems arising in one system causing reflections in the other. It is through this that we can read visceral dysfunction in the soma, via either the metamerically organized

segments or the various 'tender points'. These have a role in both diagnosis and treatment. Once again it is necessary to remember that they are in fact branches of a reflex arc, and as such are mutually dependent. Should a somaticovisceral problem have been present for more than a few weeks, and only the somatic element be resolved with treatment, it is probable that the visceral branch will reinstate the original dysfunction but now as a viscerosomatic reflex.

Korr's concept of the neurophysiological basis of the osteopathic lesion is essentially based on the aberrant bombardment of the spinal segment from the proprioceptors disturbed by the somatic dysfunction. This increase in neural input causes facilitation at the affected spinal segment, making it proportionately more easily excitable. As such it acts as a 'neurological lens', focusing passing neural activity onto that segment, causing it to respond where other less facilitated segments are unaffected. All elements supplied by that segment, be they somatic or visceral, myotome, sclerotome, viscerotome or associated connective tissues, will be subject to the same degree of change in their levels of activity. It is possible to anticipate the changes that may be occurring in a viscus by assessing its related dermatome. If the dermatome is showing signs of chronic changes it would be logical to assume that the associated viscera will similarly exhibit chronic changes.

Van Buskirk proposed a nociceptive mechanism rather than a proprioceptive one for the generation of the aberrant input. He additionally incorporates the interplay of the nervous system and immune system in the generation of local tissue changes. The more recent research on the neuroendocrine-immune system reveals that what previously were thought to be three independent systems are in fact one complex interacting system communicating bidirectionally at all levels of organization. This further supports Van Buskirk's model of somatic dysfunction by demonstrating that a nociceptive input can have a role in activating the various systems responsible for maintaining homeostasis, particularly the HPA, SNA and SAM. This can supply a rationale for the more complex systemic presentations that appear to arise as a result of dysfunction.

Central sensitization, without wanting to belittle it, is essentially central facilitation, a concept that is not difficult for an osteopath to grasp. Though the determining physiology is very complex, from a practical sense, there are psychosocial features and physical features that may indicate the possibility that a patient is passing to a more chronic pain state. Awareness of these factors will enable you to try and assist the patient, with the aim of preventing them from moving from the reversible acute state to the much more fixed chronic condition.

Little attempt has been made to discuss specific osteopathic rationale for addressing these problems. They could be approached in an infinitely varied number of ways, and it is thought that with a thorough knowledge of both the concepts discussed above, and neuroanatomy and physiology, it would be possible to devise an appropriate management plan addressing the physical and emotional elements of the problem with respect to that particular individual.

The role of the psyche in many of the more recent concepts is very apparent. This area of study is vast, and even if dealt with in a most superficial way demands a separate chapter. This is purely an attempt to keep the material as unambiguous and understandable as possible. In reality they are inseparable, as in fact are most elements discussed within this book, and you are strongly urged to reunite them in a manner that enables you to apply them as a whole within the clinical environment.

References

1. Sherrington CS. The integrative action of the nervous system. London: Constable; 1911.
2. Educational Council on Osteopathic Principles. Glossary of osteopathic terminology. Chicago: American Association of Colleges of Osteopathic Medicine; 2002.
3. Head H. On disturbances of sensation with especial reference to the pain of visceral disease. Brain 1893; 16:1–13.
4. Downing CH. Principles and practice of osteopathy. London: Tamor Pierston; 1981.
5. DeGroat WC. Spinal cord processing of visceral and somatic nociceptive input. In: Willard F H, Patterson MM, eds. Nociception and the neuroendocrine-immune connection. Indianapolis: American Academy of Osteopathy; 1994: 47–72.
6. Patterson MM, Wurster RD. Neurophysiologic system: integration and disintegration. In: Ward RC, ed. Foundations for osteopathic medicine. Baltimore: Williams and Wilkins; 1997.
7. Loeser JD, Butler SH, Chapman R et al, eds. Bonica's management of pain, 3rd edn. Baltimore: Lippincott, Williams and Wilkins; 2001.
8. Korr IM. The neural basis of the osteopathic lesion. In: Peterson B, ed. The collected papers of Irvin M. Korr. Newark: American Academy of Osteopathy; 1979: 120–127.
9. Korr IM, Thomas PE, Wright HM. Patterns of electrical skin resistance in man. In: Peterson B, ed. The collected papers of Irvin M. Korr. Newark: American Academy of Osteopathy; 1979: 33–40.
10. Korr IM, Wright HM, Thomas PE. Effects of experimental myofascial insults on cutaneous patterns of sympathetic activity in man. In: Peterson B, ed. The collected papers of Irvin M. Korr. Newark: American Academy of Osteopathy; 1979: 54–65.
11. Korr IM, Wright HM, Chace JA. Cutaneous patterns of sympathetic activity in clinical abnormalities of the musculoskeletal system. In: Peterson B, ed. The collected papers of Irvin M. Korr. Newark: American Academy of Osteopathy; 1979: 66–72.
12. Korr IM. Sustained sympatheticotonia as a factor in disease. In: Korr IM, ed. The neurobiologic mechanisms in manipulative therapy. New York: Pleniun Press; 1978: 229–268.
13. Van Buskirk RL. Nociceptive reflexes and the somatic dysfunction: a model. JAOA 1990; 90(9):792–809
14. Watkins A, ed. Mind body medicine. New York: Churchill Livingstone; 1997: 6.
15. Selye H. The Stress of Life. New York: McGraw-Hill; 1976.
16. Aston-Jones G, Valentino RJ, Van Bockstaele E et al. Brain noradrenergic neurons, nociception and stress: Basic mechanisms and clinical applications. In: Willard FH, Patterson MM, eds. Nociception and the neuro-endocrine-immune connection. Athens: University Classics; 1994: 107–147.
17. Gold P. Neurobiology of stress. In: Willard FH, Patterson MM, eds. Nociception and the neuroendocrine-immune connection. Athens: University Classics; 1994: 4–17.
18. Arendt-Nielsen L, Graven-Nielsen T. Central sensitization in fibromyalgia and other musculoskeletal disorders. Curr Pain Headache Rep 2003; 7(5):355–361.
19. Coderre TJ, Katz J. Peripheral and central hyperexcitability: Differential signs and symptoms in persistent pain. Behav and Brain Sci 1997; 20(3):404–419.
20. Urban MO, Gebhart GF. Supraspinal contributions to hyperalgesia. Proc Natl Acad Sci USA 1999; 96(14):7687–7692.
21. Schaible HG, Ebersberger A, Von Banchet GS. Mechanisms of pain in arthritis. Ann N Y Acad Sci 2002; 966:343–354.
22. Urban MO, Gebhart GF. Central mechanisms in pain. Med Clin North Am 1999; 83(3):585–596.
23. Butler DS. The sensitive nervous system. Australia: Noigroup Publications; 2000.
24. Watkins LR, Maier SF. The pain of being sick: implications of immune-to-brain communication for understanding pain. Annu Rev Psychol 2000;51:29–57.
25. Harman K. Neuroplasticity and the development of persistent pain. Physiotherapy Canada 2000; Winter:64–71.

Recommended reading

Butler DS. The sensitive nervous system. Australia: Noigroup Publications; 2000.
This is a superb book, taking you through some of the more recent advances in neurology and neurophysiology in an immediately understandable way. It is also written for manual therapists. This is a must to read.

Peterson B, ed. The collected papers of Irvin M Korr, vol 1. Newark: American Academy of Osteopathy; 1979.

King HH, ed. The collected papers of Irvin M Korr, vol 2. Colorado: American Academy of Osteopathy; 1997.
Korr's collected works cover some of the most significant studies in the neural basis of osteopathic medicine. These are still very relevant.

Chapter 7

Psychological considerations

CHAPTER CONTENTS

INTRODUCTION

The mind is known to have quite dramatic effects on the body. Reflect on someone that is suddenly very frightened: they become pale in the face, their hands sweat and body hair is raised. A depressed person is often noticeable by their habitus. They have a stooped posture with rounded shoulders, lowered head, and even their physiological processes are slowed. Anxiety gives one 'butterflies in the stomach', and if sustained is contributory to gastric ulceration. These are all examples of psychosomatic problems. In our current society the emotional demands are great, and it is rare to meet someone unaffected by these stresses and, logically, the somatic consequences. It is interesting to note how many emotions we describe in terms of somatic sensations ('gut reaction', 'butterflies', 'visceral' response, 'in the pit of my stomach').

We are aware of many of these responses intuitively. We can recognize them within ourselves, and, perhaps more importantly, observe them in others. These easily observable features have interested philosophers and scientists alike since ancient times, for example Hippocrates (460–355 BC) and his followers based their understanding on the balance or predominance of the four 'humors': black bile, yellow bile, phlegm and blood. Excess of any would lead to emotional changes hence:

- Melancholic (*melas khole* is Greek for black bile) – depressed, sad and brooding.
- Choleric (*khole* is Greek for bile) – changeable, quick to react and irritable.
- Phlegmatic (*phlegma* is Latin for lymph) – slow moving, apathetic and sluggish.

- Sanguine (*sanguis* is Latin for blood) – warm, pleasant, active and enthusiastic.

Juvenal (60–140 AD), the Roman satirist, coined the phrase '*mens sana in corpore sano*', a sound mind in a sound body. Littlejohn had similar views:

> *we realise the fact that [the] mind is the ascendant power and that in a healthy physiological life nothing less than a healthy mind can secure that vigorous condition of body which is so much desired by all, health and happiness. We must realise that while we treat what seems to be purely body diseases, we must not overlook the fact that psychopathy opens up the field of mental disease and reveals certain mind conditions without the removal of which it is impossible to cure bodily diseases.[1]*

However, with the progress of science, there has been a trend to separate the mind from the body. Descartes (1596–1650) is the individual usually cited as being responsible for separating the mind from the body. He envisaged the body as a mechanical structure able to function in a manner similar to some large mechanical manikins that he had observed, independent of the mind. This division is termed 'Cartesian dualism' and has exerted a profound influence on the understanding and practice of healthcare until very recent times.

However, it would appear that recently, healthcare generally has been undergoing a slow but steady revolution. The Cartesian reductionist approach is being challenged, and the body systems are being 'put back together again'; hence the adoption of such terms as the neuromusculoskeletal system, and the neuroendocrine-immune system.

Interest in the role of the psyche has persisted, even during the apparently reductionist and dualist period of history. As one can imagine there are as many theories as there are interested people. In this chapter, the role that the psyche plays in these processes will be addressed. We will initially look at some of the earlier and often more empirical models, then explore some of the key concepts of the emerging science of psychoneuroimmunology. This study is beginning to find rational explanations for those long observed phenomena relating stress to illness. The physiological processes behind it are understandably horrendously complicated and as yet not fully understood, but the results so far offer very tempting insights into the human condition. Osteopathy, as one of the many holistic approaches to health, is ideally suited to finding an application for these new and exciting discoveries. This chapter will conclude with a look at some of the mind–body approaches and their interpretation of disease.

PSYCHOSOMATIC CONCEPTS

Within this discussion the term psychosomatic will be used in its broadest sense (and almost certainly with opprobrium from certain quarters) for the relationship between the mind and body. The term psychosomatic was first utilized in 1818 by the German psychiatrist Heinroth,[2] but it was not until 1935 that it was used in its now generally accepted form, appearing in HF Dunbar's publication *Bodily Changes: A Survey of Literature on Psychosomatic Interrelationships: 1910-1933*.[3]

Taber's Medical Dictionary defines psychosomatic as: 'Pertaining to the relationship of the mind and body'. It continues with a brief discussion on one of the key problems within this area of study:

> *Disorders that have a physiological component but are thought to originate in the emotional state of the patient are termed psychosomatic. When so used the impression is created that the mind and body are separate entities and that a disease may be purely somatic in its effect or entirely emotional. This partitioning of the human being is not possible; thus no disease is limited to only the mind or the body. A complex interaction is always present even though in specific instances a disease might on superficial examination appear to involve only the body or the mind.*

All of the concepts discussed below could be conceived as elements of psychosomatic medicine, or perhaps more importantly the psychological modelling of the holistic continuum that defines health and disease.

There is a vast array of psychological concepts that have a relevance to psychosomatic medicine. In an attempt to simplify this, three major conceptual shifts have been recognized, each having applications within the osteopathic paradigm:

1. The psychoanalytic and psychodynamic models that originated in the work of Sigmund Freud from 1895, and which were later modified and related directly to the body by the somewhat eccentric Wilhelm Reich. These have continued to be developed and variations of these concepts are applied currently.
2. From the 1950s onwards there was a shift to more holistic models, looking at the changes the

body makes in response to its environment. This was rooted in the earlier work of Walter Cannon on homeostasis, and the then current work of Hans Selye and the General Adaptation Syndrome (GAS). External/environmental features became more important, leading to a more psychosocial concept of health.

3. The most recent shift has occurred in the last 20 years. It has been supported by the rapid advances in technology permitting a more accurate assessment of the brain and its physiological responses. This has led to new areas of study: psychoneuroimmunology (PNI) and neuroimmunomodulation (NIM). Even though this is delving ever deeper into the brain, far from being a reductionist approach, it is reuniting the mind and body and offering physiological findings to account for the previously inexplicable. The model has returned to a more holistic perspective and a biopsychosocial outlook.

The aim of this is chapter not to encourage you to become psychologists, but just by touching the surface of psychosomatic medicine to expose you to a few different perspectives on health and disease that may have a relevance to you in your clinical practice.

PSYCHOANALYSIS AND THE ROOTS OF PSYCHODYNAMICS AND MIND–BODY WORK

Sigmund Freud (1856–1939), the Austrian psychiatrist, is the founding father of psychoanalysis. The foundations were laid in 1895 with the publication by Freud and Breuer of *Studies on Hysteria*.[4] This theorized that the symptoms of hysteria derive from the suppression and repression of painful or otherwise emotionally disturbing memories, often of events that had occurred in early childhood. These have subsequently manifested themselves in the soma, a process they called 'conversion'.

From these roots, psychoanalysis developed, analysing many somatic problems from an unconscious emotional level, thus laying the groundwork for psychosomatic medicine. The broader application of these concepts became known as psychodynamics, and can be defined as a study of the interrelationship and actions of the various parts of the mind, personality and motivations.

There are so many aspects of Freud's work, and the later Neo Freudian psychodynamics, that would

be of interest and possible benefit to an osteopath – however, there are also numerous excellent texts available on his work so this chapter will briefly look at Freud's view on personality as his terms are used regularly within many of the mind/body approaches.

THE PSYCHODYNAMIC MODEL OF PERSONALITY

Freud's view of personality was that it was comprised of three interacting parts: the id, the superego and the ego.

The id

This is the totally subconscious element. It is present from birth and strives for immediate gratification of basic drives, such as thirst, hunger and desire for sex. It cannot distinguish reality from fantasy.

The superego

This is often viewed as the opposite to the id. This is the moralist attempting to curb the 'gratification at all costs' id. Part conscious and part subconscious, it tries to enforce the moral dictates of society, social grouping or family. It is often in conflict with the id.

The ego

This is the part that has to mediate between the conflicting id and superego, and function on a conscious level in the actual world. It provides the sense of self, it is the integrator of personality. Due to the conflict within the ego's role, Freud's model of personality accepts that conflict is a fact of life in personality.

The different roles are well illustrated by the following example:

> *a teenage boy sees an exotic sports car sitting parked, with the keys visible within. Id will see an opportunity to race around in a fast and powerful vehicle. Superego will insist that such behaviour would be stealing, and is morally wrong. Ego may note that people are walking on the street, and therefore the chances of getting caught are very high. Thus, in this case, the outcome would probably be not to steal the car.*[5]

We will see later that the biodynamic model applies these three elements of personality to the body.

Another significant individual at this time was Wilhelm Reich (1897–1957), also Austrian, who is said to have worked with Freud. He made a radical departure from the basic principles of classical psychoanalysis; he attempted to relate significant psychological events to patterns of responses within the body, addressing them with actual physical contact with the patient. In view of his obvious significance in the field of mind–body work we will look at his earlier concepts in some depth.

WILHELM REICH (1897–1957)

Wilhelm Reich, a psychiatrist and a sexologist, is often cited as the founder of mind–body work. In his early years he worked closely with Sigmund Freud, and he was undoubtedly influenced by Freud's theories but he developed them in a radically different way. He developed an approach that incorporated somatic, neuromuscular aspects and psychoanalysis; this eventually was termed Orgone Therapy. Fundamental to this approach was the idea that a natural energy flowed through the body. He called this energy Orgone (this may have a parallel in chi, the CRI, prana, etc.). Orgone could be blocked at various points, often as a response to some trauma or suppressed impulse or emotion. A typical example could be a child's habitual inhibition of impulses and expressions of feeling that arise from being in a difficult or unpleasant situation, such as when exposed to the disapproval of its parents. The child learns to tense the muscles to hold back the movement or feeling. When this is done repeatedly, the muscular holding pattern becomes chronic and unconscious. This would then become part of the child's character and structure.[6] Within this structure there would be palpable changes, often hypertonic, but also hypotonic. The areas of muscle rigidity became known as muscular 'armour'. This is the somatic equivalent of the ego's binding of unacceptable impulses. Release of these restrictions by bodywork, which for Reich would involve working with the somatic and the psychological systems simultaneously, would release this energy and result in a greater structural and emotional harmony.

Reich recognized the importance of the ANS acting as an interface for bodily and emotional processes. It is directly involved with the functions of the internal organs, but it also serves as a messenger for emotional perception via blood and plasma streams, and is linked to the cerebral areas which represent emotion through connections in the CNS. Impaired function of the ANS, via the central connections with the WDR neurones, manifests itself in chronically tense muscles.[7] The 'muscular armouring' or chronic muscular tension impedes the flow of body fluids and energy.

Reich's work has fostered numerous mind–body practices:

- Gerda Boyesen (Biodynamic)
- David Boadella (Biosynthesis)
- Alexander Lowen and John Pierrakos (Bioenergetics)
- Stanley Kelman (Emotional Anatomy)
- Ron Kurtz (Hakomi)
- Ida Rolf (Rolfing)
- Jack Rosenberg (Gestalt Body Psychotherapy)
- Mosche Feldenkrais (Feldenkrais method)

… to mention just a few of the more well-known ones.[8]

The biodynamic model has some interesting osteopathic parallels in its modelling of the body. Amongst other concepts it utilizes Freud's id, ego and superego and relates them to the body. The 'motoric ego' acts almost as the structural aspect of the ego, which is the regulator of the antisocial id. It is horizontally organized and it is related to the ability to translate ideas into action, to interacting in and with the world. The muscles can function to act, to hold back, to express, to repress. In them we can interject parental models, prohibitions and cultural styles as unconscious identifications with the body attitudes and postures of others. Where we are in harmony with ourselves, the muscles can embody grace, physical skills and vitality. When we are in conflict, this is directly reflected in patterns of muscular tension as the different impulses and inhibitions pull against each other. Chronic conflict reduces blood flow and creates the hardening and fixedness of muscle tension we call armour.[6] Also recognized in the biodynamic model is the alimentary canal or 'id-canal'; vertically organized, it is the instinctual force of feeling and impulse. This represents our visceral sensation; much emotion is expressed or repressed in the viscera, a point that is worth being aware of when addressing the viscera with any body work.

There are some osteopathic models that, though not perhaps directly influenced by Reich, echo some of his concepts. However, many individuals do not like having their approaches likened to Reich's work. His methods of application were often fairly strong and imposing. With most of the patient-centred practices, including the indirect and biodynamic approaches in osteopathy, they are non-imposing, permitting space for the vital force, breath of life, etc. to create the change. Also it is principally his early work that the approaches are based on, not the whole *oeuvre*. However, the caveat having been stated, there are areas of similarity between these early Reichian concepts and the biodynamic work of Jim Jealous and Rollin Becker, and the work of Robert Fulford, and from the muscular guarding aspect, Philip Latey (see the recommended reading at the end of this chapter for references).

A PSYCHODYNAMIC AND A BIOENERGETIC INTERPRETATION OF LOW BACK ACHE

To illustrate the way that these models may be applied to something that is commonly seen in osteopathic practice, there follow two examples of the possible interpretations of low back pain, firstly from a psychodynamic perspective and then a bioenergetic view.

Dave Heath, an osteopath, explains lower back-ache from a psychodynamic perspective:

Examination of these patients usually identifies tense muscles in the region of the lower back, pelvis, and thighs. Additionally, many of them have concomitant bowel dysfunction such as constipation or irritable bowel syndrome. A common pattern with many of these patients is that they give a lot of themselves sometimes to the point of feeling resentful, their problem being a difficulty in striking a balance between pleasing themselves versus pleasing others. Looked at in Psychodynamic terms the production of muscular tensions in the lumbo-pelvic area can relate to the anal stage of development; much of the dynamics of this stage being about battles of wills. This stage is typified by toilet training when the child can offer his gift of faeces of which he may be proud or ashamed, dependent on the parent's reaction to it. He can also learn that he can not only exercise self-control but control over the parent by withholding of his product through the tensing of anal sphincter and pelvic muscles. I think with some of this patient group an eruption of pain results from an archaic protest of withholding leading to increased tonus in already taut muscles and a likely explanation for bowel symptoms that sometimes coincide with lower back pain.[9]

Contrast that with Heike Buhl's bioenergetic interpretation.

The expression 'holding back' demonstrates the correlation between a muscular 'holding of the back' and the restraint on the emotional level. An immobile spinal column can be a sign for mental immobility and lack of flexibility. It mirrors an inner state of mind which requires 'backbone'. Aggressions, especially kicking impulses, are frequently suppressed in the lower back. Moreover, the back stands for support in life: a lack of necessary 'backing' results in back pain. Fear of softness and surrender lead to tension in the lumbar region: the hollow back lessens the pelvis' mobility, and with it the experiencing of sexual pleasure.[10]

When confronted with material like this many students either laugh at it or disregard it. This is very easy to understand, as both descriptions are couched in unfamiliar terminology, and discuss concepts that may at first appear strange, such as a child offering his 'gift of faeces'. Also there is a tendency now to think that Freudian concepts are no longer valid, especially as there is a discussion about the possibility of his falsifying some of his research. This, however, is throwing the baby out with the bath water; his research methods may have been dubious but his concepts are still strikingly original and have been applied for a century to good effect. We also have a tendency to analyse things from an adult perspective (not surprisingly), so the 'gift of faeces' appears laughable. However, that child is offering something of himself, and it has been rejected, and sometimes with apparent revulsion. Imagine the hurt.

It is interesting to reflect on where frustrations and emotional hurt do 'go'. Most people are aware of tension going to their shoulder muscles when they are stressed, or can tell by the set of someone's jaw that they are angry. But we often do not look beyond these obvious areas. Philip Latey[10,11] explores the role of muscles as sensory organs from a very pragmatic and jargon-free perspective. He considers the changes that may occur within muscles as a result of trauma, both physical and emotional, and offers an insight to how to approach them. His work is briefly discussed later in the chapter. These concepts do, however, permit one to look at the interplay of suppressed emotions, often from the early stages of life, and the possible somatic concepts that may arise from this.

HOMEOSTASIS, THE EFFECT OF THE ENVIRONMENT, AND STRESS

By the 1950s attitudes began to shift away from the somewhat introspective position of the psychoanalytic or psychodynamic models, toward more outward looking approaches, emphasizing objective observation and experiments. It is possible to trace the ideas of keeping physiological processes within normal limits back to the 19th century when Claude Bernard spoke of 'The ability of living beings to maintain the constancy of their internal milieu'.[12] In the early 20th century, Walter B Cannon (1871–1945) proposed the idea of 'homeostasis' and described the 'fight or flight response' initiated by the sympathetic nervous system mobilizing the body, preparing it to respond to any real or perceived threat.[13] He also apparently coined the much less used phrase 'rest and digest' as the opposite process overseen by the parasympathetic nervous system, replenishing its stores of energy when no threat is present.[14]

Then in 1936 a Viennese physiologist named Hans Selye coined the term 'stress' and eventually became known as the 'father of stress'. Selye noted that the stressors, as he called them, may be biochemical, physical or psychological in origin and he proposed the General Adaptation Syndrome (GAS) as the body's way of reacting to the stressor, irrespective of its origin.[15]

The GAS was described as consisting of three phases (alarm, resistance/adaptive and exhaustion) that formed a continuum, which to a certain extent, at least in the first two stages, is reversible. See Figure 7.1.

According to Selye, during the alarm phase, the body is mobilized in order to defend itself against the stressor and there is high arousal. The physiological processes include:

- increased cardiac rate and output
- increased respiratory rate

- vasoconstriction in the skin and certain visceral blood vessels
- increased activity in the liver
- decreased salivary production
- decreased enzymatic activity in the gut
- contraction of the spleen.

This series of actions flows into the resistance phase which is an adaptation to the stressor, where, in addition, the following processes begin:

- Increased nervous activity in the hypothalamus leads to an increase in the output of various hormones within the body, e.g. corticotropin-releasing factor (CRF), adrenocorticotropin hormone (ACTH), growth hormone-releasing hormone (GHRH), and thyroid-releasing hormone (TRH).
- This may lead to diseases of adaptation in the form of hypertension, ulcers, impaired immune function and asthma.

Finally, the exhaustion phase may occur, in which the body's resources become further compromised and the ability to resist further may collapse, resulting in disease or death. Symptoms include:

- decreased potassium in the blood: aldosterone retains sodium in exchange for potassium and hydrogen ions;
- depletion of glucocorticoids;
- over-activity of the cardiac vasculature and of the adrenal cortex;
- immunosupression and poor wound healing.

If the end result is death, it would at first glance appear that this is not a very useful defensive action to utilize! However, this is essentially a short-to-medium term process enabling the body to resist or avoid threats. The alarm phase responds to immediate threats and when these have passed, allows the body to return to its natural harmony. The resistance phase attempts to moderate the effects of longer-lasting threats, a sort of 'damage limitation' stage which, if successful, as with the alarm phase, will then permit the body to return to its normal balance. The exhaustion stage occurs when the body has been unable to resolve the threat and therefore represents the end stage and failure of this homeostatic mechanism.

At this point it would be of benefit to reflect back on the general adaptive response (GAR) and its mediating elements, the hypothalamic–pituitary–adrenal (HPA), sympathetic adrenal axis (SAM) and sympathetic neural axis (SNA), which were discussed in the previous chapter. It can be

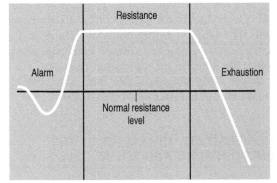

Figure 7.1   A schematic representation of Selye's General Adaptation Syndrome. (Modified after Selye H. The stress of life. New York: McGraw-Hill; 1976.)

seen that the alarm stage of the GAS is, in essence, the fight and flight response governed principally by SAM and SNA. In the resistance stage the HPA axis becomes the primary system. The GAS is thus a model of the effects that may arise as a result of protracted stressors affecting the hypothalamus via its many and varied connections, and its actions in activating and perpetuating the action of the HPA, SAM and SNA.

This triphasic general adaptation syndrome can also be perceived as representing the continuum of normal physiology, through pathophysiology and on to abnormal pathology (see Fig. 7.2). In the right circumstances, whether by the body's intrinsic self-healing factors or some form of external treatment, pathophysiological changes are able to revert to normal physiological function. The physiological and pathophysiological changes occur in the alarm and resistance phases respectively. Exhaustion represents the onset of irreversible pathological changes. Recognition and appropriate management of an individual who is in one of the first two stages will prevent their continuation to the pathological stage. The theory of the total osteopathic lesion (TOL) explores the concept of summation and compound action of multiple stressors of varied origins (see Ch. 9). Applying the TOL within this context would enable one to obtain an holistic view of the contributing factors, and help the practitioner realize that to achieve good results they have to help lighten the body's summative load. In a patient who is subject to numerous stressors, it is not always necessary to remove all of them (not that that would be possible anyway), but by addressing some of them, the body itself will then perhaps be able be restore homeostasis and enable the patient to pass back to normal healthy function, whereas without this 'lightening' the sheer load would make that an impossibility.

Tom Dummer related the GAS concept to possible findings in the body that would perhaps be more immediately observable in the musculoskeletal system (Table 7.1).

It should perhaps be pointed out at this stage that not all stress is detrimental. Selye used the term 'eustress' for stressors that are of benefit. Without some level of stress it is unlikely that many of us would achieve as much as we do. Our experience of stress is also a very personal thing. The stress of a big competition or a major event will be beneficial to some individuals, enabling them to perform at their best (i.e. eustress), but to others it can be disabling and decidedly not eustress. This is perhaps well illustrated by sportsmen: many of the top level competitors 'on paper' are performing at the same high level, and in qualifying rounds perform equally well. However, often it is the manner in which they deal with the emotional stress of the final competition that determines who ultimately wins, and not just their physical prowess.

The fact that sustained stress or the summative action of numerous stressors is detrimental to health is illustrated by the Social Readjustment Rating Scale developed in the 1960s by Holmes and Rahe[16] which relatively accurately correlated the potential illnesses someone may suffer proportionate to the amount of stress to which they have been exposed.

SOCIAL READJUSTMENT RATING SCALE

Holmes and Rahe were able to correlate, with considerable accuracy, the number of stress points a person accumulated in any 2-year period, with the degree of seriousness of the disorder which that person was then likely to suffer. From this they created the Social Readjustment Rating Scale (SRRS) which gave numerical values to many different types of stressful situations. The ratings for some of the common life stressors are shown in Table 7.2.

The number of points is calculated over a 2-year period; the results are variously described as:

- less than 150 life change units: 30% chance of developing a stress-related illness;
- 150–299 life change units: 50% chance of illness;
- over 300 life change units: 80% chance of illness;

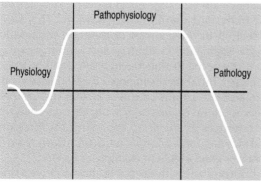

Figure 7.2   An adaptation of the GAS to demonstrate the physiology, pathophysiology, pathology continuum. (Modified after Selye H. The stress of life. New York: McGraw-Hill; 1976.)

Table 7.1   The possible consequences on the musculoskeletal system related to Selye's three stages of the general adaptation syndrome. (After Dummer T. A textbook of osteopathy, vol 1. Hadlow Down: JoTom Publications; 1999: 171)

Stage	Possible consequences
Alarm stage Acute state of reaction and defence	Muscular hypertonicity resulting from an exaggerated nervous stimulus, and local tissue changes in reaction to trauma, voluntary physiological contracture (CNS), involuntary (ANS) visceral origins, or psychological stress. This leading to decreased range of movement (ROM) due to spasms and contractures
Resistance stage +/- adequate adaptation, compensation (subacute on top of chronic symptomatology, but not uncommonly asymptomatic)	Muscular hypertrophy, fibrosis, limitation of ROM due to fibrous tissue accumulation with diminution of muscular fibres due to long-term adaptation to stress Decreased local circulation Acidic and toxic deposits Beginning of osteoarthritis
Exhaustion stage Lack of adaptation and compensation Disease Degeneration	Fibrosis and muscular atrophy, which is the result of atonia and replacement of the muscular fibres by fibrous tissue, coming generally from: • acidic saturation, circulatory and nutritive deficiency • under adaptation to chronic stress • osteoarthritis

Table 7.2   Selected examples of the life change units attributed to stressful situations from the Social Readjustment Rating Scale. (Modified from Holmes TH, Rahe RH. The social readjustment rating scale. Journal of Psychosomatic Research 1967; 11: 213–218)

Stressful situation	Units
Death of a spouse	100
Divorce	73
Marital separation	63
Death of a close family member	63
Marriage	50
Marital reconciliation	45
Retirement	45
Change to a different line of work	36
Sexual difficulties	39
Trouble with your boss	23
Change in residence	20
Taking out a mortgage or loan for a lesser purchase (e.g. for a car, TV, freezer)	17
Major change in sleeping habits (significant increase/decrease, or change in pattern)	16
Vacation	13
Christmas	12

Or:

• more than 250 points is likely to be followed by a life-threatening illness;
• 150 points by an illness which may be serious, but not life-threatening;
• 20–50 points, recurrent bronchitis, headaches, cold sores or other illnesses may result.

Though this scale is not without its detractors it would appear that stress is cumulative and that it can have a predictable effect on various systems in the body and therefore homeostasis. This has a reflection in the concept of the total osteopathic lesion, segmental facilitation and central sensitization. The Social Readjustment Scale is still occasionally used, but it has been noted that it does not take into account certain pertinent factors such as people's appraisal of the stressor, nor their mechanisms or resources available to cope with the stressors, and so other tools are now more frequently used. It is however an excellent example of its kind.[17]

Concomitant with the publication of Selye's findings and other similar research, a plethora of self-help books appeared, all addressing methods of stress reduction. Practitioners, both allopathic and other, developed and incorporated relaxation techniques within their patient management. An example of this is biofeedback, a process where information concerning the individual's own physiological responses is conveyed to them (via some sort of recording device, depending on the responses being monitored) to enable them, with practice, to alter their ANS responses through conscious techniques and therefore minimize the deleterious effects. Another example is progressive relaxation training (PRT) involving selective muscle contraction and relaxation, allowing people to become aware of focal muscle tension in their bodies as a possible indicator of stress. This differs from the often used relaxation system of progressively contracting and relaxing the muscles throughout the body: with PRT the focus is on the small muscles to create a specific awareness. It is more difficult to learn but ultimately more likely to achieve the desired effect. Yoga, transcendental meditation, and other mind–body approaches also became more widely practised. Thus the clinical emphasis had shifted from the introspective psychodynamic approach to a more outward looking one which attempted to try and control the environmental contributory factors. Associated with this was a greater tendency for the individual patient to be involved with their own therapeutic management.

MODERN PERSPECTIVES: ALLOSTASIS

Due to the possibility of normal physiology passing eventually to pathology, numerous researchers have looked more closely at the effects of stress and what occurs when the body does not fully recover. Sterling and Eyer[18] studied the effects on the cardiovascular system in its change from resting to active states. They proposed a new term, 'allostasis' to describe 'maintaining stability or homeostasis through change' (Fig. 7.3). They proposed that there were three possible outcomes to a cycle of allostasis:

1. Normal equilibrium is restored after the stress has passed.
2. The body becomes 'stuck' in an overactive state.
3. The body becomes 'stuck' in an underactive state.

Since the body is constantly exposed to numerous forms of stressors throughout every day, these repeated cycles of allostasis may go in any of the above directions. Furthermore, since the body is not indestructible, there is a price to pay for the overuse of these systems and that has been termed 'allostatic load'.

Thus allostasis relates to the short-term, protective effects and allostatic load relates to the longer-term changes and the resulting damaging effects. It appears that these changes occur in all systems of the body.

Professor Bruce McEwen[19] has offered four possible causes of allostatic load:

1. Repeated hits from multiple novel stressors.
2. Lack of adaptation.
3. Prolonged response due to delayed shutdown.
4. Inadequate response that leads to compensatory hyperactivity of other mediators.

See Figure 7.4. (A) represents the normal allostatic response. In the case of (B) an example could be a 'normal' working day: the car will not start; when it does the petrol tank is on the low mark; there is a traffic jam so you are late for a meeting with the boss … and so on throughout the day. It represents a series of different and relatively minor hindrances which each create a stress response.

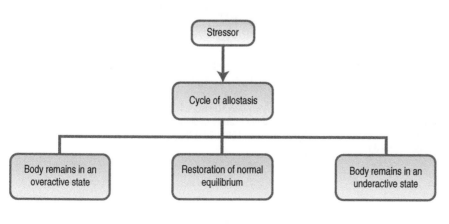

Figure 7.3   Cycle of allostasis. Cycles of allostasis may go one of three different ways. All create allostatic load but under- or overactive responses increase the load.

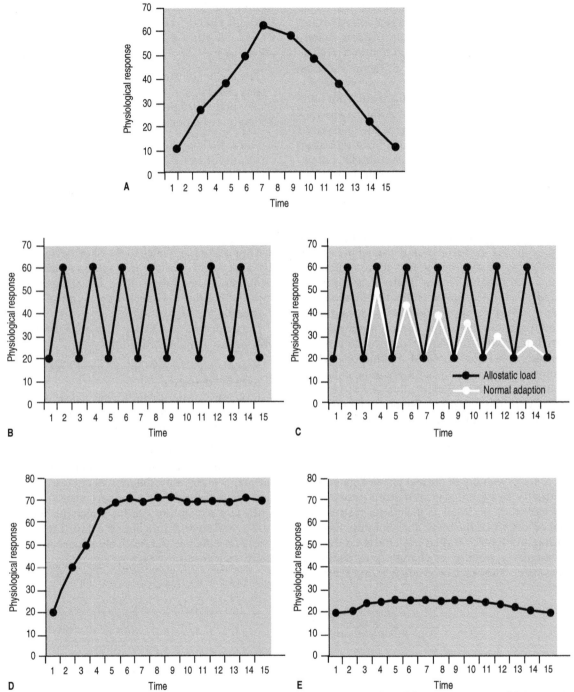

Figure 7.4 **(A)** A normal allostatic response. **(B)** Repeated hits from multiple novel stressors. **(C)** Lack of adaptation. **(D)** Prolonged response due to delayed shutdown. **(E)** Inadequate response that leads to compensatory hyperactivity of other mediators. (Reproduced with permission from McEwen BS. Three types of allostatic load. New Eng J Med 1998; 338(3):171–179. Copyright © 1998 Massachusetts Medical Society. All rights reserved.)

In the second case (C), it could be that every morning the car will not start and normally the body should dampen its response to a repeated stress, but for some reason, every morning provokes the same stress response.

In the third case (D), the normal response should be followed by a relatively rapid return to the normal resting state, but for some reason the response takes longer to return to normal.

Finally, in case four, the body does not produce an adequate response and so there may be insufficient levels of glucocorticoids which normally counter regulate the cytokines, resulting in increased levels of the latter.

McEwen states:

> When the brain perceives an experience as stressful, physiologic and behavioural responses are initiated leading to allostasis and adaptation. Over time, allostatic load can accumulate, and the overexposure to neural endocrine and immune stress mediators can have adverse effects on various organ systems leading to disease.[20]

It is the persistent exposure to over-secretion of naturally produced stress hormones and other endogenous factors that may result in a number of pathological states such as atherosclerosis, coronary heart disease and type II diabetes as well as pain, inflammation and reduced mobility.[21-25]

Although stress seems to be taking the blame for a wide number of disease states, a large number of individuals are exposed to it and a certain number of individuals seem to emerge unscathed. It is how the body reacts that determines an individual's susceptibility to the different possible outcomes. It could be argued that there is a certain genetic predisposition to the effects of stress resulting in disease state, but studies of asthma in identical twins reveal low levels of concordance so it appears not to be the complete answer.

Furthermore, it could be argued that personality, as in the classic type A or B, would predispose the type A person to a greater damaging effect, since their volatile behaviour is creating a risk of greater allostatic load. However, a type B person could also run a risk by falling into the 'inadequate response' group of McEwen's four types of allostatic load. All these points are in need of further investigation. It is also very probable that the way one perceives stress, or in fact perceives life, will have a great influence on this system.

PSYCHOSOCIAL FACTORS HELPING TO IDENTIFY RISK FACTORS THAT INCREASE THE PROBABILITY OF LONG-TERM DISABILITY

In this discussion it has been mentioned that the individual response to the GAS and the allostatic cost of stressors is dependent on the psychoemotional makeup of that individual and their environment. The New Zealand government commissioned research into the psychosocial factors that are likely to increase the risk of an individual with acute low back pain developing prolonged pain and disability causing work loss, and associated loss of quality of life. Published under the title of 'Guide to Assessing Psychosocial Yellow Flags in Acute Low Back Pain', it is freely available on the internet (see ref. 26). The following is taken from Table 2: 'Clinical assessment of psychosocial yellow flags', from this paper. They defined acute low back problems as activity intolerance due to lower back or back and leg symptoms lasting less than 3 months, and chronic low back problems as activity intolerance due to lower back or back and leg symptoms lasting more than 3 months.

They utilized the term 'Yellow Flags' for these psychosocial risk factors in contrast to 'Red Flags', which are physical risk factors.[26]

A person may be at risk if:

- there is a cluster of a few very salient factors, or
- there is a group of several less important factors that combine cumulatively.

The risk factors are discussed under the headings: attitudes and beliefs about back pain, behaviours, compensation issues, emotions, family and work.

Attitudes and beliefs about back pain

- *Belief that pain is harmful or disabling resulting in fear-avoidance behaviour, eg, the development of guarding and fear of movement*
- *Belief that all pain must be abolished before attempting to return to work or normal activity*
- *Expectation of increased pain with activity or work, lack of ability to predict capability*
- *Catastrophising, thinking the worst, misinterpreting bodily symptoms*
- *Belief that pain is uncontrollable*
- *Passive attitude to rehabilitation*

Behaviours

- Use of extended rest, disproportionate 'downtime'
- Reduced activity level with significant withdrawal from activities of daily living
- Irregular participation or poor compliance with physical exercise, tendency for activities to be in a 'boom–bust' cycle
- Avoidance of normal activity and progressive substitution of lifestyle away from productive activity
- Report of extremely high intensity of pain, eg, above 10, on a 0–10 Visual Analogue Scale
- Excessive reliance on use of aids or appliances
- Sleep quality reduced since onset of back pain
- High intake of alcohol or other substances (possibly as self-medication), with an increase since onset of back pain
- Smoking

Compensation issues

- Lack of financial incentive to return to work
- Delay in accessing income support and treatment cost, disputes over eligibility
- History of claim/s due to other injuries or pain problems
- History of extended time off work due to injury or other pain problem (eg., more than 12 weeks)
- History of previous back pain, with a previous claim/s and time off work
- Previous experience of ineffective case management (eg, absence of interest, perception of being treated punitively)

Diagnosis and treatment

- Health professional sanctioning disability, not providing interventions that will improve function
- Experience of conflicting diagnoses or explanations for back pain, resulting in confusion
- Diagnostic language leading to catastrophising and fear (eg, fear of ending up in a wheelchair)
- Dramatisation of back pain by health professional producing dependency on treatments, and continuation of passive treatment
- Number of times visited health professional in last year (excluding the present episode of back pain)
- Expectation of a 'techno-fix', eg, requests to treat as if body were a machine
- Lack of satisfaction with previous treatment for back pain
- Advice to withdraw from job

Emotions

- Fear of increased pain with activity or work
- Depression (especially long-term low mood), loss of sense of enjoyment
- More irritable than usual
- Anxiety about and heightened awareness of body sensations (includes sympathetic nervous system arousal)
- Feeling under stress and unable to maintain sense of control
- Presence of social anxiety or disinterest in social activity
- Feeling useless and not needed

Family

- Over-protective partner/spouse, emphasising fear of harm or encouraging catastrophising (usually well-intentioned)
- Solicitous behaviour from spouse (eg, taking over tasks)
- Socially punitive responses from spouse (eg, ignoring, expressing frustration)
- Extent to which family members support any attempt to return to work
- Lack of support person to talk to about problems

Work

- History of manual work, notably from the following occupational groups:
  - Fishing, forestry and farming workers
  - Construction, including carpenters and builders
  - Nurses
  - Truck drivers
  - Labourers
- Work history, including patterns of frequent job changes, experiencing stress at work, job dissatisfaction, poor relationships with peers or supervisors, lack of vocational direction
- Belief that work is harmful; that it will do damage or be dangerous
- Unsupportive or unhappy current work environment
- Low educational background, low socioeconomic status
- Job involves significant bio-mechanical demands, such as lifting, manual handling heavy items, extended sitting, extended standing, driving, vibration, maintenance of constrained or sustained postures, inflexible work schedule preventing appropriate breaks
- Job involves shift work or working unsociable hours
- Minimal availability of selected duties and graduated return to work pathways, with unsatisfactory implementation of these

- *Negative experience of workplace management of back pain (eg, absence of a reporting system, discouragement to report, punitive response from supervisors and managers)*
- *Absence of interest from employer*

It is not intended that you learn this verbatim, but it is included to give a general overview of the possible psychosocial contributory factors. This research was based on factors contributing to chronic low back pain; however, it seems reasonable that similar factors will be contributory to most musculoskeletal problems, and a large element of them to any chronic painful condition.

THE OSTEOPATHIC CONSEQUENCES

The model offered by the GAS and the more recent concepts of allostasis have a great relevance to the osteopathic practitioner. The key stage of the GAS is the adaptive stage. This is where the body is showing signs of pathophysiological change, but is not yet pathological. The body is working hard and it is drawing heavily on its reserves: drawing an analogy to a battery, there is not a lot of charge left. The individual will be facilitated emotionally, physiologically and somatically. The concept of the total osteopathic lesion is discussed in Chapter 9. Simply stated, it is a concept of summation of stressors. Each stressor, regardless of its origin, will have an effect on the individual across all aspects of their being, however you choose to describe them: mind, body, spirit, or emotion, physiology, soma. The majority of the patients that are treated within the osteopathic clinics in Europe are either at the alarm or adaptation stage, and though they may be presenting complaining of a somatic problem, all other systems will be similarly under strain. By thoroughly exploring their health and psychosocial situations it should be possible to gain an understanding of the stressors to which they are exposed. These may be cataclysmic (affecting several people or whole communities at the same time), personal (small and large), or background (the daily hassles of life, bearing in mind the cumulative effect this may have allostatically). Also it is important to assess the individual's coping strategies and their stress resistance resources (SRRs). SRRs are all of the factors that we have available to us that enable us to cope with life's stresses. They include resources of different types:

- Material: money and all the things it can buy – food, shelter, etc.
- Physical: strength, health and attractiveness.
- Intrapersonal: inner strength, based largely on self-esteem.
- Informational and educational.
- Cultural: the sense of coherence or of belonging to a community or race.[17]

Many of these elements will be interrelated.

It is now possible to create a management plan that can be patient specific, addressing as many of their stressors as possible. Where necessary, consider referral to other practitioners better suited to deal with particular aspects of the whole.

When presenting this material in lectures it tends to make osteopaths appear to be omniscient, omnipotent and to possess infinite reserves of energy. This is obviously not the case. However, many of these elements can be addressed at a very basic level and have a surprisingly good effect. Let us look very briefly at some of the levels where we may be able to help.

From a material perspective, if someone is unable to work because of long-standing pain, they will generally be less financially stable, and if unemployed perhaps have low self-esteem. Chronic pain will lead to suppression of the immune system and thus a greater susceptibility to disease. The high cortisol levels that will occur as a result of over-action of the HPA have been implicated in the aetiology of depressive disorders.[27] Resolving their pain will allow them to return to work and will ameliorate all of the above elements. Perhaps more importantly, by resolving problems before the pain passes from physiological to chronic, these complications will not arise. Hence the need to recognize the signs and symptoms of someone teetering on the cusp between the adaptive and exhaustion stages of the GAS, and by addressing the multiple factors that have brought them to that point, bring them back from the brink. The psychosocial factors, or 'yellow flags' that may help predict the likelihood of someone passing to a chronic pain state have been discussed above. Selye offers the following list of many of the physical features that he considers are possible signs of the adaptive phase:[28]

- *General irritability, hyperexcitation or depression*
- *Pounding of the heart*
- *Dryness of the throat and mouth*
- *Impulsive behaviour, emotional instability*

- *The overpowering urge to cry or run away and hide*
- *Inability to concentrate, flights of thoughts and general disorientation*
- *Predilection to become fatigued, and loss of 'joie de vivre'*
- *'Floating anxiety', that is to say we are afraid but not exactly sure what of*
- *Emotional tension and alertness, 'keyed up'*
- *Trembling, nervous ticks*
- *Tendency to be easily startled*
- *High pitched, nervous laughter*
- *Stuttering and other speech difficulties frequently stress induced*
- *Bruxism*
- *Insomnia, often as a consequence of being 'keyed up'*
- *Hypermotility, or hyperkinesia. The inability to be relaxed and rest quietly*
- *Sweating more in stressful situations*
- *The frequent need to urinate*
- *Diarrhoea, indigestion, queasiness in the stomach, and sometimes vomiting*
- *IBS*
- *Migraine headaches*
- *Premenstrual tension, or missed menstrual cycles*
- *Pain in the neck or low back*
- *Loss of, or excessive appetite*
- *Increased smoking*
- *Increased use of legally prescribed drugs*
- *Alcohol and drug addiction*
- *Nightmares*
- *Neurotic behaviour*
- *Psychoses*
- *Accident proneness.*[31]

A combined awareness of both the physical signs and symptoms and the psychosocial predictive factors should alert the practitioner to this possibility.

The practitioner's interpersonal skills are often highly significant, such as when communicating with an individual who is overweight. These individuals often have a poor self-image: telling them that they are obese or that the problem is due to their being overweight will reinforce this negative image. The term 'obese', though medically correct, to the lay person is pejorative; a more thoughtful use of language can lessen this impact. Obesity does contribute to many aspects of poor health, but is usually one of many aetiological factors: why not address these other factors first rather than putting everything down to obesity? This is not advocating avoiding the issue but presenting it in a constructive rather than destructive manner.

Someone who is well educated and articulate will have the ability to explore problems and obtain information about their condition easily. However, not everyone is that fortunate. Not knowing the cause of something, or how to go about discovering what it is, is remarkably stressful. Explaining to an individual what is occurring in lay terms and being able to offer advice around systems and procedures (especially medical) will allay the fear of the unknown.

An awareness of the compound aspects of all problems will lead to a quicker and more effective recovery and, perhaps most importantly, prevent them from getting to the irreversible exhaustion stage.

PSYCHONEUROIMMUNOLOGY

Research has been directed at trying to understand the physiological basis for the effects of stress on the immune system, as it has been observed that stress, and particularly psychoemotional stress, influences the state of health of an individual. Empirically, this phenomenon has been known for years, but the complexity of the human body, and particularly of its brain, make a full understanding of this difficult. Any stress affects the psychological state of an individual, and at the same time the psychological state influences the body function.

Research has in the past concentrated on the immune system, as it is this system that is principally responsible for the health of an individual. Studies revealed that depression, loneliness, unhappiness, anxiety and hostility all have the effect of lowering the function of the immune system, resulting in the development of minor diseases such as herpes labialis.

The effects of bereavement and marital disruption have been shown to have a similar action on the immune system: they are known to increase morbidity and mortality. However, these results are more difficult to analyse, as in such situations there is a possibility of other factors intervening, such as loss of appetite, increase in alcohol consumption or decrease in sleep, which are also factors that can influence the immune system.

More recent research is revealing a much greater interdependence between the psyche, nervous system and immune system than was previously appreciated. They are so interrelated that it seems that it is not possible to disentangle them. In the last 20 years, largely due to advances in technology and imaging techniques, the emphasis has passed to the neurophysiological processes of the CNS. Concomitant with this research was the emergence of the new field of research known as psychoneuroimmunology (PNI), (the term neuroimmunomodulation (NIM) is sometimes used in place of PNI or sometimes refers to a slightly different branch of the same study). Of fundamental significance to this area of study is the realization that the immune and neuroendocrine systems are in fact in close bidirectional communication and, indeed, 'talk' to each other all the time, ensuring a coordinated defence of the body and maintenance of homeostasis. Interruption of this communication, whether genetic, surgical or pharmacological, has led to an increased susceptibility to disease.

The demonstration of 'cross-talk' between the immune and neuroendocrine systems provides a scientific basis for understanding how emotions can influence the onset, course and remission of disease. The physiological basis is exceedingly complex; however, most of the processes behind this have already been discussed.

DEEPER EXPLORATION OF PNI

We will start by reviewing some of the key points so far discussed.

The neuroendocrine-immune system has been described as a complex interwoven series of processes that behave in a coordinated manner. There is bidirectional communication between the systems via a receptor-mediated mechanism, with neuroregulators, hormones and immunoregulators acting not just on 'their own' system, but also on the other two. At the centre of this is the hypothalamus and its numerous afferent and efferent connections with other areas of the nervous system.

The physiological changes that occur in response to noxious stimuli are mediated via the HPA, SAM and SNA axes and have been discussed elsewhere.

The descending autonomic pathways supply all of the lymphoid tissue and therefore have an immunomodulatory effect, as do certain hormones secreted by the neuroendocrine system.

The nervous system, in response to a noxious stimulus, has been shown to secrete neurotransmitters such as somatostatin and substance P which act as vasodilators and chemical attractors for tissue macrophages and lymphocytes and encourage the release of cytokinins such as IL-1 and TNF; these in turn pass to the CNS and activate the HPA.

Key to the function of all of this is the hypothalamus.

To relate this to emotions it is necessary to briefly discuss the emotional areas of the brain with reference to the above. The emotions appear to be represented in the limbic system of the brain. Of particular importance are the limbic forebrain structures, the amygdala and the hippocampus. The hypothalamus has direct connections with the limbic forebrain–limbic midbrain circuitry.[29] It is via these connections that the emotions will be able to affect the hypothalamus and therefore influence all of the elements of the neuroendocrine-immune system discussed. Thus an emotion or psychological stressor can, via the limbic-hypothalamic-brain stem circuitry, activate the HPA and the SAM, resulting in increased cortisol release and sympathetic activity, and stimulating the physiological changes already discussed. See Figure 7.5.

However, it is even more complex than this. Previous experience, cultural attitudes, individual coping strategies and a near infinite number of elements of personality, conscious and unconscious, will modulate the limbic-hypothalamic-brain stem circuitry. Consider the case of a person who has had an emotionally traumatic childhood. This person will have developed a heightened vigilance and preparedness for flight. This will possibly result in an increase in unconscious emotional response to a stressor. This in turn will lead to an increased physiological response to stress and an increase in production of immunosuppressive neuropeptides and hormones, and submissive behaviour.[30] The converse can also work, where a 'positive' mind state will moderate the response to a stressor.

Melzack and Wall,[31] in analysing pain perception, illustrate the complex interplay of psychosocial concepts that may influence the interpretation of a noxious stimulus. They state that cultural expectations surrounding the meaning of pain reflect differences in pain tolerance. Certain cultures or ethnic groupings demonstrate a more stoic attitude to pain, while others demonstrate less tolerance and allow greater expression of their emotions. Additionally, the quality and intensity of pain is determined by a number of other factors such as an individual's early experiences, their level of anxiety, and the attention that is focused on the pain.

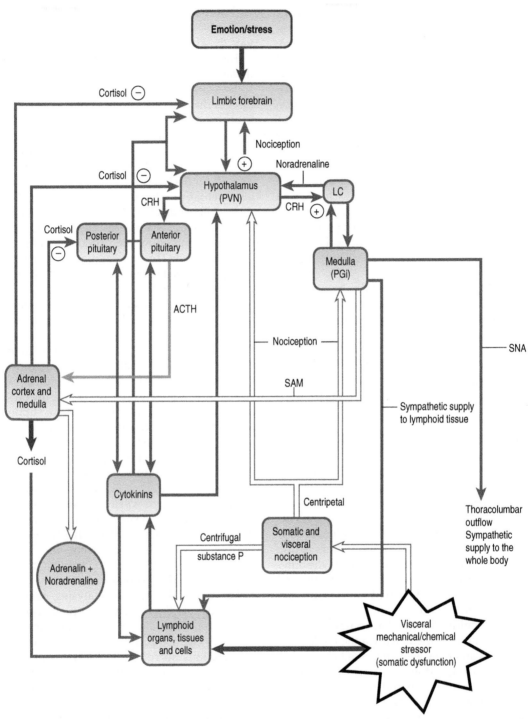

Figure 7.5   A schematic representation of the PNI process.

From this it is possible to comprehend the complexity of both the physiological processes underpinning the PNI process and the enormous range of psychosocial factors that will modulate their effects. The task for the practitioner of trying to synthesize all of this complexity appears to be insurmountable. It is easy to get buried under the constant deluge of current research, but it is important not to lose sight of fundamental concepts such as effective and empathetic communication with patients and concepts such as 'structure governs function' and *vis medicatrix naturae*. These go a long way to addressing elements of this complexity, and the intellectual concepts should be there to inform our actions, not dictate them.

THE PHYSICAL EXPRESSION OF EMOTION IN THE BODY

So far the discussion has largely been concerned with the physiology behind the psychoemotional contribution to ill health. This section will address some of the total body concepts, the physical manifestation of the emotions within the body.

Being able to assess people's emotional state is an innate skill that is present in all of us. It is possible to see anger, fear, sorrow, love, hate, in fact all of the emotions, in people's faces. Emotions are also visible within the body as a whole. Some are obvious: consider the upright, open body of the happy and confident individual, and the bowed head, closed body posture of someone who is depressed. There are also more subtle, complex patterns of emotions present within the body which are more difficult to read. We can all recognize many of these patterns but, paradoxically, it often seems that the moment many practitioners enter their clinics, these exceptionally useful skills are disregarded. Good observation of an individual will give an enormous amount of information. The way an individual stands and moves gives a detailed history of their physical and emotional life:

Body shape and patterns of movement simultaneously tell three stories, each relating to the way we experience gravity:

- *An evolutionary history, representing the millions of years that our ancestors adapted to life in the gravity field of our planet*
- *A shorter history of personal traumas and adaptations during our lifetime*

- *The history of our present emotional state, including the effects of our most recent experiences.*[32]

The muscular system carries our ego identity in the broadest sense. How we use our muscle, our characteristic posture, gait, gesture reflects and communicates a great deal about our gender, class, race, culture, and lifestyle, as well as our developmental history. Embedded in our muscles are all the skills, habits, expressions and defences we have acquired. The range of our learning includes normal development skills, such as feeding, and walking; specific skills – such as weaving, carpentry, juggling, driving; character attitudes, such as defiance or deference; patterns stemming from trauma, including birth trauma; and identifications made with others.[6]

PHILIP LATEY'S PATTERNS OF POSTURAL LAYERING, REGIONAL TENSION

The osteopath Philip Latey has spent many years looking at the sensory functions of the musculature, and exploring the relationship between the emotions and the patterns of postural layering and regional tensions that are observable within various different layers within the body. The following has been compiled from his work published in the *Journal of Bodywork and Movement Therapies*.[11,33]

He describes four layers of posture: the image, slump, residual and inner tube postures.[11]

The image posture

This is the social posture, the one that is utilized when one is aware of being observed. The body is held in an overtly 'correct' posture by the generally overtense large superficial muscles. This will give an indication of the persona that the patient expresses socially. As the patient begins to be more comfortable they begin to relax into the second posture, the slump posture.

The slump posture

This represents the individual's more habitual posture, the way that it functions in response to gravity. This is maintained by the action of the key postural muscles including the popliteus, tensor fascia lata, adductors and deep external rotators of the hip, lumbosacral muscles, serratus posterior inferior and superior, suboccipital muscles, sternomastiod, temporalis and the pterygoids. The third posture will be revealed when the patient is lying down, relaxed on the couch.

The residual posture

This is the pattern of residual tone and activity left after minimizing the effects of the social interaction and gravity. Some of the postural muscles may remain hypertonic, particularly the deep erector spinae muscles. There will also be a background tone and activity that is present in all of the musculature, this is the resting state of muscles maintained by the unconscious control of the higher centres. As such Latey considers that it is closer to the involuntary processes of the body than would be usually expected of skeletal muscle, and therefore very significant in a psychophysical context. In health the tissues should exhibit a relatively rhythmical motion; this can be affected by, and therefore indicative of, different emotions or physical influences. In chronic exhaustion or illness the movements become generally feeble and flaccid. In areas subject to extreme physical or emotional shock the tissues can feel static, lifeless, rigid, stringy or numb.

This has strong similarities to the psychodynamic concepts and the more recent interpretations of it, such as Reich's body armouring and the suppression or repression of emotions.

The inner tube

This consists broadly of the involuntary visceral and vascular smooth muscle. The gastrointestinal system lies at its centre, combined with the respiratory system. It is closely linked to emotional processes, and it is here that Latey places the senses concerned with the generation and perception of bodily and cerebral emotion, depth of meaning and mood.[33]

To describe the effects that can occur within these muscles he utilizes the analogy of a clenched fist:

A clenched fist represents the closing down of open interaction and engagement; it may be rage, fear, defiance or defensiveness; it might be a recoil in shock and denial when something awful has happened. The clenching may be enclosing something very precious; could be simply expressing tenacity and determination or enforcing stillness.

Unclenching of an area of the body, after an initial stage of weakness, vulnerability, ache and unsteadiness, should bring physiological relaxation. Warmth, breathing and involuntary motions are restored.[11]

He describes three main areas on which the tensions of the body focus: the pelvic girdle; the lower ribs and the upper abdomen; and the head, neck and shoulder girdle. When these are subject to tension, the fist analogy can be utilized with these areas being termed the lower, middle and upper fists respectively. Contraction of each of these fists in response to any of the emotions listed above will result in a series of changes that may lead to musculoskeletal and/or systemic dysfunction.

The lower fist may lead to problems with the low back, pelvis and lower extremities, creating mechanical imbalances and musculoskeletal pain. Changes in the control of the pelvic musculature and perineum may initially lead to the generation of sensation and, if sustained, its eventual obliteration. The chronic state will lead to stasis, inflammation or congestion of the bowel, bladder and genitalia, with innumerable possible clinical consequences.

The middle fist will have an effect on the muscles of respiration. This area is important in the expression (or suppression) of emotion, e.g. laughing, crying, sighing. Chronic contraction of the middle fist compresses the thoracolumbar region of the spine, possibly having an aetiological role in juvenile osteochondrosis. Mechanically this is a significant area, disturbance of which will have numerous musculoskeletal consequences. On a visceral level it may affect respiration, contributing to such conditions as asthma, recurrent chest infections or digestive system problems such as gastric reflux, ulcers and hiatus hernia.

The upper fist is involved with the perception, response and restraint of response to the outer world. Tightening of the upper fist muscles can contribute to such complaints as tension and migraine headaches, temporomandibular problems, sinusitis, and ear, nose or throat problems.

This is a very brief overview of the foundations of Latey's concepts. He has developed a broad approach which encompasses aetiological, diagnostic and therapeutic elements, all based on the interdependence of the mind and the body. It is not possible to do his work full justice within the confines of this text; for a more complete understanding you are referred to the references cited in the recommended reading at the end of this chapter.

EMOTIONAL ANATOMY

Another whole body psychoemotional approach that has a particular resonance for many osteopaths is that devised by Stanley Kelman, termed Emotional Anatomy.[34] One of the strengths of his approach is that his book, of the same name, conveys the concepts in a very visual manner. It is possibly this which perhaps makes it more obviously understandable in clinical terms. This benefit will be lost to an extent in this discussion – however, a brief overview follows.

As with the psychodynamic model, Kelman divides the body into three layers:

- The outer layer consists of the nervous system and the skin and represents our interaction with the world.
- The middle layer encompasses the muscles, bones and connective tissues.
- The inner layer consists of the internal organs of digestion, assimilation, respiration and distribution.

(The biodynamic equivalents of these would be the skin ego, the motoric ego and the id canal respectively.)

He also divides the body into three compartments, the head, chest and abdomen. For health there must be balance between the layers and pouches and good fluid exchange throughout.

This harmony, and therefore the posture, are affected by stress or 'insults'. Depending on the intensity, duration and frequency of the stresses the body will pass through a series of postural changes. Initially they become larger and expand outwards, passing progressively from a rigid cautionary stance to a threatened bracing one and then finally to a turning pose as if getting ready to run away. The next three postures involve getting smaller, shorter and becoming fixed. These represent a freezing type response. The postures evolve through the stages of a contracted bracing, to a withdrawal, submission and finally a downward collapse in defeat.

With time the tissues become thickened, the compartments shift and the fluid exchange is perturbed. Kelman describes the end result of the changes by using four types:

- Rigid and controlled
- Dense and shamed
- Swollen and manipulative
- Collapsed compliant.

Each type has its own possible sequelae physically, socially and psychologically.

Kelman believes that because of the reciprocity between emotive states and physical well-being it is possible to reverse the processes, strengthening the physical self. This involves correct breathing, nutrition and 'mindful' living. The parallels between this model and many of the osteopathic principles are clear.

SOME OSTEOPATHIC EMPIRICAL MIND–BODY CONCEPTS

There are many osteopathic concepts that have been tacitly accepted. One of these is the emotional release. Simply stated, this is the application of an osteopathic technique with the specific intention of resolving the stress patterns manifest in the body. Resolution of the pattern is often associated with some form of emotional release, ranging from crying or laughing to a complete recall of all the elements of the situation that caused the pattern.

As has been discussed, the model of a rigid 'hard wired' central neurological pathway is being questioned.

Memory is a complex phenomenon. Though not fully understood, it is probable that sensory information is passed to the higher centres as bundles of information and despite the fact that different types of information pass to separate sections of the cortex for interpretation, in some manner the information is still united. An example of this, that most people have experienced, is that of catching a waft of a particular scent and suddenly recalling a particular time, place or situation. Your memory is complete – as well as the olfactory component, it will often include the visual surroundings, an impression of sounds or recall of words, and associated emotions.

Thus, when a trauma occurs, be it physical or emotional, it is possible to hypothesize that it will create a pattern of somatic changes in the tissues of the body, including the neuromusculoskeletal and visceral systems, but at the same time the visual, auditory, olfactory and emotional sensations will be 'bundled' with it. Just as in the above example, stimulating one aspect of that bundle will have the possibility of evoking complete recall.

Patterns of dysfunction can occur as a result of purely emotional stimuli, in the absence of physical trauma. The somatic patterns may be created preferentially in certain areas of the body. Fulford[35] describes 'shock' held in the diaphragm and solar plexus. Structures like the diaphragm are easy to conceive as an area where emotion can be 'fixed'; just recall a situation where you have been suddenly frightened and how the diaphragm was felt to contract. Some other common somatic sites where this may occur are the upper fibres of trapezius, the masseter muscles and the pelvic floor. The actual distribution depends on the causative nature of the stress – any area of muscle has the potential to be emotionally charged.

The viscera are also affected by emotion. Though not as physically obvious as the above examples, most of us will have experienced the sense of certain viscera being affected emotionally. Many will know that 'gut wrenching' feeling associated with emotions of loss or jealousy, or the hollow, empty feeling that accompanies the death of someone very dear. These are acute manifestations of the emotion felt within the deep visceral structures (Latey's inner tube, Kelman's inner layer, the biodynamic id canal). Chronic emotional disturbances will have similar effects though these effects will not necessarily be felt on a conscious level. Empirical osteopathic anecdotes also describe emotional reaction to treatment at the umbilical area, the liver, gallbladder, lungs and uterus.

The fascia as a whole appears to have the ability to retain a memory of both the physical and emotional aspects of a trauma, both possibly being re-experienced as the fascial pattern is treated.

As well as the neurological explanation for the emotional charge of particular areas, some concepts appear to be rooted in a blend of Eastern and energetic concepts. The sternum, the fourth thoracic vertebra and the cardiac plexus are often considered to be emotional centres, possibly due to their relation to the heart chakra, also in this area. Another example is the relationship between shoulder dysfunction and parental disagreements, or home or work conflict.

Whatever the underpinning mechanism, empirically there is a relatively high incidence of emotional releases occurring when working in areas such as these. An awareness of this will allow you to appreciate the subtle interplay between the mind and the body. It will enable you to be prepared for the possible emotional release that may occur when treating someone with emotional or shock patterns. This will help you establish an appropriate time to effect the release; it will not be appreciated if it is performed when the patient is unprepared, or not strong enough to cope with it at that time, or just prior to an important occasion without leaving sufficient time for the effects to wear off.

It will also prevent you from further traumatizing an area by attempting to release it directly, when it would respond more effectively to an indirect approach.

From a diagnostic perspective, it is thought to be possible to distinguish the feel of tissue affected by emotional shock as opposed to physical trauma. If this is the case then it may be appropriate to gently enquire about possible traumatic occasions that may have precipitated it. Uniting the emotion with its physical manifestation in the body, prior to treating the somatic element, is thought by many to be more powerful in resolving it completely.

We, as osteopaths, do not need to know specific information on what has caused the particular psychological disturbance; as long as the patient is aware of it, that is sufficient. Should the patient wish to discuss it, that is their choice, and it is up to you as a practitioner to establish your own boundaries around this. A note of caution should be introduced at this point. Most osteopaths are not psychologists, and there are times when appropriate referral to someone more qualified in this field may be more beneficial for the patient and for you, the practitioner, too.

CONCLUSION

This chapter was intended to reinforce the concept that the mind and body are inextricably related. It aims to build on some of the elements brought up in the earlier section on biotypology, most notably the work of Sheldon and Kretschmer. These biotypical models attempt to express the potential or predisposition of an individual both somatically and emotionally. They analyse the whole body morphology, rather than responses to particular events. This potential is then moulded by the environment and situations to which they are exposed to create a unique combination of mind and body.

It is the outcome of effects of the moulding from other sources that is explored here. Some of the concepts that have been utilized over the last century to rationalize this relationship were introduced. The chapter has focused most particularly on the mechanisms through which this relationship occurs, as opposed to the manner in which one would treat such situations, because the approach of this book is primarily conceptual rather than practical. The link between the concepts and their application is something that will have to be experienced clinically with the supervision of a tutor.

The theories explored were discussed with regard to their chronology. However, just because one approach has been superseded by another does not mean that the earlier one is now redundant. Most conceptual models can be kept 'current' by incorporating the new levels of understanding as they arise. In the practice of medicine in its broadest sense, there are very few absolutes, and this appears to be particularly true in the approach to the psyche. Currently there is an enormous range of different therapeutic psychological approaches, each having a degree of success. It has been the aim of the author to scratch the surface of some of the major approaches, in the hope that you will find one that resonates with you as a person and as a practitioner, and which will enable you to formulate some ideas behind the psychoemotional contribution to the whole.

In the author's opinion (JSP) the most important skill that can be learned within this field is that of listening. This is not just hearing the words, and then jumping in with your ideas of how any problems can be solved, but listening with the intent of understanding. You need to create an environment in which the patient feels comfortable in expressing what they want to express, and thereby allow them to create their own associations and answers. Where they are having difficulties in doing this, rather than telling them what they need to do, ask them a question that will start their minds thinking again.

Whatever way you choose to apply this knowledge, helping someone to evolve emotionally as well as physically is perhaps one of the most rewarding aspects of our job.

References

1. Littlejohn JM. Psychology and osteopathy. J Osteopath 1898; July:67–72.
2. Lipowski ZJ. What does the word 'psychosomatic' really mean? A historical and semantic inquiry. Psychosom Med 1984; 46(2):153–171.
3. Dunbar HF. Bodily changes: a survey of literature on psychosomatic interrelationships:1910–1933. New York: Colombia University Press; 1935.
4. Breuer J, Freud S. Studies on hysteria. In: Strachey J, ed. The standard edition of the complete psychological works of Sigmund Freud, vol 2. London: Hogarth Press; 1955.
5. Glassman WE. Approaches to psychology. Buckingham: Open University Press; 2001.
6. Carroll R. The motoric ego, thinking through the body. 1999. Online. http://www.thinkbody.co.uk/papers/motoricego.htm 13 July 2003.
7. Buhl HS. Autonomic nervous system and energetic medicine: bioenergetic and psychosomatic causes for health and illness. Online. http://www.orgone.org/articles/ax2001buhl-a.htm 5 July 2003.
8. Eiden B. The use of touch in psychotherapy. Self & Society Magazine 1998; 26(2):3–8. Online. http://www.chironcentre.freeserve.co.uk/articles/useoftouch.html 7 July 2003.
9. Heath D. Bodywork and the psyche, psychotherapy and the body. Online. Available: http://www.uktherapists.com/articles/lifestream/1998/7/03.htm 5 July 2003.
10. Latey P. The muscular manifesto, 2nd edn. London: Philip Latey; 1979.
11. Latey P. Feelings, muscles and movement. Journal of Bodywork and Movement Therapies 1996; 1(1):44–52.
12. Bernard C. Les phenomenes de la vie, vol 1. Paris: J-B Baillière; 1878.
13. Cannon WB. The wisdom of the body. New York: Norton; 1932.
14. Butler DS. The sensitive nervous system. Australia: Noigroup Publications; 2000.
15. Selye H. The stress of life. New York: McGraw-Hill; 1976.
16. Holmes TH, Rahe RH. The social readjustment rating scale. J Psychosom Res 1967; 11:213–218.
17. Sheridan CL, Radmacher SA. Health psychology, challenging the biomedical model. New York: Wiley; 1992.
18. Sterling P, Eyer J. Allostasis: A new paradigm to explain arousal pathology. In: Fisher S, Reason J, eds. Handbook of life stress, cognition and health. New York: John Wiley; 1988.
19. McEwen BS. Protective and damaging effects of stress mediators. New Engl J Med 1998; 338:171–179.
20. McEwen BS, Stellar E. Stress and the individual mechanisms leading to disease. Arch Intern Med 1993; 153:2093–2101.
21. Akerstedt T, Gillberg M, Hjemdahl P et al. Comparison of urinary and plasma catecholamine responses to mental stress. Acta Physiol Scand 1983; 117:19–26.
22. Karasek RA, Russell RS, Theorell T. Physiology of stress and regeneration in job related cardiovascular illness. J Human Stress 1982; 8:29–42.
23. Manuck SB, Kaplan JR, Adams MR et al. Studies of psychosocial influences on coronary artery atherosclerosis in cynomolgus monkeys. Health Psychol 1995; 7:113–124.
24. Rozanski A, Bairey CN, Krantz DS et al. Mental stress and the induction of silent myocardial ischaemia in patients with coronary artery disease. New Engl J Med 1988; 318:1005–1011.
25. Seeman TE, McEwen BS, Singer BH et al. Price of adaptation – Allostatic load and its health consequences. MacArthur Studies of Successful Ageing. Arch Intern Med 1997; 157:2259–2268.
26. Kendall N, Linton S, Main C. Guide to assessing psychosocial yellow flags in acute low back pain: Risk factors for long-term disability and work loss. Wellington: ACC and National Health Committee; 1997. Online. http://www.acc.co.nz/injury-prevention/back-injury-prevention/treatment-provider-guides or http://www.nzgg.org.nz/library/gl_complete/backpain2/purpose.cfm#contents 16 Sept 2003.

27. Gold P. Neurobiology of stress. In: Willard FH, Patterson MM, eds. Nociception and the Neuroendorine-Immune Connection. Athens: University Classics; 1994.

28. Selye H. The stress of life. Revised edn. New York: McGraw-Hill; 1978.

29. Willard FH, Mokler DJ, Morgane PJ. Neuroendocrine-immune system and homeostasis. In: Ward RC, ed. Foundations for Osteopathic Medicine. Baltimore: Williams and Wilkins; 1997.

30. Watkins A, ed. Mind body medicine. New York: Churchill Livingstone; 1997.

31. Melzack R, Wall P. The challenge of pain, 2nd edn. London: Penguin Books; 1988.

32. Oschman JL. Energy medicine. Edinburgh: Churchill Livingstone; 2000.

33. Latey P. Maturation – the evolution of psychosomatic problems: migraine and asthma. Journal of Bodywork and Movement Therapies 1997; 1(2):107–116.

34. Keleman S. Emotional anatomy. Berkeley: Center Press; 1985.

35. Comeaux Z. Robert Fulford DO and the philosopher physician. Seattle: Eastland Press; 2002.

Recommended reading

Brooks RE, ed. Life in motion: the osteopathic vision of Rollin E. Becker, DO. Portland: Rudra Press; 1997.

Brooks RE, ed. The stillness of life: the osteopathic philosophy of Rollin E. Becker, DO. Portland: Stillness Press; 2000.

Comeaux Z. Robert Fulford DO and the philosopher physician. Seattle: Eastland Press; 2002.

Glassman WE. Approaches to Psychology, 3rd edn. Buckingham: Open University Press; 2000.
A good basic introduction to the various theories in psychology, very readable.

Kline N. Time to think, listening to ignite the human mind. London: Cassell Illustrated; 1999.
An excellent book that explores how to listen effectively, very strongly recommended.

Latey P. The muscular manifesto, 2nd edn. London: Philip Latey; 1979.
Almost impossible to obtain, hence all of the journal references below:

Latey P. Feelings, muscles and movement. Journal of Bodywork and Movement Therapies 1996; 1(1):44–52.

Latey P. Maturation – the evolution of psychosomatic problems: migraine and asthma. Journal of Bodywork and Movement Therapies 1997; 1(2):107–116.

Latey P. Basic clinical tactics. Journal of Bodywork and Movement Therapies 1997; 1(3):163–172.

Latey P. The balance of practice. Journal of Bodywork and Movement Therapies 1997; 1(4):223–230.

Latey P. Complexity and the changing individual. Journal of Bodywork and Movement Therapies 1997; 1(5):270–279.

Latey P. The pressures of the group. Journal of Bodywork and Movement Therapies 1998; 2(2):115–124.

Latey P. Curable migraines: part 1. Journal of Bodywork and Movement Therapies 2000; 4(3):202–215.

Latey P. Curable migraines: part 2, upper body technique. Journal of Bodywork and Movement Therapies 2000; 4(4):251–260

Watkins A, ed. Mind body medicine. New York: Churchill Livingstone; 1997.
A good introduction to PNI.

Chapter 8

The respiratory–circulatory model of osteopathic care

INTRODUCTION

'The rule of the artery is supreme' is one of Still's most often cited principles. It was later modified to the more globally inclusive 'The movement of the body fluids is essential to the maintenance of health'. Fluid bathes our whole body. Many of us tend to think initially of the blood in the arterial and venous system as the major fluid system in the body. This, however, accounts for only 8% of the total body fluid. Body fluid accounts for 60% of the total body weight of a human, which is 42 L of fluid. Of this, 40%, or 28 L, is intracellular fluid and 20%, or 14 L, extracellular fluid. The blood represents just 5 L.[1]

The fluids serve a multiplicity of tasks. They carry the nutritional requirements such as oxygen and glucose to all of the tissues of the body, and then bear away the waste products such as lactic acid and carbon dioxide.

They can be seen as the mediator of the humoral communication systems that are essential for the defence of the body and the maintenance of homeostasis. The cellular elements of the immune system are conveyed within the vascular system and can pass into the extracellular fluid when required. The humoral communication messengers of the neuroendocrine immune system, the hormones, neurotransmitters, cytokinins, etc., are all transmitted via the fluid systems.

The lymphatic system, though often seen as a separate entity, is also a part of the total fluid system. It has two major roles. It transmits the fatty fluids from the gastrointestinal tract (GIT), and the interstitial fluid that escapes from the capillaries, back into the cardiovascular system. It also has a major role in the defence of the body, with mobile 'surveillance' elements, such as the lymphocytes, circulating the body and destroying or producing antibodies to any foreign substances; and static organs through which the fluids have to pass and through which medium foreign substances are removed.

It also has a role in support and protection. Fluid fills the fascial cavities, 'inflating' them, and thereby offering structural support to the area both locally and to the body globally. These fluid-filled cavities act as tensegrity structures, offering protection by causing any forces acting on them to pass equally to the entire surrounding structure, diminishing the overall effect. It can also be seen as a hydraulic support system which can buffer the supported structures from any external forces, such as the cerebrospinal fluid (CSF) protecting the central nervous system.

MOVEMENT OF FLUIDS

Fluid passes to every cell, even when there are no vessels or obvious passageways for it to get there. The only obvious pump for the circulation of the fluids is the heart, which acts on the arterial system. Circulation of the extra- and intracellular fluids, lymph, venous blood and CSF depend on a complex interplay of the soft tissues and the resulting pressure changes in the body. On a gross scale the contraction and relaxation of the thoracic diaphragm in respiration creates a constant cycle of pressure changes throughout the body. As the diaphragm moves inferiorly on inspiration there will be a relative increase in pressure below the diaphragm and a relative decrease above. Increase in pressure tends to 'squeeze' fluids out of tissues; as the pressure is decreased it will cause fluids to be 'sucked' into the tissues. This helps the perfusion of these tissues. Similarly any movement of the body will be transmitted through the extracellular tissue matrix, torsioning and shearing the planes of the tissues, creating 'wringing out' effects on the tissues right down to a cellular and intracellular level.

To aid these two actions the body is organized into a series of fascial compartments on both a local level, creating multiple small spaces, and a global level with the cranial, thoracic and abdominopelvic cavities. Transmission between these fascial compartments, or even from extracellular to intracellular, is dependent on pressure gradients. Where the appropriate pressure gradient is disturbed there will be a disturbance in the flow of fluids, resulting in a relative decrease in perfusion in areas of high pressure, and stasis in areas of low pressure. Thus an increase in the pressure of the abdominopelvic cavity will result in a relative hypoperfusion in the organs and tissue contained therein, but as the pressure gradient between the lower extremities and the pelvis has increased, there may be insufficient pressure within the lower extremity return mechanisms to overcome this gradient. Consequently, fluids will tend to pool in the lower extremities, both in the venous system and in the tissues and extracellular spaces, and stasis will ensue. With decrease in perfusion there will also be a reduction in all of the physiological effects of the fluid: nutrition, communication, elimination, etc.

Other mechanisms of aiding the return of fluids are the contraction and relaxation of striated muscles and of the smooth muscle of the alimentary canal in peristalsis. As they are contained in a fascial envelope, this will cause an alternating pressure within the envelope, moving the fluids along. There will also be an effect on the neighbouring soft tissue structures in their envelopes, creating similar changes in the fluids. The movement of fluid is assisted by the valves in the lymphatic system and parts of the venous system. When the pressure is increased in a cavity, fluid will be pushed along the vessel, but it will be prevented from dropping back with the following decrease in pressure, by the action of the valves.

The inherent motility of cells, tissues and organs will also have an effect on the fluid dynamics.

The various diaphragms are also thought to have a great influence on the circulation of fluids. The thoracic diaphragm has already been mentioned. The plantar fascia is thought by some to act as a gentle pump, being active when walking. The remaining diaphragms, the pelvic floor, the thoracic inlet (Sibson's fascia), and the tentorium cerebellae with or without the diaphragma sella, are more generally seen as possible areas of restriction to fluid flow if dysfunctioning.

It will be noted that fluid movement is dependent on pressure and movement of tissues. If a local somatic dysfunction occurs, it will often result in local hypomobility and an increase in tension in the associated soft tissues. This will automatically result in a local decrease in tissue perfusion which will result in relative hypoxia and decrease in all of the physiological functions mediated by the constituents carried in the fluid.

Gross disturbances of the body, such as postural problems, will disturb the balance of pressure between the cavities and will therefore have a dramatic effect on the circulation of all of the fluids of the body, and consequently a global physiological effect. This is described by Littlejohn in the anterior and posterior weight types, Goldthwait in *Body Mechanics* and Kelman in *Emotional Anatomy*.[2,3,4]

Pressure and mobility are not the only factors affecting fluid exchange. Others include osmolar gradients and the electrical potential of particles,[5] to mention just two; however, the obvious importance of the factors discussed earlier and their accessibility to manual therapists make them predominantly important.

Inherent in many treatment approaches is the concept of restoring mobility and thereby restoring fluid exchange. The general osteopathic treatment (GOT) is an approach that cites this as one of its key aims, and this is discussed in the next section. Some of the approaches within the involuntary mechanism are based on fluid movement, such as the CV4 which is thought of as a compression of the fourth ventricle which encourages CSF exchange, amongst other stated benefits. The osseous structures themselves may be visualized as being composed of a sea of molecules rather than as a rigid structure, permitting work on an intraosseous level; again the rationale behind involuntary approaches is discussed in Section 3.

Another approach that is perhaps more conceptual than practical is that of Gordon Zink's Respiratory–Circulatory Model of Osteopathic Care. The practical application of this draws on a series of approaches including articulation, high velocity thrust (HVT) and indirect work such as fascial unwinding, or cranial techniques. It can be seen as a conceptual model, the application of which can be adapted by the practitioner depending on the patient's needs, biotype, state of health and the practitioner's abilities.

THE RESPIRATORY–CIRCULATORY MODEL OF OSTEOPATHIC CARE

J Gordon Zink was an American osteopath and educator based at the Des Moines College of Osteopathic Medicine and Surgery in Iowa (until he died in 1982).

It would appear that he was influenced by the strong emphasis that AT Still placed on the role of the body fluids and particularly the lymphatics: 'your patient had better save his life and money by passing you by as a failure, until you are by knowledge qualified to deal with the lymphatics'.[6] Another great influence was FP Millard who developed a systematic approach to evaluate and treat the lymphatic system.[7] Zink's respiratory and circulatory model can be seen as an expansion of Millard's work. The other major influence was WG Sutherland, most notably his work on the primary respiratory mechanism and fluid fluctuations.

The key feature of Zink's model is that for health (or homeostasis) there must be good circulation of all of the body fluids; this will ensure that there is proper nutrition and drainage of the tissues right down to a cellular level. This represents the circulatory part of the name.

In order to achieve this, the respiratory processes must be working efficiently. Of prime importance is the 'respiratory suction pump', by which he means the action in respiration of the thoracic diaphragm, the thorax and the lungs. He describes it as a 'three way' suction pump; air, venous blood and lymph being aspirated by it.[8] This pump is therefore working synergistically with the 'pressure pump' of the heart to ensure the circulation of the body fluids. This is the respiratory aspect of the title.

The concept as a whole is best described in Zink's own words.

Respiration and circulation are unifiable functions. The need for establishing 'normal respiration', which is diaphragmatic when the patient is resting in the supine position, is obvious when we consider the fact that most of the volume of blood is found in the venous reservoir. This low pressure system is dependent on pressure differentials in the body cavities for effective flow, because there is no assistance from the muscles, which are aptly called 'peripheral pumps'. The cardiogenic aspect of circulation depends on the respirogenic aspect of circulation to complete the circuit. But that is not all; the most important feature is the fact that the 'terminal' lymphatic drainage into the venous system is also dependent on the effective diaphragmatic respiration when the patient is resting.[9]

Another element that was thought by Zink to be essential to the body's physiological respiratory mechanisms was the primary respiration described by Sutherland. Particular attention was paid to the freedom of movement of the cranial and pelvic diaphragms, and their relationship with the thoracic diaphragm, and articular mobility of the sacrum between the ilia. The primary respiration is therefore supporting the secondary respiration and its thoracoabdominal pelvic pump, these two working in synergy with the heart.

THE COMMON COMPENSATORY PATTERN (CCP)

The pattern as described by Zink and BA TePoorten[10] is based on the junctional areas between the three body parts, the cranium, thorax and pelvis. These junctions are the upper cervical complex, the thoracic inlet, the thoracic outlet or thoracolumbar junction, and the lumbosacral complex. These areas are mobile and vulnerable to dysfunction and they each have a diaphragm associated with them and a relationship with the ANS. This is shown in Table 8.1.

The four diaphragms are, as already mentioned, important in the movement of both body fluids and air by producing pressure differentials within the body cavities. They are considered the main rotational/torsional components in the body's compensatory pattern. Besides being connected to the junctional areas of the spine, the diaphragms are also linked with the longitudinal connective tissue continuity of the body. Distortion of the diaphragms would introduce a myofascial torsioning of the longitudinal fascial continuity, and their function as a vascular pathway of the body would be disturbed.

Thus any fascial torsion will affect the fluid circulation of the body and therefore compromise its health. The common compensatory pattern (CCP) represents a series of myofascial torsions that are compatible with physiological function. Simply stated, if the diaphragms are rotated in alternating directions it indicates compensated physiological function (Fig. 8.1).

Zink also described another physiological pattern which is a series of myofascial torsions that are rotated in alternating directions but opposite to that of the CCP; it is also compatible with physiological function. As it is relatively rare it is termed the uncommon compensatory pattern (Fig. 8.2).

If the fascial torsions are found on testing not to be rotated in alternately opposite directions it indicates a non-compensatory pattern. This is not physiological and therefore compromises the respiratory–circulatory integrity of the body and its normal function, predisposing the individual to disease. This should be resolved to restore a physiological compensatory pattern. This can be achieved by addressing the osseous attachments of the diaphragm utilizing a direct approach, or by addressing the fascia by an indirect approach, or by a combination of the two.

Table 8.1 The relationship between the junctions in the common compensatory pattern in Zink's respiratory–circulatory model

Junction	Spinal level	Related diaphragm	Autonomic action
The upper cervical complex	C0–C3	The tentorium cerebellae and the falx cerebri (also part of the RTM)	PSNS
The thoracic inlet	C7–T1	The thoracic inlet diaphragm (Sibson's fascia)	SNS
The thoracic outlet	T12–L1	The thoracoabdominal diaphragm	SNS
Lumbosacral complex	L5–S1	The urogenital or pelvic diaphragm	PSNS

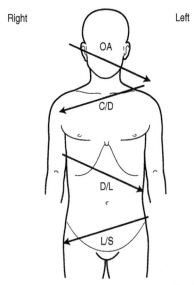

Figure 8.1 The common compensatory pattern (CCP), the specific finding of alternating fascial motion at the diaphragms of the junctional areas of the body as described by Zink. (Modified after Glossary of osteopathic terminology. Chicago: American Association of Colleges of Osteopathic Medicine; 2002.)

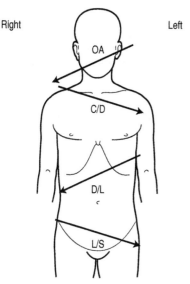

Right   Left

Figure 8.2   The uncommon compensatory pattern: the specific finding of alternating fascial motion at the diaphragms of the junctional areas of the body opposite to that of the CCP. (Modified after Glossary of osteopathic terminology. Chicago: American Association of Colleges of Osteopathic Medicine; 2002.)

BA TePoorten describes the structural pattern of dysfunction that is to be found in the CCP.[10] He advocates that these dysfunctions should be resolved and suggests that, once this is achieved, most of the associated problems should be resolved.

1. Pelvic torsion with the left inominate being posterior and the right anterior with a consequent left elevated pubic tubercle.
2. The sacrum is in a left on left torsion.
3. Right rotation and left side-bending of the lumbosacral articulation.
4. The thoracolumbar junction is left rotated and side-bent.
5. The tenth rib is held in inspiration, being inferior and posterior.
6. Rib five is in inspiration and anterior to its left equivalent. The fifth thoracic vertebra is in extension and right rotation.
7. The third thoracic vertebra is right rotated causing the left rib to be anterior.
8. The first rib is elevated on the left.
9. The first and second thoracic vertebrae are rotated to the right.
10. The upper cervical complex (C2) is in side-bending right and left rotation.

A BRIEF DISCUSSION OF THIS MODEL

Using Zink's (and TePoorten's) compensatory and non-compensatory patterns in evaluation and management of patients has many advantages. First of all, it is inclusive, which means that your approach to the patient is global, not focal. It is relatively descriptive: the sequencing allows you to approach patients who are acutely ill or hospitalized. Where, after your examination, you do not understand the chaos of findings, following the descriptors will take care of approximately 80% of the body's dysfunction. The model focuses on respiration and circulation, crucial factors in restoring and maintaining health. It acts as a sort of American GOT.[11]

Within Europe many would find this prescriptive treatment approach anathema. However, that does not invalidate the fascial torsion patterns and the consequences that this will have on the fluid exchange. Perhaps a more flexible treatment approach will enable this useful conceptual model to be applied more widely.

CONCLUSION

This is a very short section, in essence dealing purely with Zink's Respiratory–Circulatory Model of Osteopathic Care. This is included here as the model has at its roots a very simple concept, that of correct breathing being of great importance in completing the cardiac cycle and thus ensuring the optimum perfusion of the body's tissues. At first glance it appears to be somewhat naïve and, with TePoorten's model, prescriptive. However, if you take on board the concept underpinning the model, and then incorporate it into the conceptual models that you already have, it becomes an interesting and important and perhaps different perspective that will add to the efficacy of your treatment. An immediate example that is cited about Zink's treatment is that he utilizes a HVT to ring the fluid out of the tissues, not a thought that would immediately have sprung to mind.

Little has been said here about CSF circulation and cranial treatment. It is addressed slightly in Section 3, but as there is a plethora of articles currently available on this subject, and the concepts are changing very rapidly, a search on the web for the most recent concepts would be more appropriate than anything written here.

References

1. Guyton AC, Hall JE. Textbook of medical physiology. In: Royder JO. Fluid hydraulics in human physiology. J Am Acad Osteopath 1997; 7(2):11–16.
2. Wernham J, Hall TE. The mechanics of the spine and pelvis. Maidstone: Maidstone College of Osteopathy; 1960.
3. Goldthwait JE, Lloyd T, Loring T et al. Essentials of body mechanics in health and disease, 5th edn. Philadelphia: JB Lippincott; 1952.
4. Keleman S. Emotional anatomy. Berkeley: Center Press; 1985.
5. Royder JO. Fluid hydraulics in human physiology. J Am Acad Osteopath 1997; 7(2):11–16.
6. Still AT. Philosophy and mechanical principles of osteopathy. Kirksville: Journal Press; 1902: 105.
7. Millard FP. Applied anatomy of the lymphatics. Kirksville: Journal Printing; 1922.
8. Zink JG. Applications of the holistic approach to homeostasis. AAO Yearbook; 1973.
9. Zink JG. Respiratory and circulatory care: The conceptual model. Osteopathic Annals 1997; March: 108–112.
10. TePoorten BA. The common compensatory pattern. The Journal of the New Zealand Register of Osteopaths 1988; 2:17–19.
11. Fossum C. Personal communication; 2003.

Recommended reading

Little is written on Zink's model other than the articles referenced here; these are of interest. For an historical perspective Millard's book makes interesting reading.

Millard FP. Applied anatomy of the lymphatics. Kirksville: Journal Printing; 1922.

Chapter 9

The total osteopathic lesion

INTRODUCTION

The total osteopathic lesion is a concept that underpins the entire practice of osteopathy. It is founded on the humanist perception of care, looking at the patient as a whole person, the sum of their mind, body and spirit, and being aware of all of the influences, both internal and environmental, to which they are subject in everyday life. Then by assessing their import and impact on the patient, trying to determine how these factors may be contributing to the specific complaint that the individual has consulted you about and their response to these influences generally.

HISTORICAL PERSPECTIVE/ORIGINS

It is possible to see in the writings of AT Still that he saw humankind from more than just a somatic perspective. He stated that 'man is a triune when complete',[1] a triune being an integration of the mind, body and spirit, and that the duality of the mind and body was an intellectual fabrication.[2]

We know from his students that Littlejohn's teaching was based on this more global perspective from as early as 1905. He taught that 'adjustment was the fundamental principle of osteopathy, [and] that its application embraced every conceivable form of structural, functional or environmental maladjustment that might affect the human organism'.[3] The structural element included all of 'the skeletal and articular problems, and also to include the soft tissues, the intercellular and intracellular structures in an attempt to affect the tissues on an atomic level'. Functional was the 'chemical change in the structures', and as these structures are made up of biochemical elements there must be adequate nutrition. The environment included the 'air, sunshine and psychic stimuli'. He believed that 'biochemistry or nutrition, psychology and environment [were] equally important links of the chain of osteopathic theraperutics'.[3] It is fascinating to reflect on the breadth of his conception and how advanced his ideas were.

The total lesion concept was reified by HH Fryette in 1954.[4] He studied at the Littlejohn College in Chicago, and was therefore exposed to Litlejohn's ideas. He also drew on the concept that Dr AD Becker had originated in the late 1920s which he termed the 'total structural lesion'. This consisted of 'the primary structural lesion plus all of the resulting mechanical complications and compensations, and that all of these related mechanical factors should be thought of as one mechanical lesion and should be considered en masse'.[4] This definition is very much rooted in the structuromechanistic approach that was current at that time.

Fryette expanded on Becker's total structural lesion, incorporating a broader range of factors. He dropped the word structural from the name, being content just to use 'total lesion'. The total lesion is 'the composite of all the various separate individual lesions or factors, mechanical or otherwise, which cause or predispose to cause disease from which the patient may be suffering at the moment. These factors may vary from corns to cholera, from "nervousness" to insanity'.[4] This clear statement reiterated those concepts that are tacit in the writings of Still, and placed osteopathy firmly in the realms of holism.

THE TOTAL OSTEOPATHIC LESION

The word osteopathic became incorporated some time later, so that now it is generally referred to as the total osteopathic lesion. It is often represented schematically by a Venn diagram (Fig. 9.1).

The terms utilized in such a Venn diagram vary from author to author. A selection of commonly occurring ones are listed below; however, whatever terms are used, the principle of the triune is the same.

- Mind, body, spirit
- Psychology, biomechanics, physiology
- Emotional, physical, chemical
- Neural, mechanical, chemical.

As can be seen from Figure 9.1, the terms psychological, mechanical and physiological have been used, with some degree of subdivision. The central area, where all three circles overlap, represents the combined influence of these three factors to which the individual is subject. The circles can be perceived as the internal expression of these groupings. The whole of this is surrounded by the environment. This exerts an overruling influence, which can affect the individual via any or all of the three groupings. We will now look at each of these aspects in greater depth.

THE ENVIRONMENT

The environment is perhaps one of the most influential elements. Reflecting on the concepts expressed in biotypology, there are certain characteristics of a biotype that are immutable, referred to as the 'constitution' or 'somatotype'. However, the 'temperament' defines those aspects that can change. Vannier states that it is the dynamic state of an individual 'which represents the sum of all the possibilities of the subject – physical, biological, psychological, psychic and dynamic. During the life of the human being their temperament alters, either getting better and better, or, thwarted by environment or illness, becoming progressively weaker until the characteristic signs of disease appear whether physical, biological, mental or psychological'.[5] It can be seen from this that Vannier shared the holistic approach that underpins the total osteopathic lesion and understood the key role that the environment performs in sculpting the individual in health and disease.

Our interaction with the environment occurs on several different levels. On the physical level, this includes the manner in which the body is used at work or recreationally, and what traumata, micro and macro, acute and chronic, it is exposed to through these and other sources.

Psychosocially, we all exist in a collection of settings, i.e. family, work, racial, religious and recreational settings. Each of these will shape our psychoemotional attitude, and will be overlain by the influence of the current zeitgeist. Elements of these will be constructive, such as an excellent support network of friends and family, and others destructive: divorce, trouble with the boss. Early

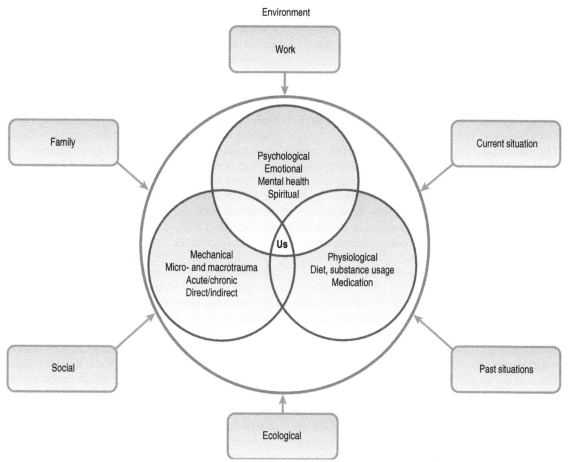

Figure 9.1 The total osteopathic lesion. The central portion represents the individual and the spheres of experience to which she is exposed.

influences are often critical as they are the foundations on which we are built. An obvious and extreme example of this is the changes that occur as a result of child abuse. Abused children develop defensive behaviours to keep them safe in the threatening environment, but these learnt behaviours are generally not discarded and continue into adult life. This has ramifications socially, in their interactions with others, physiologically, affecting the neuroendocrine function, and structurally, with actual structural changes occurring in the brain.[6] Abuse is an extreme example, but any stressor will have an effect physiologically and if protracted, structurally, as demonstrated by Selye's GAS.

Our spiritual interaction with the environment, both religious and non-religious, has dramatic effects on our bodies and minds. Anyone who has

cared for the terminally ill will have observed the profound difference in behaviour, on all levels, between those 'at one' with the world, their God or their belief system, and those who are not. Again, this is an extreme example but it illustrates the point and can be applied to less extreme situations accordingly.

Many of these elements shape the way that things are perceived. Someone brought up in a rural environment will have different perceptions of life from someone in the city. In the city, the pace of life is very fast; in the country the pace is generally slower (though this distinction is becoming less marked). People working on the land are in tune with the seasons, whereas many city workers are more in tune with the opening of the Stock Market. The authors, having lived and worked as osteopaths in both environments, became aware that the expectation in the city is of an immediate response; in the country they are generally happy to wait for it to mature. Though a sweeping generalisation it merits consideration.

THE INTERNAL ENVIRONMENT

Three groupings have been utilized: mechanical, physiological and psychological.

The mechanical grouping generally reflects the musculoskeletal system and its prime coordinator the nervous system. Causes of dysfunction can be direct via trauma and posture, or indirect, by psychological or physiological problems. Dysfunction in this area will be reflected in changes in these systems, be they pathological processes, functional disturbances or habitual posture. It is subject to such aspects as biotype, age and gender. Problems here will also have an effect on the other two groupings, at the most basic level via the reflexes, i.e. somaticovisceral, and somaticopsychic, or through the much more complex communication systems that exist, as were discussed in the earlier chapters on psychology and neurology.

Physiology is reflected in the endocrine and immune systems and their interaction with the visceral and nervous systems. The function of these systems may be affected by diet, intake of alcohol/cigarettes, exposure to invading pathogens, psychoemotional state/stress, genetic predisposition, etc. Similarly there are innumerable interconnections between this grouping and the other two.

Psychological factors arise from a multitude of sources. They can often be linked to external events such as stress from home/work life. However, there is some evidence for endogenous disturbances or attitudinal factors contributing to a psychological well-being (or not). 'Spiritual' has also been included within this group – it is a difficult element to define, but having a philosophical belief system does appear to influence people's way of being, and therefore, in many subtle ways, their health. It is also worth reflecting that some of the more rigid spiritual systems may actually have detrimental rather than beneficial effects.

APPLICATION OF THE MODEL

This model can be applied aetiologically, in the sense that it can make one look at the causative and maintaining factors, such as somatic dysfunction, poor diet, or a recent divorce. Or it can be applied more in a functional way, to explore the changes that will be occurring in each of these areas as a result of a certain situation, such as an increase in catecholamine secretion, panic attacks or premature osteoarthritis.

The more you look at this, though, the more these boundaries blur. For example, a hypertensive individual will have internal mechanical factors such as the loss of elasticity of the arterial walls due to increasing age. However, these changes will probably have been accelerated by the stress arising from a demanding job. Is the problem internal or external? In actuality, each problem is multifactoral, and with the hypertensive there will be physiological and psychological factors, but with effects arising from both internal and external sources. This, however, is the strength of this model. It causes one to explore any problem from several perspectives and in doing so it will make explicit the complex interplay and influences that are at work.

This blurring of the boundaries is reflected in contemporary research (discussed earlier) which is tending to 'put the systems back together again'. Terms reflecting the interdependence of the systems are being used, such as the neuromusculoskeletal system, neuroendocrine-immune system, and psychoneuroimmunology.

Bearing the above in mind, problems with either structure or function, internal or external influences, psychological, physiological or mechanical will possibly lead to somatic dysfunction within that individual. The challenge presented to the osteopath is to work out what is the principal cause of this dysfunction. To do this one has to have as full a knowledge as possible of the patient's medical history in its broadest sense including illness, trauma, emotional state, and a full picture of their biomechanical state.

The Venn diagram representing this has one major failing, in that it just represents a moment in time, inadvertently tending to focus one's mind on the *current* situation. However, the individual's whole life is important. This should include past stresses occurring in any of the groupings, with an understanding of the duration (short or long term) and the possible consequences, to try to establish possible lasting effects that may have occurred, thus creating a clinical temporal profile (i.e. a profile of the insults to which the body has been subject, chronologically organized). Figure 9.2 is an attempt to illustrate this concept.

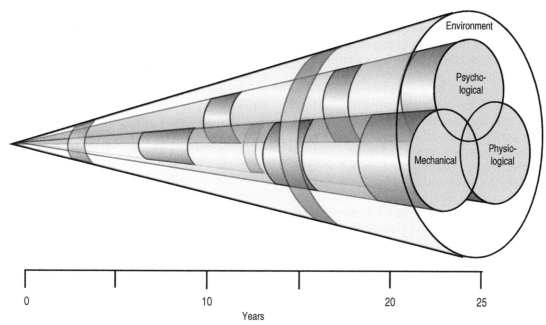

Figure 9.2 A schematic representation of the total osteopathic lesion over time. The shaded areas show periods of stress in each of the possible areas over the individual's lifetime.

FRYETTE'S ILLUSTRATION OF THE SUMMATIVE EFFECTS OF THE TOTAL OSTEOPATHIC LESION

Fryette demonstrated one method of interpreting this model. He utilized a very simple but useful example to illustrate the clinical consequences of a constellation of essentially minor problems, affecting different spheres of an individual, and how the summation of these might result ultimately in death![4] He also posed the profound question, what was the cause of death? Before attempting his illustration he stated that every individual will have their own particular ability to deal with various types and amounts of stressors. Then he set out the concept that each individual has a resistance point, a point beyond which they will die. For the purpose of discussion he chose 1000 units as the critical point. An individual who suffers a tooth infection may suffer 100 units as a result of this. However, the worry over this costs him 200 units, and the medication100 units (Fryette, like many of the early osteopaths, was against the use of medication).

This long-suffering individual was also subject to a sacroiliac strain, causing lumbago and sciatica, at a cost of 200 units, and for good measure he was docked 50 units for dietary deficiencies and 50 units for endocrine deficiencies. So at this point in time his total lesion is 700 units.

A final 200 units of fatigue and 200 units of pneumonia cause him to exceed his 1000 unit limit and, sadly, he dies. The death certificate states that he died of pneumonia. Fryette proposes that he did not really die of pneumonia, but of the summation of each of the contributing factors.

If the individual in question had received treatment from a psychologist, homeopath, osteopath, allopath, etc., each would have 'looked for their own pet lesion', but in so doing, if even one practitioner was able to relieve even part of the load, it might have been sufficient to enable the body's self-healing faculties to return him to relative health without further help.

COMPARISONS WITH OTHER CONCEPTS AND MODELS

One very simple analogy can be drawn between the above and the concept of the facilitated segment. To summarize briefly, the facilitated segment depends on the concept of 'all or nothing'. For a neurone to transmit an action potential a stimulus needs to be sufficient to exceed the threshold potential of that neurone. If it is not sufficient, even by the smallest of amounts, there will be no response. However, background neural activity can elevate the resting potential of the neurone, so that a lesser stimulus is required to elicit a response. Thus it has become facilitated or potentiated. With regard to the total osteopathic lesion, the summation of stressors is 'facilitating' the body. As a consequence, something that would normally be a relatively insignificant problem may, in the facilitated individual, be most detrimental to their health.

Selye's triphasic model of stress also offers an interesting comparison (Fig. 9.3). Fryette's example is terminal, which would equate to Selye's exhaustion phase; this is associated with frank disease, irreparable system damage and eventual death. However, Fryette alludes to the fact that if intervention occurs at an appropriate time the whole process can be reversed. This would equate to the adaptive stage. This stage is characterized by diseases of adaptation such as hypertension, ulcers, impaired immune function and asthma.

In this phase, homeostasis is still able to return the individual back to normal. The majority of patients that European osteopaths see are in this adaptive stage. Therefore anything we can do to reduce their 'load' will enhance their chances of recovery. We can utilize any of the osteopathic tools and approaches, but also aspects that may not be thought of directly as 'osteopathic treatment', such as compassion, listening, dietary advice. It is not uncommon when treating a patient who has multiple problems for them to return after a treatment, amazed at the fact that you have resolved one of their problems which, in their mind, is unrelated to the problem for which they consulted you. It may have actually resolved, but often it has only been silenced by taking one level of stress out of the system, which will have an effect on 'global stress'. Drawing on the facilitated segment analogy, this global reduction in stress may allow some of the coexisting complaints to drop below their 'symptomatic thresholds' and therefore become asymptomatic. However, they are still potentiated and unless the body is now able to continue to defacilitate itself, or further treatment is applied to reduce other elements of the individual's total lesion, the problem will recur the next time a stressor affects the body.

Fryette's interpretation could be seen as a rather pragmatic illustration of the concepts of A-Bechamp and C-Bernard, generally termed the Cellular theory (compare with Pasteur's Germ theory). This proposes that we are exposed to potential pathogens at all times, but that they only become pathogenic due to the effects of stressors such as somatic dysfunction, psychological or social problems, or poor diet affecting the 'terrain' of the body, adversely lowering its inherent resistance to the pathogen. Thus the summation of the stresses leads to a greater vulnerability to illness, which further increases the demands, leaving the patient more vulnerable.

A final analogy that is sometimes useful in the conceptualization of the total osteopathic lesion is that of a battery. We, like a battery, have a quantum of energy; it is rechargeable but not inexhaustible. In a normal healthy state there are processes that sustain life and a regular pattern of behaviour that demand a certain amount of the available energy. These include all of the vital functions, and those activities that we do in everyday life: working, socializing, in fact all of those aspects of day-to-day living. This requires only a certain amount of energy, so the remaining or 'spare' energy is available for general well-being and any exceptional demands. This is, in fact, the ideal situation. This individual will exhibit good health and has the capacity and interest to respond to new situations and challenges as they arise. Even if the body is occasionally 'pushed hard' by working long hours and playing hard, they still have reserves. The atypical demands of a particularly heavy session would be absorbed within the physiological processes described in Selye's alarm stage. Homeostasis, however, would still be achieved (see Fig. 9.4).

If we draw on Fryette's example, and this individual gets a tooth infection, the defence processes are mobilized to counter the infection, but they do so at the expense of the spare energy. Continuing with Fryette's example, the associated worry and the toll taken by the medication will further deplete

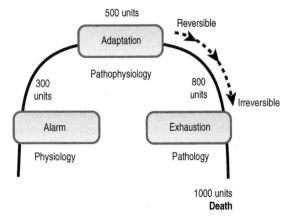

Figure 9.3 The total osteopathic lesion compared with Selye's general adaptation syndrome.

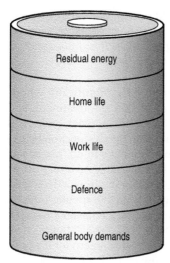

Figure 9.4   The battery in the ideal situation. Plenty of residual energy is available for unusual demands and to enjoy life and its challenges.

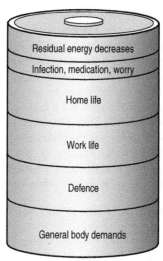

Figure 9.5   Additional demands of worry, infection and medication reduce the residual energy.

the spare energy. This individual will still appear relatively healthy; however, they will be more easily fatigued, and will be less open to challenges or spontaneous suggestions. They will also be more susceptible to passing infections and be more aware of their own problems on somatic and emotional levels. If this situation continues, and they do not modify their habits, they will enter a downwardly spiralling cycle of behaviour. This stage would equate to Selye's adaptive phase. See Figure 9.5.

If another stressor is added, for example a work promotion, increasing the pressure of work, this will use up the remaining spare energy. The person can still function, but they have now become potentiated – if there is another demand, this person will have insufficient energy to cope with it, and their systems will fail generally. They will not necessarily die, as in Fryette's example, but may suffer a debilitating problem. Postviral syndrome, chronic fatigue or myalgic encephalitis are classic examples of such a problem. Centralized sensitization would also fit in with this scenario. Anything requiring an effort, be it physical or emotional, would be avoided, and if they were unavoidable the individual would expend what would appear to be a disproportionate amount of energy. If this continued it would represent Selye's exhaustion phase. See Figure 9.6.

As with many of these examples this has been exaggerated to illustrate a point. In the above example the nature and number of stressors is unlikely to result in the dire consequences we have penned for

our subject. However the principle is the relevant point.

THE PRACTITIONER AS PART OF THE TOTAL OSTEOPATHIC LESION

It is of interest to reflect on our role as practitioners in the therapeutic situation. As people, we too have our own total osteopathic lesions, and though the

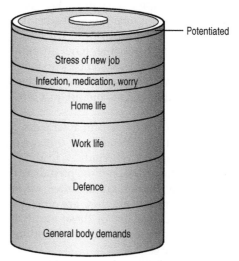

Figure 9.6   Potentiated. This is on the cusp of the exhaustion phase: another stressor may result in serious pathological change.

contractual agreement is that we are paid to treat the patient, in reality the position is not quite so clear cut. We cannot fail to interact with the patient. Healing does not occur in a vacuum – it is an exchange between two (or more) individuals, each contributing in subtle ways to the ultimate outcome. When it works well it is a fantastic and invigorating experience for both. However, it is possible, if you are not careful, for the patient to get no better *and* to cost you vital energy. It is important to acknowledge that practitioners are humans, and as such, are as vulnerable as any other humans.

FACTORS THAT MAY INFLUENCE THE THERAPEUTIC OUTCOME

Before looking at the deficit side of the equation, it is perhaps better to look at the ideal situation, and for a change to look at it principally from a therapist's perspective. For a good therapeutic exchange to occur, the environment should be one in which the practitioner feels comfortable. This will differ from practitioner to practitioner. One example could be an environment that is not too clinical and that has been personalized in some way, such as with family photographs, or choosing the paintings for the walls.

The practitioner's health, both physical and emotional, is important. Just as the patients can be seen as 'batteries' with charge left or not, so too are practitioners. If your battery is running flat, you will run the risk of harming yourself and generally will not even be helping the patient. Without wanting to sound like a popular guide to good health, it is important to have a fulfilling life outside of osteopathy. Also, if possible, have an emotional support network, or at least someone to whom you can say *'Bloody patients!'* and they understand that you *do* care for the patients but are just letting off steam.

It is also beneficial to have an awareness of ourselves as individuals. We all have our own belief systems and prejudices. Prejudices in themselves are acceptable, but acting on those prejudices causes them to become discrimination. Often we are not aware of our prejudices, they are unconscious. Trying to be more aware of these and bringing them to a conscious recognition will help us to be non-discriminatory.

Wherever possible we should be able to have an 'unconditional positive regard' for our patients. Carl Rogers writes:

the therapist experiences a warm caring for the client – a caring which is not possessive, which demands no personal gratification. It is an atmosphere which simply demonstrates 'I care'.[7]

This is particularly significant when 'intention' is being used within the treatment, as in some involuntary mechanism work, where there is no direct contact with the dysfunction being treated, but rather the practitioner's mind 'reaches in' to achieve the effect. This is working on a very deep level within the patient, and coming from a deep level within the practitioner. If your therapeutic intention is to, for example, release the mediastinal fascia, the patient's body will 'hear' *'relax, relax'*. But if you do not have unconditional positive regard for the patient the message may be mixed with a background grumbling of *'I don't like you'* or possibly worse. Whatever we think or feel about patients will be unconsciously conveyed, often giving their bodies mixed messages. If there is a true antipathy between the patient and practitioner, which is very rare, it is probably better to make the clinical decision not to treat that individual, as it will rarely benefit patients to treat them under such circumstances, plus the attempt will probably cost the practitioner a lot in energy.

Another aspect of self-awareness that is interesting to explore, is 'Why do you want to practise as an osteopath?'. Or, perhaps more directly, 'What do you get out of it?'. There are an infinite number of worthy reasons. We shall briefly explore just one aspect and look at both the positive and negative aspects of it.

Carl Jung discussed the archetype of 'The Wounded Healer'. Its imagery immediately caught the imagination of many writers and philosophers, with the concept often being applied to those in the caring professions. The imagery originates with the Greek myth of Chiron, a centaur who was unable to treat an incurable wound in his own knee, and by way of overcoming the pain of his own wounds he became a compassionate healer, physician and teacher. Many of us have incurable wounds, be they physical or emotional, and we will perhaps seek some solace in helping others. This can have truly beneficial effects, perhaps giving a greater level of empathy and compassion that will ultimately enhance our practice of osteopathy. However, it can occasionally have a less beneficial side. An example of this is the 'need to be needed'. This can develop insidiously with both patient and practitioner feeding it. To know you can make someone better is a great feeling; however, the clue to the problem that can arise is in the preceding sentence. We do not *make people better*, the patients make themselves better, we just help by signposting the way. If we take responsibility for someone's health, we are not helping the patient, we are creating a dependency. The patient becomes dependent on you as a practitioner. The fact that you are needed and respected by someone can be intoxicating, but will not in the long term help the patient. The patient needs to understand the problem and its ultimate resolution as their own problem. We are there to help them, and their body, to this. Conveying this to the patient does not have to be done in hushed and reverent tones, it can be conveyed with humour and with the use of metaphors and examples, usually the more bizarre the better. As cited above we need to demonstrate a 'caring which is not possessive, which demands no personal gratification'. We want our patients to get better, but there should be no personal investment in the outcome. This will be better understood as you progress in clinical experience.

PRACTICAL APPLICATION OF THE TOTAL OSTEOPATHIC LESION

With the massive amount of potential elements to consider within a total osteopathic lesion approach, it is possibly difficult to see how it can be applied. This section will attempt to address this to some extent.

The importance of a well-taken case history cannot be exaggerated. It is necessary to observe and note the patient's gender, biotype and habitual posture, ask their age and then obtain information on the presenting complaint. In addition they should be asked about their current state of health, reviewing all of the major systems, and their social situation, such as family situation, work, hobbies and stresses. Sensitive topics do not have to be broached in the initial case history session, but can be explored whilst treating or later when trust has been established. With this we can begin to construct a 'picture' of their current stressors.

This establishes the present situation; however, to get a more complete picture it is necessary to include past stresses, both somatic and psychic. Explore the nature, severity and duration of each incident, and discover whether it was a one-off situation or intermittently recurring, and by doing so to try to establish any possible lasting effects that may have occurred.

This will eventually result in a clinical temporal profile of the patient's somatic and psychic insults. With this it is possible to begin to estimate the total osteopathic lesion of the patient and their potential vitality; additionally it will begin to give some understanding of the aetiology of the presenting complaint and possible avenues open to address them.

It is worth reflecting on the fact that we rely on the self-healing nature of the body to respond to the guidance of our treatment – this in itself is going to demand energy from the body. In one whose total osteopathic lesion is 'potentiated', the treatment needs to be sufficiently non-demanding of energy so as not to destabilize the patient and cause adverse reactions to the treatment. In such cases it may be appropriate to firstly address secondary issues that are less demanding energetically. This could be resolving the secondary compensation for the primary rather than addressing the primary directly; reducing global stresses by giving advice about posture and the set-up of computer work stations; or refer to another practitioner such as a counsellor to resolve psychological stress before undertaking the course of treatment.

This will potentially 'free up' some energy to permit the primary problem to be resolved safely without further stressing the patient.

The concept of the total osteopathic lesion allows us to understand how a combination of load factors or stressors contributes to the overall state of health. The role of a competent practitioner is to recognize these and to address as many of these problems as possible, being aware of our own skills and limitations and making appropriate referral where necessary. This aspect of treatment can also be considered to be preventive medicine, in that correct application of the model will mean that treatment is not just symptom-led but actually aiming to improve the health of the patient. Symptoms are poor indicators of health; the fact that a symptom resolves does not mean the problem has resolved, but that it has gone below its symptomatic threshold. Awareness of this will mean that treatment should be aimed at resolving the total osteopathic lesion as far as possible, thereby improving their health and leaving them less vulnerable to future stressors.

This really does highlight the importance of understanding the problem holistically, and making an accurate diagnosis. TE Hall states that a 'fundamental point which is often overlooked in our teaching is that seventy-five percent of technique is diagnosis'. From this point of understanding we can begin to unravel the complex interrelated problems and chip away at them bit by bit.

CONCLUDING THOUGHTS

The body is slowly being put back together. It is now more than 350 years since René Descartes offered his mechanistic basis for the philosophical theory of dualism. Slowly this has been challenged. JC Smuts (1870–1950) was the founding father of holism; he derived the word from the Greek 'holus' meaning 'whole'. He first wrote about holism in 1912 in his unpublished book *Inquiry into the Whole*. With the advances in theoretical physics, such as Einstein's theory of relativity and quantum mechanics, he was able to root the philosophical concepts of his early writings in this new science. The results of this were published in 1926 in *Holism and Evolution*.[8] He saw the world as an organic unity, a web of relations, where the transitions between matter, life and mind became fluid.[9] His concepts are often summarized somewhat simplistically as, 'the whole is more than the sum of its parts', and 'if one part of the whole changes, this will have an effect on the whole'. Also implicit within this concept is that by examining the parts it is not possible to understand the parts.

These concepts were taken further by Ludwig von Bertalanffy (1901–1972). He developed the general systems theory (GST), describing it as

A general science of wholeness ... The meaning of the somewhat mystical expression, 'The whole is more than the sum of its parts' is simply that constitutive characteristics are not explainable from the characteristics of the isolated parts. The characteristics of the complex, therefore, appear as 'new' or 'emergent'.

The strength of this system is that the methodology is valid for all sciences. 'There appears to exist general system laws which apply to any system of a particular type, irrespective of the particular properties of the systems and the elements involved.'[10] The GST focuses on the complexity and interdependence of elements within systems.

Bertalanffy described the body as being an open rather than a closed system. A closed system is self-sustaining and can exist independent of the environment. The human requires sustenance from the environment, such as food and oxygen, and is such an open system. We are also dependent on innumerable other elements within our environments including physical and emotional elements. Health is dependent on a correct balance of all of these factors. Open systems are naturally entropic; however, this tendency is resisted by the homeostatic mechanisms. When these mechanisms fail, possibly due to an imbalance between the factors, entropy prevails and illness results.

Systems are organized hierarchically, and are mutually interdependent: cells are dependent on all of the systems of the body for nourishment but the systems are dependent on the cells; the individual is dependent on the environment, but we have control of our environment. Changes in one affect the other. This is reflected in the synergistic concepts within tensegrity, and perhaps more importantly the understanding that humans are just a point on the tensegrity continuum passing from the level of atoms through societies and eventually to the universe. We cannot view ourselves as apart from all of these systems, and as such, there will be a mutual interdependence between us and them.

As the notion of an independent physical entity has become problematic in subatomic physics, so has the notion of an independent organism in biology. Living organisms, being open systems, keep themselves alive and functioning through intense transactions with their environment, which itself consists partially of organisms. Thus the whole biosphere – our planetary ecosystem – is a dynamic and highly integrated web of living and nonliving forms. Although this web is multileveled, transactions and interdependencies exist among all its levels.[11]

The total osteopathic lesion (TOL) is the osteopathic way of attempting to express elements of this, and to relate them to the onset of disease. Perhaps the diagram should be modified to include the hierarchical levels of systems with which we interact, to remind us of the various levels within which we interact. Children seem to be more aware of their place in the grand scale of things. The author can remember writing in his school books, 'Jon Parsons, Sexey's Boys School, Bruton, Somerset, England, UK, Europe, The Earth, The Universe'. Adults often appear to lose this awareness, and focus on only that which is immediately accessed. This lack of awareness of these system superstructures and the reciprocal relationships may account for the current ailing state of society, and the ailments caused thereby. For osteopathy to be truly effective in the pursuit of health these concepts need to be considered.

This book has split up the osteopathic concepts and rationale in an attempt to facilitate the understanding of the ideas contained within. However, the clinical application of these concepts should make an attempt to bring the concepts to bear as a united whole. Treatment, stated simply, is just an attempt to reverse diagnosis. We construct a diagnosis from all of those aspects of the total osteopathic lesion, current and past. Then we model the dysfunction from our structural, neurophysiological and fluidic understanding of somatic dysfunction, and try to understand the complex physiological mechanisms that may be perpetuating the problems via the PNI or neuroendocrine immune systems. By understanding the needs of the patient, their biotype and general state of health, an appropriate treatment approach can be considered, including referral if necessary. The treatment is 'just' to assist in reversing all of the above!

References

1. Still AT. Philosophy of osteopathy. Indianapolis: American Academy of Osteopathy; 1899: 11–42.
2. Still AT. Osteopathy research and practice. Reprint 1910 edn. Seattle: Eastland Press; 1992:xvii, 13–14.
3. Comstock ES. The larger concept (editorial). Journal AOA 1928; (Feb):463–464.
4. Fryette HH. Principles of osteopathic technic. Reprint. Colorado Springs: American Academy of Osteopathy; 1980: 41.
5. Vannier L. Typology in homoeopathy. Beaconsfield: Beaconsfield Publishers; 1992: 3.
6. Teicher MH. Scars that won't heal: the neurobiology of child abuse. Scientific American 2002; March: 68–75.
7. Rogers CR. On becoming a person. London: Constable; 1967.
8. Smuts JC. Holism and evolution. Cape Town: N&S Press; 1926.
9. Benking H, van Meurs M. History, Concepts and Potentials of Holism. Online. http://www.newciv.org/ISSS_Primer/asem09js.html 7 Feb 2004.
10. Bertalanffy L von. General system theory: foundations, development, applications. New York: George Braziller; 1968.
11. Fritjof C. The turning point. New York: Simon & Schuster; 1982.

Recommended reading

Little is written directly on the total osteopathic lesion; the texts below are included as possible sources of information that may inform the concept rather than describe it.

Brooks RE, ed. Life in motion: The osteopathic vision of Rollin E. Becker, DO. Portland: Rudra Press; 1997.
Brooks RE, ed. The stillness of life: the osteopathic philosophy of Rollin E. Becker, DO. Portland: Stillness Press; 2000.
Comeaux Z. Robert Fulford, DO and the philosopher physician. Seattle: Eastland Press; 2002.
Fryette HH. Principles of osteopathic technic. Reprint. Colorado Springs: American Academy of Osteopathy; 1980.

Oschman JL. Energy medicine. Edinburgh: Churchill Livingstone; 2000.

Systems theory has much to offer in terms of a global model and for dealing with complexity – which with some effort and interest could be beneficially applied to the conceptualisation of osteopathy within the scientific world and, in fact, the world in general. It is easy to find information on the internet though the most useful site I have found is the Principia Cybernetica website, http://pespmc1.vub.ac.be. This has many easily understandable notes plus fundamental books and articles that can be freely downloaded.

SECTION 3

Introduction to models of diagnosis and treatment

In this section the more commonly used models of osteopathic treatment will be described. It is not intended that these descriptions are by any means a 'comprehensive licence to practise' but merely an outline guide as to the basics and variations between them. At the end of many of the treatment model discussions is a suggested reading list to take the reader into a full and deeper understanding of these approaches.

TREATMENT APPROACHES

The broad range of treatment modalities available is there to enable you to be selective in your treatment approach. There is a way to treat everybody and every complaint, not necessarily to resolve it, maybe just to palliate in some conditions. The diagrams in Figures S3I.1 and S3I.2 attempt to demonstrate the range of approaches available, and that to an extent, they are on a continuum. Within this approach continuum, each modality is also on its own continuum, being able to be applied differently depending on the desired effect, shifting along the structure, function, energy continuum of Figure S3I.1 as necessary. The change can be via a physical change in the way of applying an approach, or it may be in the intention behind the approach.

Another way of conceiving technique approaches and their application is demonstrated in Figure S31.2. This, once again, expresses the continuum or variation of application of the two broadest means of classification of osteopathic technique: direct and indirect or structural and functional. Each can be applied either maximally or minimally according to the patient's requirements and the desired outcome. The treatment approaches themselves will be discussed in the following section and a brief discussion on factors determining their choice is to be found in Chapter 33.

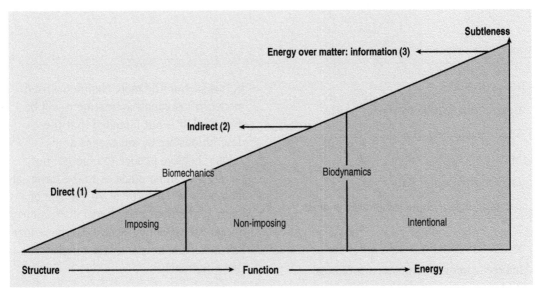

Figure S31.1   The treatment continuum. This diagram expresses the full range of treatment approaches available. The following section focuses primarily on the left two-thirds of the diagram. This is because a thorough grounding in these approaches is necessary before attempting to work at the energetic level, and though touched on within this book, many of the energetic approaches would be considered postgraduate and therefore beyond the immediate scope of this book. (With permission from Fossum C. Lecture notes. Maidstone: Unpublished; 2003.)

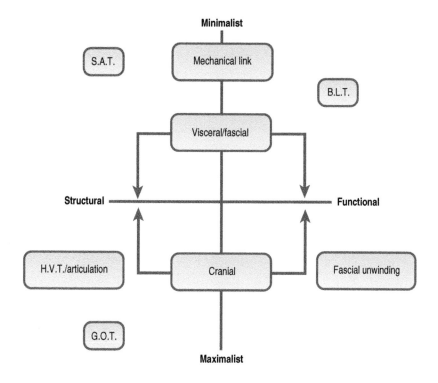

Structural
Involve taking the dysfunctional unit in the direction towards the restricted motion barrier until a state of pretreatment tension is obtained, followed by some degree of force to overcome the restriction (thrust, articulation, muscle force)

Often referred to as direct techniques
Minimalist
Treating the whole through its parts. Embraces the concept of finding the 'primary' or 'Still' lesion as the source of all the other compensatory and adaptory lesions, and correcting it with minimal intervention

Functional
Involve taking the dysfunctional unit in a direction away from the restricted motion barrier until a state of balanced tension is obtained

Often referred to as indirect techniques

Maximalist
Treating the parts through the whole. Several areas, or often the whole body, are treated to integrate the functional, mechanical and neurogenic / physiological functions of the body

Figure S31.2 The structure/function, minimal/maximal treatment axis. (With permission from Fossum C. Lecture notes. Maidstone: Unpublished; 2003.)

Chapter 10

General osteopathic treatment

INTRODUCTION

The general osteopathic treatment (GOT) is a system of treating the body of the patient as a whole. It allows the osteopath to perform a total body treatment, hence its alternative name, the total body adjustment (TBA). For the purposes of this book, it will be referred to as GOT. However, the name 'general osteopathic treatment' is misleading in that it tends to imply that the treatment is non-specific which, in reality, could not be further from the truth.

The GOT as practised currently in the UK and much of the rest of Europe was first introduced by some of the early British pioneers of osteopathy, JM Littlejohn, TE Hall and J Wernham, and as a technique routine it has developed and continued more in Europe than in America. However, some of the early American osteopaths used a system of working through the whole body, mobilizing every joint from head to toes. Unverferth[1] wrote of the realization that the general treatment enabled the treatment of 'hayfever, asthma, various allergic conditions, goiter, and various gynaecological conditions by manipulative measures alone'. He stated that the objective of the general treatment was 'to normalise the haemopoietic system' and 'to normalise the machinery of elimination'. Unfortunately, the early osteopaths using this general treatment felt that it was almost an admission of inferiority, as Unverferth states 'its greatest value lies in the fact that it can be used by the physician who has not yet mastered the art of skilful, specific adjustive treatment' and that until that mastery is reached 'it were best if we stuck to intelligent general treatment'. However, he goes on to state 'Dr AT Still was osteopathy's foremost artist in the application of specific adjustment, nevertheless, in all his writings he strongly urged general treatment'. It should be noted here that the references to 'specific adjustment' is not referring to 'specific adjusting technique' which will be discussed later.

Over the years, like any good method of treatment, the general osteopathic treatment has been adapted with progress, but the underlying principles remain more or less the same. Obviously, the body has not changed in structure or function since the initial inception of the GOT but our knowledge of the body's physiological functioning has improved.

Tom Dummer,[2] in his *Textbook of Osteopathy*, defined the GOT as follows:

> *The underlying principle is expressed in the words Mechanical Organic Adjustment and osteopathy may be described as a system of treatment that uses the natural resources of the body in the corrective field for the adjustment of structural conditions in order to stimulate the proper preparation, and distribution, of the fluids and forces of the body, and to promote cooperation and harmony in the body as a mechanism. We believe that healthy tissue depends on the correlation of blood and nerve supply. We believe that practically all pathological conditions are associated with interference, or obstruction, to nerve and blood supply. The osteopathic lesion is represented by anything that gives rise to interference, or obstruction to these great and major forces in the body, involving misplacement of structure, alteration in the relation of one structure to another, or change in the condition of the cells.*

The GOT is a routine of treatment that encompasses the complete structure of the body with respect to its physiological function. In other words, it uses a corrective articulatory force in order to influence the aforementioned correlation of blood and nerve supply. When talking of blood supply we can extend this further to include the venous and lymphatic drainage systems. To many there seems no better way to treat the structure and function of each individual patient than a total body routine.

ARTICULATORY TECHNIQUE

This is sometimes called simply 'articulation' though this may confuse the reader with the alternative name for joints of the body or articulations. In contrast to high velocity low amplitude (HVLA) techniques (described later) this is a low velocity high amplitude (LVHA) technique. It involves taking a joint through its complete range of motion in a fairly slow but controlled manner. It is aimed at restoring joint mobility and reducing soft tissue tension around the joint being 'articulated'. In addition, it promotes drainage of the soft tissues and thus reduces inflammation. Furthermore, it is said to have a positive feedback effect on the proprioceptive mechanism of the joint concerned, restoring better biomechanical balance. As with an HVLA technique it is performed actively by the practitioner whilst the patient has a passive role.

There is a continuum within the principles of the GOT that permits examination, diagnosis and treatment to blend together (Fig. 10.1).

With respect to the aforementioned continuum, if we articulate the foot, we begin our procedure as a general articulation that allows us to test the foot, i.e. examination. By assimilating the information gathered from this examination we are able to make a diagnosis of the structures articulated. If, for example, we find that there is a restriction between the talus and the navicular, further specific articulation at this joint will then become treatment. It is in this fashion that the GOT loses its generality and becomes a highly specific treatment that can then be applied to the whole body. Nevertheless, the important case history, examination and diagnosis related to a particular presenting complaint with respect to differential diagnosis and possible contraindications to treatment will not be overlooked.

Unfortunately, some practitioners who use the GOT have demoted it to a kind of warm-up before the 'real treatment' begins. It is often used as a general loosening preamble to the high velocity thrust (HVT) techniques.

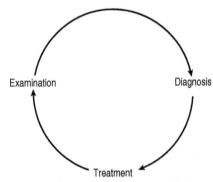

Figure 10.1   Examination – diagnosis – treatment.

HIGH VELOCITY THRUST (HVT)

This is a manipulation technique used by many practitioners of manual medicine and its roots certainly date back to Hippocrates (400 BC) and probably to ancient Thailand and Egypt possibly 4000 years ago.[3,4] This particular technique has been seen throughout many osteopathic texts under various names. In Britain and Europe for many years it was known as high velocity thrust technique or HVT and it was performed in order to 'manipulate' or 'correct' a lesion – thus it was often referred to as a correction or manipulation technique. However, in the USA and more recently in other parts of the world it is referred to as HVLA technique or 'high velocity low amplitude technique', which describes it better. *The Foundations for Osteopathic Medicine*[5] text book terms it HVLA or 'high velocity low amplitude' technique and describes it as 'a direct technique which uses high velocity/low amplitude forces; also called mobilization with impulse treatment'.

The aim is to restore normal joint mobility to a restricted joint, vertebral or otherwise. This is achieved by the careful application of a force by using either long or short levers. An example of a long lever technique would be using the limbs in order to assist force localization at a particular lumbar vertebral level; 'short levers' may be induced by the manipulator's hands working directly about a restricted joint.

An audible 'click' or 'pop' is often heard and is considered by some to be an indication of a successful manoeuvre. Though pleasing for the manipulator and sometimes also for the patient alike, it seems to many that the sound is irrelevant and that the true indicator of a successful technique is a palpable change in the range of motion, usually accompanied by a reduction in sensitivity of the region concerned.

The origin of the 'click' is also open for discussion and the latest theories tend to agree that it is due to a cavitation or vacuum phenomenon taking place within the synovial cavity of the joint. In other words, there seems to be a brief, transitory change of synovial fluid from the liquid to a gaseous state. Radiographic examination of joints undergoing manipulation does tend to support this idea.[6,7]

In fact, if the GOT is performed accurately and specifically there may be less need for HVTs, if any at all. Furthermore, it could be considered that HVTs without adequate soft tissue and joint preparation are a little barbaric, as could be the overuse of HVTs. It would be, like trying to run a marathon or play a game of tennis without first doing some stretching to prepare the tissues, potentially harmful. Therefore, if the GOT is used by some only as a warm-up, then at least not all is lost. However, the authors are of the opinion that the GOT is a highly specific treatment in its own right that may or may not be augmented by other modes of treatment depending on the individual patient's needs and the appropriate clinical decision making of the individual practitioner.

John Wernham was a student of John Martin Littlejohn and wrote of Littlejohn's proposed 10 principles of the general osteopathic treatment.[8,9] They are:

- routine
- rhythm
- rotation
- mobility
- motility
- articular integrity
- coordination
- correlation
- stabilization
- mechanical law.

Routine

The treatment follows a regular procedure that allows both the patient and the practitioner to relax. Having a routine to the treatment means that the whole body may be treated without neglecting areas. By following a routine, the practitioner is able to measure the progress or decline of the patient's condition. It also allows preparation and education of the body's tissues.

Rhythm

The practitioner must be aware of the presence of rhythms within both the body of the patient and his/her own body. By working with the patient's own individual rhythm, the practitioner is able to easily notice any alterations of rhythm. These may present as tension, rigidity, oedema, toxicity or altered function in joint muscles or other bodily tissues. It is considered important to locate arrhythmia and to normalize rhythms without imposing the practitioner's own rhythm onto the patient. Having stated this, the GOT may be used to stimulate or to inhibit, and this may be achieved by an increase or decrease in the applied rhythmic articulatory technique.

Rotation

All movements of the articulations are in a rotatory fashion and by using the limbs as long levers it is possible to work in a rotatory manner by circumducting the joints through their full range of normal motion.

Mobility

Mobility is essential at both a cellular and a gross level and it follows that any loss or reduction of mobility sets up the process of reduced function, altered structure and therefore a diseased state. Mobility testing is a method of uncovering dysfunction and the articulatory techniques rely on the introduction of mobility to the restricted areas. This form of movement is considered to be under a voluntary control.

Motility

This is a form of movement that is considered not to be under voluntary control. Although Littlejohn did not speak directly of the 'cranial rhythmic impulse' he was aware that there was an underlying involuntary movement to the brain and spinal nervous tissues.[10]

Articular integrity

The shape of the joint, muscle tone and ligamentous tension all contribute to the integrity of an articulation. The muscles are generally under voluntary control whereas the ligamentous tension is not. The key to the restoration of articular integrity is through mobility and motility.

Coordination

This refers to the ordered balance of the various systems which brings unity to the body. There is also the coordination of the practitioner and patient during the treatment.

Correlation

This is more subtle than coordination and refers to the interdependence of structures upon one another whether they are organs or regions within the musculoskeletal framework. In order to function, a structure requires a nerve supply but in addition, it needs to be 'fed and cleaned' and so the correlation of innervation, nutrition and drainage is considered important.

Stabilization

It is the coordination and correlation that provide the stabilization of the body with respect to homeostasis. The normalization of homeostasis is one of the primary aims of the GOT.

Mechanical law

These are the laws established from the scientific study of motion and force and refer to Littlejohn's system of body mechanics.

When viewed from a purely mechanical standpoint, the GOT aims to restore mobility to articulations that have reduced movement, which should be of benefit to the body's overall functioning. However, when we consider the effect that we may have on the neural reflexes, we can see that the treatment offers far more than an improvement in mobility. When we consider the effect of improved vascular and lymphatic function, it is clear that the treatment will not just affect the musculoskeletal system.

The rhythmic, rotatory techniques employed in the GOT routine are aimed at improving mobility of fluids within the body, and reducing stasis. The long lever articulatory techniques are directed from the periphery towards the centre to improve lymphatic and venous drainage. When working on the axial skeleton, the leverage is focused to each vertebral level, including the pelvic articulations, in order to improve mobility to specific restrictions. An area of restriction in the spine may be having an effect on the neural reflexes at that level and so particular attention is paid to the levels important in the autonomic outflow.

SPINAL CORD LEVELS AND VERTEBRAL LEVELS

Due to the development of the central nervous system, the spinal cord and vertebral column are much the same length until the third month of fetal life, after which the vertebral column lengthens more rapidly than the spinal cord.[11] At birth, the tip of the spinal cord or conus medullaris lies at about the L3 vertebral level and, in the adult, at about L1/2[12] (see Fig. 10.2). As an example of this difference, the nerve roots exiting from the eighth thoracic spinal cord segment level remain within the vertebral canal and descend slightly therein to their vertebral exit level of T8. Those nerve roots from the lower part of the

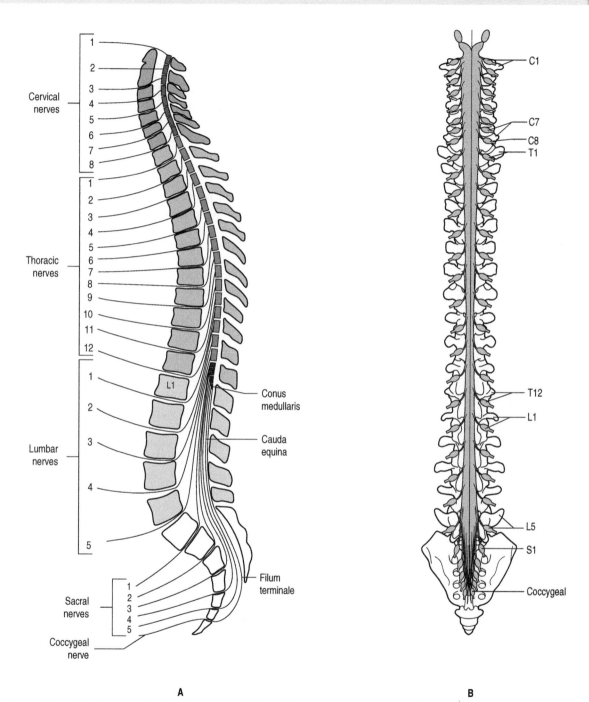

A   **B**

Figure 10.2   (A) Lateral view showing spinal nerves. (B) Dorsal view showing spinal ganglia. The lateral view of the vertebral column shows the relative length of the spinal cord in the adult. Note how on descending the vertebral column, the spinal nerves have to descend within the vertebral canal to reach their corresponding exit levels. The dorsal view of the vertebral column has the vertebral arch removed to reveal the dural sac. (From Kahle W, Leonhardt H, Platzer W. Colour atlas of human anatomy, vol 3. Nervous system and sensory organs. New York: Thieme Medical Publishers; 1993. Reprinted by permission.)

spinal cord, i.e. from L2 and below, form the cauda equina (horse's tail) descending within the vertebral canal to their respective vertebral exit levels. If this was not confusing enough, although it is accepted to speak of spinal cord segments, in actual fact, the spinal cord is not truly segmented. It is a continuous structure and it is only the clumping together of the nerve rootlets to form nerve roots that exhibits the remaining marks of embryonic segmentation. Nevertheless, a nerve root originating from the second lumbar spinal cord 'segment' will descend in the cauda equina and exit from the vertebral canal at the second lumbar vertebral level and will supply, amongst other structures somatic and visceral, the paravertebral musculature corresponding to its exit level.

Much of the GOT is aimed at restoring vertebral mobility. The pelvis is considered to be the seat of normal vertebral function and, in some ways, rightly so. Let us now consider the effects that the GOT may have on improving pelvic function. By articulating the sacroiliac (SI) joints to improve sacral and innominate mobility, not only are we going to make locomotion freer and more fluid but we will in turn affect the structures contained within the pelvis. The pelvic splanchnic nerves of the parasympathetic nervous system exit from the sacral foramina, their spinal cord level origin being the second to fourth sacral segments. The SI joints lie at approximately these levels (first to third bony sacral segments), so any mechanical disturbance may have a feedback to the same spinal cord segments, and cause disturbed neural reflexes at these levels by setting up facilitation from somatic dysfunctions.

There has been a lot of discussion as to how to begin the GOT and many practitioners will start by comparing the levels of the posterior superior iliac spines (PSIS). It has been suggested that if the PSIS on one side is higher, this indicates an anterior rotation of that particular innominate and posterior rotation of the other. In actual fact it could be that the whole innominate is merely shifted up on one side or down on the other, and so it is necessary to check the anterior superior iliac spines (ASIS) to confirm a rotation. For example, if the PSIS on the right side appears higher and the ASIS appears lower on the right side than their corresponding counterparts on the left side, then it may be assumed that there is a forward rotation of the right innominate bone with a corresponding backward rotation of the left innominate. The abbreviated terminology describes this situation as 'anterior right, posterior left' when viewed from behind, which is the normal point of view when testing these structures. Once this diagnosis has been made, the treatment may begin. With the patient supine, many practitioners will begin by circumducting the hip on the higher PSIS side, in other words, on the anterior innominate side. The movement is into an external rotation direction in order to 'posteriorize' the anteriorly rotated innominate. The movement is encouraged by focusing the forces made by the long lever of the leg at the SI joint. This is achieved by placing the fingers of one hand into the sulcus of the SI joint and palpating the movement whilst at the same time encouraging the movement locally with the palpating hand. The opposite movement is performed on the other side, circumduction into internal rotation in order to 'anteriorize' the posteriorly rotated innominate. Some practitioners are less concerned about the direction of circumduction and are more interested in focusing the movement at the SI joint and then allowing the body to take care of the dysfunction rather than forcing or encouraging a particular direction. Some feel that the freeing up of a particular articulation gives the body the 'space' to self correct.

The next stage is to continue the circumduction movement of the hip and to combine the effect of the long lever and the focusing hand to work segmentally throughout the lumbar and lower thoracic spines. This combination of movements aims to 'tease' the tissues into releasing, thereby permitting better segmental mobility.

A similar procedure is then applied to the upper body, this time using the arm as the long lever and focusing with the other hand to enhance mobility to the thoracic spine and costal articulations. The typical ribs articulate posteriorly with the vertebral bodies at the costovertebral joints and the transverse processes at the costotransverse joints. Lying juxtaposed to these articulations are the sympathetic ganglia of the paravertebral ganglionic chain. Anteriorly, the typical ribs articulate with the costal cartilages and thence to the sternum. A variety of handholds allows the practitioner to focus on both the anterior and posterior articulations of the ribs as well as the intercostal muscles. Attention is paid to the articulations of the pectoral girdle and the muscles attached there.

The next procedure is to then apply a series of articulatory and soft tissue techniques to the neck and in particular to the suboccipital region which is considered important for the exit and route of the vagus nerve.

Better purchase and access is afforded to different joints and soft tissues in different positions and so the routine is normally performed in supine, prone and both side-lying patient positions, and on occasions sitting.

The fact that some practitioners neglect the foot and lower extremity, preferring to begin the treatment at the SI joint, would appear to be the cardinal sin of a complete general treatment. The whole idea of the treatment is to treat the whole body and since the lower extremities constitute a part of the body and, furthermore, play an important role in locomotion, it is considered by some that they are doubly important.

One might well ask, how does this series of articulatory procedures to the musculoskeletal system affect the person as a whole and thus constitute a total body treatment? It is apparent that the treatment uses the medium of the musculoskeletal system and in doing so may have a positive effect on its functioning. Osteopaths using GOT will suggest that the rhythmic movements will have an effect on muscle tone and thus affect venous and lymphatic drainage as well as arterial supply throughout the body. Furthermore, specific techniques within the routine are aimed at fluid movements in the body by pumping mechanisms in the region of the lower extremities, diaphragm and pectoral girdle; all are aimed at improving venous and lymphatic return. Attention is paid to the major sites of restriction to lymphatic return, the inguinal regions, the iliac and lumbar lymph nodes and notably the cisterna chyli at around the level of the diaphragm. As the lymph has to pass through the thorax, particular attention is paid to all the attachments of the diaphragm and to the subclavicular region where the lymph rejoins the venous circulation. Likewise, as the lymph descends from the head, specific techniques are applied to the routes of the deep and superficial lymph channels.

With respect to the neurological system, the GOT is aimed at restoring mobility to restricted areas and thus reducing unwanted proprioceptive feedback in the form of neural circuits from hypertonic muscles and over-tense ligaments. Furthermore, the specific articulation applied to each of the vertebral segments is aimed at reducing the neurological effects of somatic dysfunctions. In particular, the aim is to normalize the functioning of the sympathetic and parasympathetic nervous systems and thus restore homeostasis. The exit of the vagus in the suboccipital region and its route through the carotid sheath in the cervical region, the thoracolumbar sympathetic outflow from the levels of T1–L2/3 and the pelvic splanchnics in the sacral region are all considered to be affected in the GOT routine.

It has been suggested by some practitioners that the fact that the patient has consulted a so-called holistic practitioner in the first place would indicate that they are expecting a treatment that resembles, at least in the patient's mind, a holistic approach. The GOT will provide a treatment that is not only physiologically holistic but in addition, psychologically so. It is difficult to quantitatively measure the psychological effects of treatment but it is generally accepted that there is an effect of improved 'well-being', to a greater or lesser extent. Although the treatment is a passive patient form of treatment, it does require a certain amount of patient participation after the treatment has been administered. This means that the input made by the practitioner does not stop with the end of the treatment but continues as the body adapts to the changes made. GOT practitioners must, then, take the vitality of the patient into account when performing the treatment (although this should be considered by all practitioners no matter what their preferred approach). Assessing the patient's vitality is important because if vitality is low, too great an input by too demanding a treatment may 'overload' the body's energy resources and create an adverse reaction.

References

1. Unverferth EC. The value of the general osteopathic treatment. Digest by TL Northup. American Academy of Osteopathy Yearbook 1939; 1:11–13.
2. Dummer TG. Textbook of osteopathy, vol 2. Hove: JoTom Publications; 1999: 35–38.
3. Schiötz EH, Cyriax J. Manipulation past and present. London: Heinemann; 1975: 5–14.
4. Greenman P. Principles of manual medicine. Maryland: Williams and Wilkins; 1996: 3–11.
5. Kappler RE. In Ward R, ed. Foundations for osteopathic medicine. Maryland: Williams and Wilkins; 1992: 661–666.
6. Greenman P. Principles of manual medicine. Maryland: Williams and Wilkins; 1996: 99–103.
7. Lewit K. Manipulative therapy in rehabilitation of the motor system. London: Butterworths; 1985.
8. Wernham J. The Littlejohn Lectures, vol 1. Maidstone: Maidstone College of Osteopathy; 1999.

9. Reeve AC. Lecturer of GOT. European School of Osteopathy, Maidstone, Kent. Personal communication; 2004.
10. Littlejohn JM. The physiological basis of the therapeutic law. J Sci Osteopath 1902:3(4).
11. Crouch JE. Functional human anatomy, 4th edn. Philadelphia: Lea and Febiger; 1985: 288–302.
12. Kahle W, Leonhardt H, Platzer W. Colour atlas/text of human anatomy, vol 3: nervous system and sensory organs, 4th edn. New York: Thieme; 1993: 42–43.

Recommended reading

There has not been a great deal of material published on the GOT, and much information has come from 'hand-me-downs'. Littlejohn and Wernham have contributed much to this battery of information with additions made by Dummer and Hall. Some of the early work is written in a form that is sometimes a little difficult to understand, but when deciphered provides valuable information.

A recent book written by a French osteopath, Françoise Hématy, has a lot of the history and principles collected directly from John Wernham himself (although it is a little biased to his particular direction). It contains black and white line drawings of the various procedures and descriptions of each. However, it does commit the cardinal sin: it neglects the feet!

Hématy F. Le TOG Du Traitement Ostéopathique Général: l'Ajustement du Corps. Vannes: Sully; 2001.

A German video entitled TGO is written by French osteopath Bernard Ligner, who is co-principal of the International School of Osteopathy in Vienna.

Chapter 11

Specific adjusting technique

INTRODUCTION

This is a model of treatment that differs from the general osteopathic treatment (GOT) in the sense that it is considered a minimal approach to treatment whereas GOT is considered maximal. Specific adjusting technique or SAT takes into account the idea that there may be a 'positional' element to particular lesions. A positional lesion is one in which an excessive amount of force has caused the lesion and as such, they are usually considered to be of traumatic origin.

The origins of the present day SAT date back to the 1950s when Parnell Bradbury devised a system of treatment that he named 'spinology'. He felt that the two schools of thought at that time that he had contact with placed great emphasis on opposite ends of the spinal column. He felt that Littlejohn (British School of Osteopathy) was overly interested in the pelvis and Palmer (Palmer School of Chiropractic) placed too much interest in the upper cervicals.

History tells us that Bradbury was working in an osteopathic practice and one day, due to staff illness, found himself the only practitioner with a list of 40 patients to see. He treated the patients with a kind of minimalist approach, making only one thrust technique to what he considered the most significant lesion to the patient at that time. He noted that there was a marked improvement in the patients' conditions but especially so in those patients in whom he had addressed the pelvis or upper cervicals. From this point on he concentrated on perfecting this finding into a usable technique. Parnell Bradbury had a close association with Tom Dummer and it is through this association that the approach of SAT has evolved to its present day state. Tom Dummer cofounded the European School of Osteopathy and went on to be its principal. Until his death in 1998 he taught SAT at both undergraduate and postgraduate levels.

In his book, *Specific Adjusting Technique*, Tom Dummer[1] states that Parnell Bradbury 're-discovered' SAT in the sense that it was AT Still himself who 'taught and practised specific structural adjustment'. He goes on to say 'it would appear that SAT is not necessarily a 20th century innovation'. Still is often quoted as saying, 'find it, fix it and leave it alone' where 'it' is referring to the 'osteopathic lesion'. This is the principle underpinning minimal approach to treatment.

It has been suggested that GOT is aimed at the structural type problems whereas SAT is aimed at the functional positional type problems. The positional lesion as described earlier is usually associated with a certain amount of trauma or force, for example the result of a whiplash type injury.' Sometimes this force may be sufficient to move the vertebra beyond the normal physiological limits and then this displacement may be visible on radiographic examination. This positional disruption then becomes the most important factor of the lesion, more so than the mere immobility of the vertebra as addressed in GOT. Associated with this type of traumatic input to the body, there is often an emotional or psychological aspect to the lesionology that is also taken into account. It is the reversal of the components of the traumatic input that not only 'corrects' the structural aspect of the lesion but that may also reach a far deeper level on the emotional aspect.

It has been suggested that positional lesions arise due to excessive force entering the body, often due to accidents, motor vehicle or otherwise. When this force is imposed on the body, it may remain focalized at the point of entry as a type of tension within the tissues affected. Alternatively, the force may be dissipated or shunted through the spinal mechanical system and remain locked up within this system. Dummer[1] states: 'In principle it may be stated that the more traumatic force involved in a given accident the more apparently "structural" or inertia bound the resulting somatic-dysfunction will be'.

By working with the Littlejohn system of spinal mechanics, SAT practitioners have found that the principal areas of the spine that become lesioned by traumatic input are the intermediate pivots in the typical areas of the spine, notably C2, C3, C6–7,

T3–4 and the sacrum. SAT also places great importance on the soft tissue elements of traumatic lesions especially in the cervical region. The soft tissues are considered responsible for the maintenance of the positional lesion and with it the emotional trauma. In examination of the body, Dummer[2] used the three unities (Fig. 11.1) as his basis for diagnosis, examining each in turn and then assimilating the information. He described unity 1 (basically L3 down to the pelvis and lower extremities) as being important for 'locomotion', unity 2 (pectoral girdle, head and neck and down to T4) for 'doing things' and unity 3 (thorax and abdomen between the other two unities) for 'vital functions'. He looked for a primary lesion in each unity and then decided which of these three was the overall primary lesion and which secondary and tertiary.

Commonly, with the SAT approach, the use of radiographic examination is considered of utmost importance for the true assessment of the positional

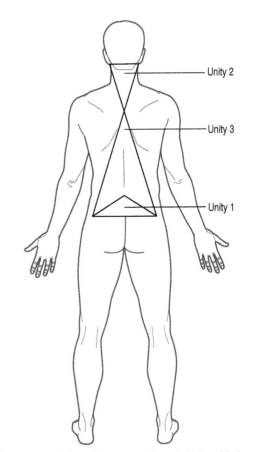

Figure 11.1   Schematic representation of the '3 unities'.

lesion. Often, osteopathy and radiography do not mix in the same way that chiropractic and radiography do. Many osteopaths will only consider radiographic examination when they suspect pathology, fracture or anomalies. Routine radiographic examination is considered by some osteopaths to be an unnecessary exposure of the patient to the harmful effects of X-rays. Furthermore, a radiograph is a static 'split second' moment in the patient's life, a life that is dynamic and progressive. One might consider that a radiograph is akin to a photograph of the inside of a clock: we can see that it is a clock from the structure but it relates nothing to us of its function. Does the clock work? Has it ever worked? Will it ever work? These are questions that the photograph cannot answer. However, radiographic examination does have its uses and one of them seems to be in aiding the SAT practitioners in their assessment of the patient's lesion pattern and, thus, the treatment of that lesion. In their analysis of positional X-rays, SAT practitioners may use rulers and dividers to measure the subtle differences of position of a single vertebra upon another. Here again, critics may say that if the differences are so small as to require measurements in this manner, how does one know that the patient was not merely tilting the head to alleviate discomfort at the moment of the radiological examination? This type of criticism seems justified for a method of assessing a three-dimensional problem with a two-dimensional diagnostic tool. Thomas Dummer answers his critics by stating:

in osteopathy positional X-rays are always only secondary to clinical, manual palpatory procedures. They usually serve the double role of (a) confirming the presence of the positional-lesion already found clinically and/or (b) adding an element of precision to the palpatory findings.[1]

Stating that X-rays are secondary to palpation and then going on to say that they add precision to the palpatory findings seems a little contradictory; nevertheless, SAT practitioners maintain that they gain valuable information from radiographic examination.

Armed with this radiographic back-up to the palpatory findings, the method of treatment is to choose the vertebra to be manipulated and to then apply a technique that will correct the somatic dysfunction. Dummer states that:

The technique employed must be capable of

(a) overcoming the very considerable inertia, typical

to this type of disturbance and

(b) reversing in an exactly opposite sense the 'lesion-pathway' (as it is called) i.e. by executing a corrective arc of movement in order to reverse and normalise the disturbed force-vectors and thus re-establish a normal arc or physiological movement and proprioceptor pattern.[1]

In contrast to traditional high velocity thrust (HVT) techniques, there is no physiological or anatomical locking of the segment to be adjusted. SAT attempts to find a neutral position in which to apply the thrust and the term 'floating field' has been used to describe this neutral point. In order to overcome the positional aspect of the lesion, the thrust applied is 'ultra high velocity' but with an absolute minimum of force. The velocity will overcome the need for force. The thrust should be 'recoil' in nature to prevent tissue damage and to allow the natural recoil of the elasticity of the joint structures to aid in the technique itself. Whilst preparing to line up the vertebra for correction, the practitioner will 'visualize' all the information he/she has regarding the patient, for example, the trauma and the X-ray information. This visualization process prior to manipulation has been termed 'loading the lesion'. This allows the practitioner to 'envisage the corrective arc of movement necessary to retrace and thus release locked-up traumatic force'. Then at the point of thrusting, the practitioner is required to empty his/her mind, allowing the adjustment to be reflex and spontaneous.

The principle behind SAT is that by adjusting the primary lesion, the body will then react to allow any adaptations or compensations that have been set up to normalize. In certain patients, termed functional types, one or very few specific adjustments may be sufficient for their own healing mechanism to react and to complete the healing process. In the more structural type of patient, a series of specific adjustments may be required to normalize any compensations. However, it is the norm for SAT practitioners to adjust only one pivot during each treatment session. After each adjustment, the patient is required to rest for 10 or 15 minutes in order for the body's healing mechanism to commence re-shuffling the complicated compensatory lesion patterns.

Dummer felt that SAT should, where possible, be used exclusive of other modes of treatment. However, he felt that it could be combined with functional or cranial technique and, on occasions, with gentle articulatory techniques. He felt that it should not be combined with the GOT method, since there is the danger of disturbing the compensatory pattern that the SAT input will be working upon. Based upon these considerations, he developed his own form of articulatory treatment, which he named the General Articulatory Treatment or GAT, which he felt could be combined safely and successfully with SAT when the practitioner had a good understanding of the SAT model.

To many casual observers, there seems little difference between the GAT and the previously described GOT. Dummer[3] describes the difference as follows: 'GOT is primarily concerned with normalising the functional–structural integrity of both the articulatory, mechanical and visceral aspects of the whole person, the emphasis in GAT is addressed rather more specifically to normalising the structural aspect, i.e. benign musculo-skeletal pathology'. This would seem to go against the principles of the structural functional relationship but it is exactly this interrelatedness that allows treatment of one system to influence the other.

The SAT routine, though working through a system of spinal mechanics, is not a prescribed 'push-button' system. Patients are reassessed at each visit and although there is often a predictive direction to the treatment it remains flexible and as such may be altered to take in new information either from palpatory findings or from the patient's account of their health since the last treatment.

References

1. Dummer TG. Specific adjusting technique. Hove: JoTom Publications; 1995.
2. Dummer TG. Textbook of Osteopathy, vol 1. Hove: JoTom Publications; 1999.
3. Dummer TG. Textbook of Osteopathy, vol 2. Hove: JoTom Publications; 1999.

Recommended reading

Tom Dummer's Specific Adjusting Technique *is the only published work to date. Dummer's book gives an account of the principles of SAT and an insight into the 'technique itself'. It gives a number of case examples in his own abbreviated form but unfortunately he does not discuss them fully, leaving the reader to sift through to find the relevant information. The text was aimed as an introduction and teaching aid and was due to be followed by a more comprehensive text, unfortunately never published before Tom Dummer's untimely death in 1998.*

Amongst Dummer's other publications, his two-volume Textbook of Osteopathy *gives an insight to SAT and GAT.*

Dummer TG. Specific Adjusting Technique. Hove: JoTom Publications; 1995.
Dummer TG. Textbook of Osteopathy, vols 1 and 2. Hove: JoTom Publications; 1999.

Chapter 12

Muscle energy technique

INTRODUCTION

Muscle energy technique (MET) as recognized by the osteopathic profession owes its thanks to Dr Fred L Mitchell Snr. His work[1] was first published in the 1958 *Yearbook of the American Academy of Osteopathy*, although he had been developing his methods for the previous 20 years. His son, Dr Fred Mitchell Jnr, has carried on his work with a team of collaborators at the College of Osteopathic Medicine, Michigan State University, USA. Even though the credit has been given to Mitchell Snr, he in turn gave credit to two other osteopaths, TJ Ruddy and Carl Kettler for the true roots of MET.

Ruddy[2] had developed a system of treatment that he named 'resistive duction' in which the patient was required to make a rapid series of muscular contractions against the practitioner's resistance. Since he was an ophthalmologist and an otorhinolaryngologist, he mainly used these techniques around the orbit and in the cervical spine. Kettler's importance[3] was to focus Mitchell's attention on the need to balance myofascial tensions around lesion sites prior to any articulatory adjustment.

Since Mitchell Snr never wrote any books or papers directly on his techniques, it was down to his son Fred Mitchell Jnr[4] to apply the science to MET and to do the work of presenting it in written form. Leon Chaitow[5] and his collaborator, Craig Liebenson, acknowledge in their book *Muscle Energy Techniques* two other important workers in related fields, Karel Lewit and Vladimir Janda, both of the former Czechoslovakia. They have both added innovations to the basic MET theme; Lewit[6] calls his method 'post isometric relaxation', whilst

Janda[7] offers 'post facilitation stretch'. Finally, another version, 'proprioceptive neuromuscular facilitation' is used in the physiotherapy profession to strengthen neurologically weakened muscles.

As to which method is preferable, undoubtedly, all will claim their own! Fred Mitchell Jnr[8] in the *Muscle Energy Manual* states some of the advantages of MET to the osteopathic profession:

1. *MET is non-traumatic.*
2. *The methods of MET can efficiently lead to discovery and correction of 'key' lesions.*
3. *Because of its conceptual scope, MET could be considered a logical first step for beginning students of manual therapy, as it provides a framework for a better understanding of other manual therapy modalities. For example, for one who has mastered MET, thrust technique becomes gentler and more precise.*

Suggesting MET as a good 'first step' may imply that it is an easy technique to master. In 1970, Mitchell Snr taught his techniques to 'seasoned osteopaths' during 5-day tutorials. By 1974, the tutorials had increased to 12 days, an indication that more time was required in order to achieve a satisfactory level of competence even to begin using MET in a clinical setting. MET should be 'nontraumatic' in the sense that if all necessary precautionary safety steps are taken, it is considered safe. There are obviously incidences when MET would not be indicated. Since it requires patient participation, uncooperative or unresponsive patients would be excluded; these may include babies and young children, or patients with a high degree of senility. It could be considered contraindicated in a patient with certain primary muscle diseases, muscle damage or excessive muscle pain. With respect to the 'discovery and correction of key lesions', Mitchell described a 'Ten Step Screening Procedure'[8] which he used in order to facilitate this (see later).

Mitchell's definition of MET is:

A system of manual therapy for the treatment of movement impairments that combines the precision of passive mobilization with the effectiveness, safety and specificity of re-education therapies and therapeutic exercise. The therapist localizes and controls the procedures, while the patient provides the corrective forces and energies for the treatment as instructed by the therapist.[8]

He states that: 'The concepts and techniques of MET unquestionably are complex, but they are also logical. Once the abstract concepts are understood, the systematic application of MET becomes simple'.[8]

VARIATIONS OF MUSCULAR CONTRACTION

Different authors[5,8–10] offer numerous types of muscular contractions that may be used in MET. There seems to be a consensus that there are four main types of muscle contraction: isometric, isotonic concentric, isotonic eccentric and isokinetic. See Figure 12.1.

Isometric muscle contraction

This is described as a contraction in which both the patient's and practitioner's forces are equally matched, resulting in no change in length of the muscle. This type of contraction is used to reset the muscle's proprioceptors and to create inhibition of the muscle's antagonist via the reciprocal inhibition pathway.

Isotonic concentric muscle contraction

This is described as a contraction in which there is shortening of the muscle. This is achieved by the practitioner providing a resistive counterforce that is just less than that of the patient's. This type of contraction is used to increase the tone of weakened muscles.

Isotonic eccentric muscle contraction

This is described as a contraction of the muscle in which at the same time there is lengthening of the muscle. This is achieved by the force of the practitioner being just greater than that of the patient. It is used to stretch tight or fibrotic muscles. It is sometimes termed isolytic because it 'lyses' or breaks down fibrosity.

Isokinetic muscle contraction

This is described as a kind of combination of isotonic and isometric contractions. It is achieved by taking the muscle through its complete range of motion whilst a resistive force is applied to maintain the same 'speed' of contraction. It achieves recruitment of all the muscle fibres in sequence. At either end of the range of movement, the resistance is reduced because the contracting force of the muscle will be minimal. During the mid-range of contraction, the counterforce has to be increased to meet

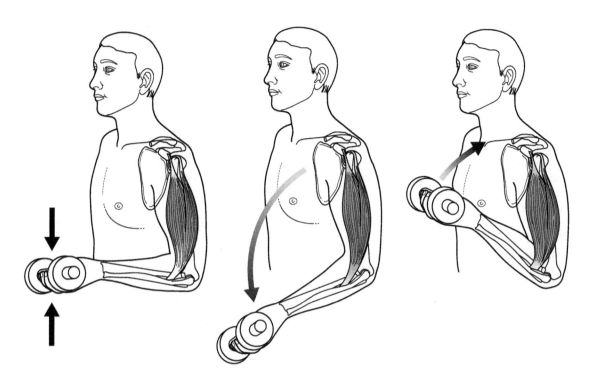

A Isometric contraction   **B** Eccentric contraction   **C** Concentric contraction

Figure 12.1 The range of motion of any articulation is limited by the anatomical motion barrier. Within this range lies the physiological range of motion that can be actively performed. In the figure, a restricted motion barrier has been placed within the physiological range of motion – this indicates a further reduction in the normal voluntarily achievable range of motion.

the strength of the larger bulk of muscle working to its best mechanical advantage. It is used to tone weak muscles, increase strength and 'homogenize' the effect of the muscle fibres.

Many osteopathic practitioners who use MET will mostly use direct techniques which are aimed at correction of somatic dysfunction via the post-isometric relaxation route. In other words, the technique is performed and then, during the relaxation stage immediately after a muscle contraction, there is a repositioning of the affected articulation by the practitioner towards a newly set up motion barrier. Repetition of the technique allows the motion barrier to be taken further towards the normal full range of motion. Indirect techniques are used much less often and they rely on the principle of reciprocal inhibition in order to correct the dysfunction. They are most useful when the main muscle affected is too tender to make the contraction and so its antagonist is utilized, resulting in the inhibition and thus relaxation of the agonist.

So, if we use the knee flexors and extensors as examples, in the direct technique if the flexor is in spasm or hypertonic, it is taken to its maximum comfortable length, i.e. until its motion barrier is felt. It is then contracted by the patient and actively resisted by the practitioner for a number of seconds. On relaxation, the practitioner then gently stretches the flexor to find its new motion barrier.

For an indirect technique acting on the same muscle hypertonicity, the contraction by the patient will take place in the extensor muscles, once again whilst actively resisted by the practitioner. This should create a reciprocal inhibition of the flexor thus allowing it to be stretched to a new motion barrier.

ASSESSMENT

Though these techniques may be applied to any muscle or group of muscles, they are particularly useful for the spine and pelvis. Mitchell described various specific techniques for 'repositioning' of vertebral or pelvic dysfunctions. The descriptions as to how they worked and which muscles are involved may not be entirely accurate but nevertheless many thousands of practitioners, osteopaths and others, have found them to be useful.

Mitchell recognized numerous restrictions possible in the pelvis including pubic shears, up and down slip of the innominates, innominate rotations, inflare and outflare of the pelvis and sacral torsions. The latter he noted as combined side-bending rotation restrictions coupled with either flexion or extension components and turning around an oblique axis.

Mitchell described the oblique axes as passing from the superior pole of one auricular surface of the sacrum to the inferior pole of the opposite side. They are named for the side of the superior pole, thus a left sacral axis passes from the superior pole on the left to the inferior pole on the right. Should the sacrum nutate around the left oblique axis, the anterior surface of the sacrum will rotate to the left. Should the sacrum become restricted in this position it is named as a left rotation on a left oblique axis or merely 'left on left sacral torsion' (L/L). The same arrangement may occur with nutation and rotation around a right axis resulting in a 'right on right sacral torsion' (R/R). However, should the sacrum counternutate around an

oblique sacral axis then it will rotate to the opposite side resulting in, for example, a right rotation on a left axis (R/L) or a left rotation on a right axis (L/R). These are shortened to right on left or left on right sacral torsions. To make things simpler (or to confuse things more) a nutated restriction is called a 'forward sacral torsion' whilst a counternutated restriction is known as a 'backward sacral torsion'. The forward sacral torsions have rotation on the same side as the axis, e.g. L/L or R/R, whilst the backward torsions have rotation to the opposite side of the axiss, e.g. L/R or R/L (Figs 12.2 and 12.3).

Movement around the sacral oblique axes takes place under circumstances which are at some stage unipedal, as in walking. The gait cycle creates a constantly changing series of movements that alternately involve the two oblique sacral axes. During the stance phase of the left leg, the left leg is weight-bearing and the movement occurs around a left sacral axis with the sacrum turning to the left (a forward sacral torsion to the left, L/L). The right leg initiates the swing phase and as it moves forwards, the right ilium rotates first slightly anteriorly then posteriorly as the whole swing takes place. At foot strike on the right, the ilium will begin to rotate anteriorly towards its neutral position and when under weight-bearing, the sacrum will begin to rotate to the right around the right oblique axis.

Figure 12.2 The oblique axes. The auricular surface with the superior and inferior surfaces marked.

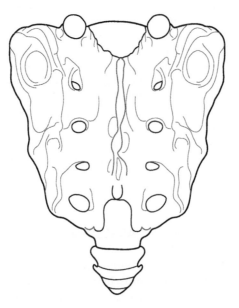

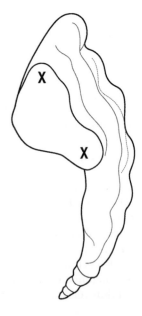

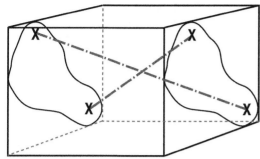

Figure 12.3 Diagrammatic representation of an oblique axis passing from one superior pole to the contralateral inferior pole, thus permitting the coupled motion of sacral torsion to take place.

Naturally, these movements do not occur in isolation, there are concomitant side-bending and rotation movements throughout the lumbar and thoracic vertebral segments.

The above series of movements occurs as a natural part of the walking cycle and, as such, restrictions in forward sacral torsion are found quite commonly, since they are within normal physiological motions. However, backward sacral torsions occur most often as a result of trauma and since the walking cycle will oppose this type of restriction, unless very restricted, they will often be rectified by the physiological movements of walking.

Anterior and posterior iliac rotations as described by Mitchell are as previously described in Chapter 10 on general osteopathic treatment (GOT) whereas, quite simply, an up or down slipped innominate is when the whole innominate on one side becomes shunted up or down. Deciding whether a left ilium is up shifted or a right ilium is down shifted will depend on the relationships to the sacrum and lumbar spine and the soft tissue findings of muscular and ligamentous tensions. This also applies in the cases of inflare and outflare which occur as a closing in or opening out of the anterior aspect of the pelvic girdle. It is beyond the scope of this text to describe all of the findings in detail and the relevant information may be found in the recommended reading list at the end of this chapter.

In addition to the standard restrictions of nutation and counter-nutation, which he termed bilateral flexion and extension respectively, Mitchell also proposed unilateral sacral flexion and extension lesions. A basic understanding of pelvic biomechanics will perplex the osteopath with regard to these two latter lesion patterns and it seems appar-

ent that either of these particular lesions may not be found in isolation. Having stated that, it is quite likely that many of the pelvic lesions will not be found alone. For this reason, some authors have proposed a protocol for treating the pelvis in order to avoid repetition of techniques. Mitchell[4] proposed the following sequence:

- Non-neutral dysfunction of the lumbothoracic spine
- Pubic or innominate subluxation
- Sacroiliac dysfunction
- Iliosacral dysfunction.

Kenneth Graham[11] in his book *Outline of Muscle Energy Techniques* has proposed the following sequence in order to treat the pelvis:

- Leg restrictors of the pelvis, i.e. major muscle groups
- Up/downslipped innominate
- Pubic dysfunction
- Lumbars and in particular an uncompensated L5 restriction
- Sacrum
- Ilia
- Iliopsoas.

However, Greenman[9] feels that any dysfunction found at the pubis should be addressed prior to proceeding with the rest of the diagnostic sequence. He reasons that since the rest of the testing procedure is performed with the patient prone, any dysfunction present at the pubis may confuse the picture. Next, he looks to innominate shears and any sacroiliac dysfunction which he feels clears the way for sacral diagnosis and treatment.

With these differences in opinions it comes as no surprise that there will be sceptics to this approach of treatment, but it has been seen that this is a problem encountered often in osteopathy. Two different osteopaths may have two different models that they stick to as 'their' preferred approach; it is down to the particular individual to decide which they prefer for their particular patient. Furthermore, in this case, it is not the techniques that are different but merely their sequence of application.

It has been proposed by Fryer[12] that it seems strange that Mitchell should have begun his work at the pelvis since there are no prime movers acting over these joints. Nowadays it seems fairly well accepted that the techniques do not work on single muscles, as was sometimes thought to be the action, but rather on groups of muscles and their connective tissues. In fact, Mitchell[1] stated clearly that 'the barrier ... means the restricting mechanism, which can be made up of one or many factors, i.e. ligamentous tension (including capsular tightening), muscular contracture, fascial restraint, pain producing muscular splinting, etc.'. It seems that he was well aware that it was probably a combination of factors that was responsible for the dysfunction and thus also had to be addressed for the technique to be effective.

When connective tissues are put under a sustained stretch, a temporary elongation takes place. This is known as 'creep' and occurs as a result of the viscoelastic properties of the tissue. Should the forces create a microtrauma within the connective tissue fibres, resulting in tearing and reorganization, then permanent plastic changes occur. A controlled combination of creep and plastic changes, such as that produced during an MET procedure, may be responsible for the increase in muscle length and other effects seen. However, MET procedures are often performed for a time span of only 3–5 seconds, and though repeated 3–5 times, still fall short of the optimum duration of 30 seconds for an effective stretch.[13] A study[14] comparing the passive stretching of a muscle against that of isometric contraction found that the latter gave a decreased passive tension. An explanation[15] for this may be that the active contraction creates tension not only in the connective tissue parallel fibres, as in passive stretching, but in addition, tenses the in-series fibres. Fryer summarizes that the biomechanical action of postisometric relaxation may be due to 'a combination of viscoelastic creep and plastic change in the parallel and series connective tissue elements of the muscle, above and beyond that obtained by passive stretch'.[12]

In an unpublished study,[16] indwelling electrodes were placed in specific muscles on a number of 'volunteers'. When the subject was asked to make a contraction of a particular specific muscle, numerous muscles were activated, creating a huge overflow of nervous stimulation. This would imply that it is nigh impossible to contract a specific single muscle and that the efficacy of Mitchell's technique relies on the contraction of muscle *groups*, utilizing the prime mover muscle required and probably many of its synergists and fixators. It is likely that the positioning of the patient for the specific technique may make certain muscles work harder, placing them in a mechanically advantageous or disadvantageous position as required.

However, MET is not used just to reposition bones of the pelvis and balance muscle tensions. In addition, it is used to mobilize joints, stretch the fascia and other connective tissues, and improve fluid movement, both lymphatic and blood. There is also an effect on oedematous or congested tissues by improving drainage and the reduction of tissue tension that thus inhibits the free flow of interstitial fluids. Furthermore, stretching of the fascia is an accompaniment to muscular contraction. As it is an active patient participation technique resulting in metabolite formation and possible microtrauma, patients may feel a slight soreness of the tissues for a day or so after a treatment. Excessive soreness or pain should not be felt and may indicate overzealous execution of the technique or, worse still, overlooked pathology.

Mitchell proposed a 'ten-step' screening examination[8] of the body to be carried out as a routine prior to treatment. It enabled the practitioner to identify a body region or regions that warranted further, more detailed examination. His screening was limited to the musculoskeletal system because that was where he was going to direct his treatment. He was well aware that, as with any examination, it might need to be adapted for the individual patient and their specific circumstances. His ten-step screening used two physical examination modalities, observation and motion testing. By motion testing, he would naturally palpate structures, but not in the full osteopathic sense of the word. He omitted the palpatory modalities such as temperature, moisture, size and shape. He knew that they were important, but felt that for this 'screening' they were too specific and detailed. He felt:

> one reason for their exclusion is that we believe it is a mistake to emphasize, or focus early attention on, the phenomena related to neurologic reflex activity ... the fact that changes in mechanical function bring about changes in circulation, reflex activity, etc., is axiomatic in the structure/function relationship, which is basic in the osteopathic theory of medicine.[4]

Mitchell's ten-step screening examination had the following format:

I   Gait and posture
II   Standing spine side-bending test
III   Standing flexion test
IV   Seated flexion test

V   Seated upper extremity test
VI   Seated trunk rotation
VII   Seated trunk side-bending
VIII Seated cervical motion
IX   Supine thoracic cage motion
X   Lower extremity motion.

Mitchell checked for asymmetry and tissue texture abnormalities and felt that by using this screening routine he had a reliable global view of each individual patient. Undoubtedly it served him well. However, many osteopaths before him and surely many after will have their own routine for globally assessing their patients; otherwise how else can a global treatment be made?

Muscle energy techniques, like many forms of osteopathic treatment techniques, have been used successfully by many practitioners for many years. The explanations for their mode of action may need rethinking but that does not negate their efficacy. It requires, like many aspects of the osteopathic repertoire, a well-researched investigation in order to validate its clinical usage, not just for the osteopath's peace of mind but also for the usage of other allied manual medicine practitioners.

References

1. Mitchell FL. Structural pelvic function. American Academy of Osteopathy 1958 Yearbook. Indianapolis: AAO; 1958:71–90.
2. Ruddy TJ. Osteopathic rhythmic resistive duction therapy. American Academy of Osteopathy 1961 Yearbook. Indianapolis: AAO; 1961:60–68.
3. Kettler C. Angina pectoris technic. American Academy of Osteopathy 1941 Yearbook. Indianapolis: AAO; 1941:31–33.
4. Mitchell FL Jr, Moran PS, Pruzzo NA. An evaluation and treatment manual of osteopathic muscle energy procedures. Missouri: Institute for Continuing Education in Osteopathic Principles; 1979.
5. Chaitow L, Liebenson C. Muscle energy techniques. Edinburgh: Churchill Livingstone; 1996.
6. Lewit K. Manipulative therapy in rehabilitation of the motor system. London: Butterworths; 1985.
7. Janda V. Muscle function testing. London: Butterworths; 1989.
8. Mitchell FL Jr. The muscle energy manual. Michigan: MET Press; 1995: v–vii.
9. Greenman PE. Principles of manual medicine, 2nd edn. Philadelphia: Williams and Wilkins; 1996:93–98.
10. Goodridge JP. In: Ward R, ed. Foundations for osteopathic medicine. Baltimore: Williams and Wilkins; 1997: 691–762.
11. Graham KE. Outline of muscle energy techniques. Oklahoma: Oklahoma College of Osteopathic Medicine and Surgery; 1985:18–30.
12. Fryer G. Muscle energy concepts. A need for a change. J Osteopath Med 2000; 3(2):54–59.
13. Bandy WD, Irion JM, Briggler M. The effect of time and frequency of static stretching on flexibility of the hamstring muscles. Phys Ther 1997; 77(10):1090–1096.
14. Taylor DC, Brooks DE, Ryan JB. Viscoelastic characteristics of muscle: passive stretching versus muscular contractions. Med Sci Sport Exerc 1997; 29(12):1619–1624.
15. Lederman E. Fundamentals of manual therapy. Edinburgh: Churchill Livingstone; 1997.
16. Shaver T. Study performed at the West Virginia College of Osteopathic Medicine. Personal communication; 1998.

Recommended reading

The Muscle Energy Manuals *is a series of three volumes aimed at the evaluation and treatment of the musculoskeletal system written by Fred Mitchell Jnr. They are weighty volumes full of relevant anatomy and deep explanations of all the techniques used by Mitchell.*
Mitchell FL Jnr. The muscle energy manual, vols 1 to 3. Michigan: MET Press; 1995.

Muscle Energy Techniques *by Leon Chaitow is not a comprehensive technique book although it does give some useful ideas.*
Chaitow L, Liebenson C. Muscle energy techniques. Edinburgh: Churchill Livingstone; 1996.

Both Principles of Manual Medicine (*Greenman*) and Foundations for Osteopathic Medicine *contain sections on MET and are well illustrated with black and white photos of most techniques.*
Greenman PE. Principles of manual medicine, 2nd edn. Philadelphia: Williams and Wilkins; 1996.
Ward R, ed. Foundations for osteopathic medicine. Baltimore: Williams and Wilkins; 1997.

Chapter 13

Cranial osteopathy

CHAPTER CONTENTS

INTRODUCTION

The credit for osteopathy in the cranial field goes to William Garner Sutherland (1873–1954) who, whilst still a student at the American School of Osteopathy, Kirksville, USA, showed an interest in the structure and function of the cranial bones.

> As I stood looking and thinking in the channel of Dr. Still's philosophy, my attention was called to the bevelled articular surfaces of the sphenoid bone. Suddenly there came a thought; I call it a guiding thought – bevelled like the gills of a fish, indicating articular mobility for a respiratory mechanism.

This oft quoted paragraph from *With Thinking Fingers* by Sutherland[1] indicates the manner in which he thought, and initiated his work in the cranial field. It is worth remembering that when Sutherland made these observations it went against the grain of all anatomy texts written at that time; the articulations between the bones of the cranium were considered immobile.

It was after many years of study and research, some actually performed on himself, that Sutherland began teaching his principles of craniosacral technique in the mid-1940s. As with any new ideas, Sutherland's were treated with a great deal of scepticism and to the present day, there are many critics of this technique. Likewise, it has many supporters.

Cranial osteopathy, cranial technique and cranial treatment are all misnomers. Although Sutherland first began his studies on the cranium, 'cranial treatment' is in no way limited to the skull. In fact, practitioners using this mode of treatment will apply their technique to the whole body, either from the cranium or pelvis, or from just about anywhere on the body. By using the principles of 'cranial technique', one is able to give a holistic treatment from a single point rather in the same way that specific adjusting technique (SAT) achieves its success. However, there has been a tendency to move away from the term 'cranial osteopathy'. Many people practising in this field tend to say that they are working with the involuntary mechanism (IVM) or involuntary motion rather than cranial treatment. Involuntary motion is motion that occurs within the body in the absence of conscious control, such as breathing, or the pumping of the heart. The motion that osteopaths are focusing on when using this method of treatment is indeed involuntary, and IVM is increasingly the phrase of choice.

Nevertheless, osteopaths using IVM techniques in the cranial field do spend a lot of time studying the anatomy of the head. This is not limited to the bony structures but also to the soft tissues and in particular the cranial meninges. In the same way that traditional osteopathy has recognized that a restriction in motion within the tissues of the body may cause 'disease', likewise, cranial osteopaths recognize the same principle within the tissues, soft and hard, of the skull. Moreover, these restrictions may be set up by trauma or systemic disease just as easily in the skull as they may in the rest of the body.

It has taken many years for the osteopathic profession to accept cranial osteopathy and to give it the recognition that it justly deserves. Sutherland and his followers have pushed relentlessly for acceptance – but then, so did Andrew Taylor Still for his ideas on the once estranged osteopathy. Cranial osteopathy is now fairly well accepted within and often outside of the profession although it may not be fully understood and, as yet, remains to be 'scientifically proven'.

In order to understand the concepts of cranial osteopathy we should look firstly at the anatomy of the skull (Fig. 13.1). We can divide the skull into three basic regions; the base, the vault and the face.

The base of the skull is comprised of the sphenoid body, the occipital condyles, basilar portions, and the petrous and mastoid portions of the temporal bones. All of these parts are derived from endochondral ossification. That is to say that the precursor to the osseous tissue is cartilage; prior to that it is mesenchymal tissue that responds to the compressive forces of the developing brain upon it by transforming into cartilage.

The vault is comprised of the parietals, the squamae of the occiput and temporal bones and the vertical portion of the frontal bone along with greater wings of the sphenoid. All of these parts are derived from intramembranous ossification. This differs from endochondral ossification in that there is no interim cartilaginous state; the forces applied to the membranes result in the laying down of bone within the membranes, hence intramembranous ossification.

The facial skeleton is comprised of the mandible, maxillae, nasals, lacrimals and zygomae, all of which are formed by intramembranous ossification. This leaves the ethmoid, vomer, inferior nasal conchae and palatines. Since the ethmoid and inferior nasal conchae are ossified from cartilage they may be considered part of the cranial base; whilst the vomer and the palatines are formed from membrane, they are often considered as part of the facial skeleton. However, the vomer is rather a strange entity and may also be considered by some as part of the base of the skull.

Another possibly simpler way of viewing the bones of the skull is to divide them into paired and unpaired bones. The unpaired bones are the sphenoid, occiput, ethmoid and vomer, all of which lie in the midline. The paired bones include the maxillae, zygomae, palatines, lacrimals, nasals, inferior conchae, parietals and temporals. The frontal and mandible may be considered as paired bones since they both develop in two halves which later fuse together. See Table 13.1.

Of the major skull articulations to consider, the temporomandibular joint (TMJ) between the condylar portion of the mandible and the mandibular fossa of the temporal bone, being a synovial joint, is the most mobile. In addition to the TMJ, there is an 'articulation' between the sphenoid and the basilar portion of the occiput at the region known as the clivus. It is formed of cartilage and ligamentous tissue and as such constitutes a synchondrosis known as the sphenobasilar synchondrosis or SBS. With the exception of the TMJs and the SBS, all other connections between the cranial bones are sutural articulations.

Table 13.1 Paired and unpaired bones of the skull

Unpaired bones	Paired bones	Oddities
Sphenoid	Maxillae	Frontal
Ethmoid	Zygomae	Mandible
Occiput	Palatines	
Vomer	Lacrimals	
	Nasals	
	Inferior conchae	
	Parietals	
	Temporals	

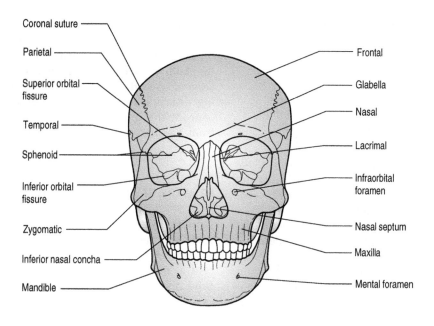

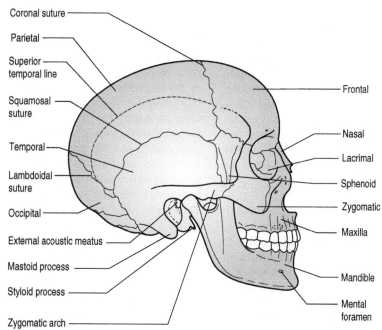

Figure 13.1 Bony landmarks of the skull.

SUTURES

These particular articulations require close attention. Hollinshead's *Textbook of Anatomy*[2] states:

in a suture, the bones are held together by a very small amount of fibrous tissue. Periosteum is contin-
uous from bone to bone, over the suture. Typically, the osseous surfaces have irregular areas of contact, such as serrations or ridges, which provide resistance to shearing forces or torsion. Sutures are essentially immovable joints. They occur only in the skull. With age, the fibrous tissue is gradually replaced by bone

and the suture becomes a completely bony union or synostosis.

Gray's Anatomy[3] states:

fusion does not even commence until the late twenties, proceeding slowly thereafter; yet it is clearly necessary that sutures should cease to function as mobile joints as rapidly as possible after birth.

Lockhart, Hamilton and Fyfe's[4] *Anatomy of the Human Body* gives a diagram that indicates the 'approximate years when union of sutures is completed' ranging from 35 to 80+ years.

Once again, it would appear that osteopaths and anatomists are not in complete accordance because, essentially, osteopaths, and followers of Sutherland in particular, feel that sutures *do* retain a certain amount of movement. Heisey and Adams[5] demonstrated that in an anaesthetized cat there is a certain amount of recordable mobility between the parietal bones. Retzlaff and co-workers[6] found the presence of several layers of tissue, nerve fibres and blood vessels within the sutural spaces. In neonatal sutures, there is the presence of membranous and/or cartilaginous tissue between the smooth edges of the bony plates. With growth and motion, the edges become serrated, providing both motion and protection of the underlying structures. Indeed, *Gray's Anatomy*[3] states that 'it is of considerable interest to find that, during the period of growth, areas of secondary cartilage formation are frequently observed in sutural ligaments'. In the early 1900s, Sperino,[7] an Italian anatomist, considered the ossification of cranial sutures in the mature human adult was pathological.

It is accepted by all that there is a need for mobility of the cranial bones, by way of the sutures, at birth. This is in order to allow the cranial plates to glide over one another as the baby passes through the relatively narrow and unforgiving pelvic outlet and the more distensible vagina. It is apparent to osteopaths that this need for mobility of the cranial bones is extended into adult life. Why should the skull become a fixed box?

It is also worthy of note that in most anatomy laboratories throughout the world, there is an example of an 'exploded skull', one in which the cranial bones have been disarticulated. The process used in 'exploding' the skull is to fill the cranial cavity with dried beans and to then immerse the whole thing in water. The result is disarticulation of the skull by the slowly expanding beans as they take up water. Importantly, the skull does not fracture but merely separates at the sutures, irrespective of the age of the skull. It would seem conceivable that the sutures serve some other purpose than merely facilitating disarticulation of the skull and it was to this concept that Sutherland devoted his life's work from his student days at Kirksville to his death in 1954.

PRIMARY RESPIRATORY MECHANISM

Dr Sutherland was convinced that the reason the sutures of the skull have their unique structure was in response to their function of accommodating the central nervous system (CNS), the cerebrospinal fluid and the attachments of the dura mater. He expressed it as a complete functional unit, and coined the term 'the primary respiratory mechanism' (PRM) to describe the involuntary motion and physiological function of the cranial mechanism. 'Primary' was used in the sense that it is in some way fundamental to our function. 'Respiration' is intended to mean physiological respiration, the nutrition and metabolic effects of the body tissues. This is distinct from what he called 'secondary respiration', which is that of the breathing movements of the thorax. This primary respiratory mechanism is a regular rhythmic cycle of 'respiration' that is a synchronous and integrated motion of the CNS, the meninges, the osseous components and the cerebrospinal fluid. The primary respiratory mechanism as proposed by Sutherland consisted of five distinct but related anatomicophysiological elements that he named 'the five phenomena'. They are:

- the mobility of the cranial articulations
- the mobility of the sacrum
- the mobility of the meninges
- the inherent motility of the CNS
- the fluctuation of the cerebrospinal fluid.

Sutherland was convinced that the primary respiratory mechanism was related to the rest of the body via the fascial connections and that the body functioned as a totality. Disruption of the PRM could manifest as a result of trauma, disease or psychological stress. In addition, it might be influenced by exercise, voluntary inhalation or exhalation and, of course, by the judicious use of treatment.

MOBILITY OF THE CRANIAL ARTICULATIONS

Sutherland noted that each of the cranial bones has an inherent motion that is permitted by the cranial articulations or sutures. The cranial bones articulate together rather like the cogwheels of a clock in a slight coupled motion. He felt that restriction of any of these movements will have a local effect on its contiguous structures as well as possible far reaching effects elsewhere in the body.

He named the movement in the midline bones flexion and extension, whilst the movement in the paired bones he described as internal and external rotation. He described the flexion and extension movements of the sphenoid and occiput as creating a type of hinge about the sphenobasilar synchondrosis (SBS). During the flexion phase (Fig. 13.2), the SBS permits the sphenoid to tip anteriorly and the occiput posteriorly. He proposed that during flexion the basilar portion of the sphenoid raised towards the vertex whilst the pterygoid processes and the greater wings moved caudally. The basilar portion of the occiput raised in the same manner towards the vertex and the condylar and squamous portions moved caudally. During the extension phase of the cycle, the opposite movements take place.

The ethmoid lying just anterior to the jugum sphenoidale is tipped in the same direction as the occiput by sphenoidal flexion. The vomer lying just inferior to the anterior portion of the sphenoid is carried caudally by sphenoidal flexion. Once again, the opposite movements take place during the extension phase.

During the SBS movement there is an accompanying movement of the paired bones. During SBS flexion, the paired bones move into external rotation, and during SBS extension the paired bones move into internal rotation. This combination of movements results in contoural changes of the cranium. During flexion of the sphenoid and external rotation of the paired bones there is a widening transversely and flattening vertically of the skull. Conversely, extension and internal rotation results in narrowing and lengthening of the skull. Due to this coordinated movement of the cranial bones it has been proposed that the anterior bones, when in dysfunction, are related to sphenoid dysfunction, whilst posterior cranial bone dysfunction is related to occipital dysfunction, although as stated earlier the effects may be further reaching than just the skull.

MOBILITY OF THE MENINGES

Sutherland also placed great importance on the meninges, the coverings of the central nervous system. The meninges consist of three layers: the innermost pia mater, the intermediate arachnoid mater and the outermost dura mater. The meninges play important roles in supporting and protecting the CNS within the bony framework of the skull and vertebral column. The outermost layer, the dura, is a tough, fibrous bag that is composed of white collagen fibres and some elastic fibres. Within the cranium it is composed of two layers adhered together in all but a few places where they separate to form the venous sinuses. The outer layer is strongly attached to the inside of the cranial vault forming the periosteal lining of the vault or endocranium. As a result of intramembranous ossification the dura is continuous through the sutures of the skull to form the periosteum on the external surface. The inner layer covers the brain and spinal cord and is termed the meningeal layer of the dura. Within the cranial cavity, the meningeal layer of dura has reduplications that project into the cranial cavity and at their attached ends house venous sinuses. These projections create a number of partitions that are named the falx cerebri, falx cerebelli, tentorium cerebelli and the diaphragma sellae. The

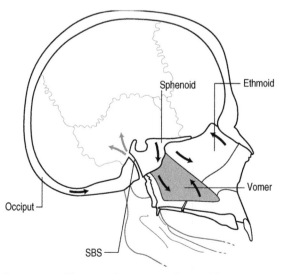

Figure 13.2 Diagrammatic representation of SBS flexion with the accompanying movements of the ethmoid and vomer.

falx cerebri separates the two cerebral hemispheres, whilst the falx cerebelli separates the two cerebellar hemispheres. The tentorium cerebelli separates the cerebrum from the cerebellum whilst the diaphragma sellae forms a 'canopy' over the pituitary fossa. See Figs 13.3 and 13.4.

The falx cerebri, falx cerebelli and the tentorium cerebelli unite at the straight sinus and extend to various cranial bones. It is this common origin of the four 'sickle shaped' projections of dura that has been named 'The Sutherland Fulcrum' in honour of its 'discoverer', and the projections extend from this point to their 'secondary attachments' on various bones of the skull.[8] The falx cerebri attaches anteriorly to the crista galli of the ethmoid before extending arc-like from the frontal, parietals and occiput in the sagittal plane to the internal occipital protuberance. Its two layers separate at their bony attachment to form the superior sagittal sinus throughout its length, whilst its free inferior border houses the inferior sagittal sinus. The falx cerebelli continues in virtually the same manner extending from the internal occipital protuberance down to the posterior margin of the foramen magnum, and it contains the occipital sinus. The tentorium cerebelli extends anteriorly around the internal aspect of the cranial vault from the internal occipital protuberance of the

occiput to the petrous ridge of the temporal bone; it houses the transverse sinus to this point. It then extends along the petrous ridge to attach to the posterior clinoid process, housing the superior petrosal sinus en route. The free innermost margin of the tentorium cerebelli sweeps around the midbrain and passes anteriorly to attach to the anterior clinoid process. It is these dural attachments that play a role in the transmission of cranial movements throughout the skull and vertebral canal.

The dura is continuous through the foramen magnum and extends down within the vertebral canal to about the level of the second sacral segment, to which it attaches. It then forms a blind ending, closing off to fuse with the pial extension of the filum terminale. On passing down the vertebral canal, the dura is attached at the level of the upper two or three cervical vertebrae before hanging relatively freely until its attachment to the sacrum. It is reported that the dura may attach in places to the posterior longitudinal ligament, the attachments being known as Hoffmann's ligaments.[9] The dura forms a sleeve-like covering to the spinal nerves as they project towards their respective intervertebral foramina. The dura surrounds the spinal nerve rootlets and the dorsal root ganglion and then becomes continuous with the

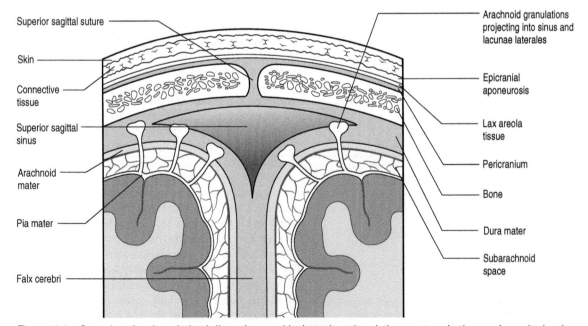

Figure 13.3   Coronal section through the skull, meninges and brain to show the relative structures in the superior sagittal region.

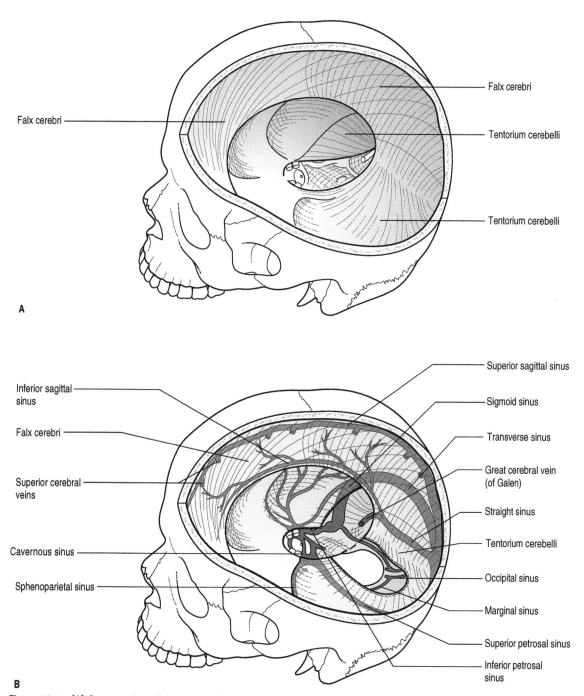

Figure 13.4 **(A)** Cutaway view of the adult skull to show the meningeal partitioning of the cranial cavity. **(B)** The same view as A but with the addition of the venous sinuses. (Reproduced with permission from Hall-Craggs ECB. Anatomy as a basis for clinical medicine. Copyright © Urban & Schwarzenberg; 1985.)

epineurium of the spinal nerves as they exit the vertebral canal. Connective tissue slips anchor the dura within the intervertebral foramina and prevent overstretching of the spinal nerves on movements of the spine. The attachments of the dura to the cranium and sacrum create what has been termed the 'core link' between the cranial and pelvic bowls.

MOBILITY OF THE SACRUM

Medical opinion at the time of Sutherland was that the sacrum was immovably fixed between the ilia. Sutherland proposed that the motion of the cranial mechanism is transmitted to the sacrum via the core link and that the sacrum moves relatively freely between the ilia. Thus the cranium and the sacrum work together as a coupled unit.

On SBS flexion, there is a raising of the SBS towards the vertex of the skull and this creates a tension through the dura that is projected to the sacrum, creating a cephalad pull on the sacral base. This results in a counternutation type movement of the sacrum that in 'cranial' terms is called sacral flexion. On SBS extension, the cephalad tension is reduced and the result is a nutation type movement of the sacrum which in cranial terms is called sacral extension. The movement of the sacrum correlates to that of the occiput (Fig. 13.5).

Sutherland named the whole unit of linkage between the dura of the cranium through the vertebral canal to the sacrum the 'reciprocal tension membrane' (RTM).

(*Note.* The terms used cranially to describe sacral flexion and extension are the complete opposite to the terms used in structural descriptions of sacral movements! When the sacral base tips anteriorly, nutation, structurally this is termed flexion whilst in a cranial sense this movement corresponds to extension).

THE INHERENT MOTILITY OF THE CENTRAL NERVOUS SYSTEM

Sutherland also proposed the idea that there is an inherent movement within the CNS. It has a rhythmic sinusoidal cycle in which the whole CNS undergoes shortening and widening followed by a lengthening and narrowing, or inhalation and exhalation, of the primary respiratory mechanism. To some, this appears to be a coiling and uncoiling of the nervous system, mimicking its embryological development. It was this movement that Sutherland considered the source of the primary respiratory mechanism. However, he was convinced that every cell in the body plays a part in the mechanism. Sutherland considered the thoracic respiration, or breathing, as secondary. He felt that the origin of

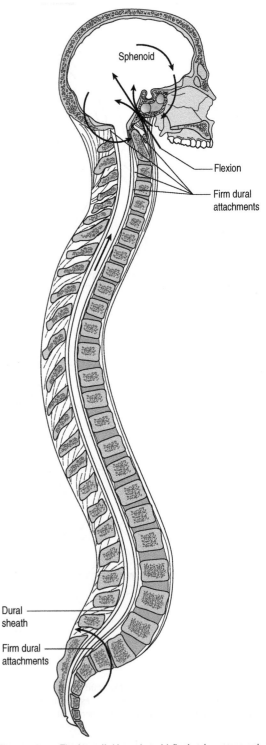

Figure 13.5   The 'core link' – sphenoid flexion is accompanied by a counternutatory type movement of the sacrum, known as sacral flexion.

the nervous system motility was in the floor of the fourth ventricle of the brain where the centres controlling breathing, circulation, digestion and elimination are found. These physiological functions are dependent on the functioning of the nervous system and, to Sutherland, this region and its movement were of prime importance.

FLUCTUATION OF THE CEREBROSPINAL FLUID

The final element that gained Sutherland's attention with respect to the primary respiratory mechanism was the cerebrospinal fluid (CSF) and he proposed that there is a fluctuation in its flow. Earlier, Still[10] had named the CSF as the 'highest known element', implying that it is the most important element among the known constituents of the human body. According to Still, it was the relationship of the 'CSF to the metabolism and well-being of the central nervous system, which controls the rest of the body'.[8]

The CSF is a clear, colourless fluid that fills the spaces in and around the central nervous system. External to the CNS, the CSF is found in the subarachnoid space that lies between the arachnoid and pia maters. Internal to the CNS, it is found in the ventricles, cerebral aqueduct and central canal of the spinal cord. It is isotonic with blood plasma although the CSF normally contains only traces of proteins.

The CSF is produced by the choroid plexuses, mostly in the lateral ventricles although the third and fourth ventricles do contribute to its production. There is also reported to be a general seepage of CSF from the whole of the surface of the brain.[11] The choroid plexuses are vascular invaginations of the pia mater that project into the cavity of the ventricles. The CSF produced in the lateral ventricles follows a particular route of flow (Fig. 13.6). It passes through the interventricular foramen of Monro to arrive in the third ventricle. From here, it passes through the cerebral aqueduct of Sylvius to reach the fourth ventricle. Additional CSF from the third and fourth ventricles is added to it. It leaves the fourth ventricle through four possible exits, two lateral apertures named the foramina of Luschka, a median aperture named the foramen of Magendie or it may continue into the central canal of the spinal cord. On leaving the fourth ventricle

via the named foramina, the CSF has now gained access to the subarachnoid cisterna. From there, it bathes the exterior of the spinal cord by passing down in the subarachnoid space to the lumbar cistern and up over the cerebellum via the tentorial notch to gain access to the external surface of the cerebrum. The CSF is returned to the venous circulation via the arachnoid granulations that are clusters of arachnoid villi that are mostly found adjacent to the superior sagittal sinus, although they may be present elsewhere. A certain amount of CSF is also returned to the venous system by draining into the connective tissue spaces around the spinal nerves as they exit their meningeal coverings.

Sutherland described a wave-like fluctuation of the CSF that was produced by the shortening and lengthening of the CNS. He referred to this fluctuation as 'the tide' and he felt that the ebb and flow of this tide played an important role in the nourishment of the body tissues. He identified a 'potency' to the mechanism that, although considered palpable, has not been fully explained. Sutherland noted that the rhythmic activity of this mechanism was normally between 10 to 14 cycles a minute. He named this phenomenon the 'cranial rhythmic impulse' (CRI). The CRI may be assessed with respect to its rate, amplitude, rhythm and quality and together they are said to give an indication of the patient's overall condition of health.

The 'frequency' is the rate of the CRI. The range of movement from flexion to extension is the 'amplitude'; optimal amplitude occurs when there is full expression of both flexion and extension. In someone who is compromised this expression is found to be limited either globally or locally. If both the flexion and extension are limited, it is usually indicative of global systemic dysfunction. Or, if one movement is preferentially affected (for example, extension is limited but flexion is full), this may indicate a local osteopathic lesion in flexion of that particular bone. (*Note.* An osteopathic lesion permits ease of movement into the direction of the lesion and limits movement away.) The 'rhythm' is simply the fluency of the movement, in the sense of regularity, equality of movement side to side, front to back, etc.

These descriptors (rate, rhythm and amplitude) represent one of the first ways to assess a patient, giving us an overall impression of the individual's health state and vitality. Simplistically stated, if the

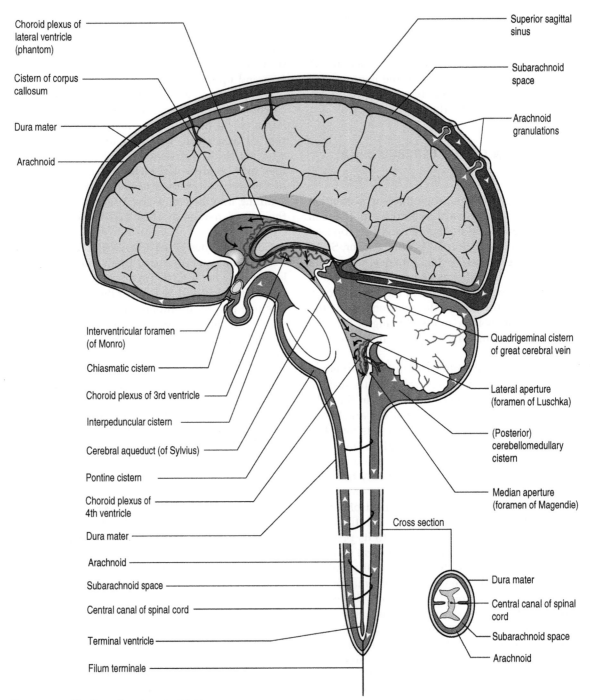

Choroid plexus of lateral ventricle (phantom)

Cistern of corpus callosum

Dura mater

Arachnoid

Superior sagittal sinus

Subarachnoid space

Arachnoid granulations

Interventricular foramen (of Monro)

Chiasmatic cistern

Choroid plexus of 3rd ventricle

Interpeduncular cistern

Cerebral aqueduct (of Sylvius)

Pontine cistern

Choroid plexus of 4th ventricle

Dura mater

Arachnoid

Subarachnoid space

Central canal of spinal cord

Terminal ventricle

Filum terminale

Quadrigeminal cistern of great cerebral vein

Lateral aperture (foramen of Luschka)

(Posterior) cerebellomedullary cistern

Median aperture (foramen of Magendie)

Cross section

Dura mater

Central canal of spinal cord

Subarachnoid space

Arachnoid

Figure 13.6   The flow of cerebrospinal fluid.

rate and amplitude are reduced or the rhythm is impaired there is dysfunction. The greater the dysfunction, the more they will be impaired.

One of the greatest problems when studying much of osteopathy is that it is almost impossible to describe the palpatory experience of any situation; this is very much the case in the above situation. Although we can describe full and limited movements and discuss their quality, these can only be appreciated after having palpated them, and thus one develops a palpatory reference of norm and variations away from the norm.

ASSESSMENT OF THE PRIMARY RESPIRATORY MECHANISM

As with most osteopathic treatment techniques, different practitioners have different approaches. Most will begin with normal case history taking, which is then followed by observation before actual handling or palpation is performed.

On 'cranial' observation, we should look carefully for any signs of cranial asymmetry from all angles. We should be aware of the normal bony landmarks of the skull and note any anomalies. At the same time we should note any asymmetry of the soft tissues, e.g. the ears, mouth, nose and nasolabial folds.

On palpation, we would usually begin by gently palpating the bone and soft tissues to confirm our observational findings. Then, with the patient comfortably relaxed in the supine position and the practitioner seated comfortably at the head, we can commence the 'true' cranial assessment.

The practitioner will usually place his/her hands in the position of the 'vault hold' (Fig. 13.7). This permits assessment of the overall motion of the cranial bones and, in particular, the motion of the cranial base. In this position, the index finger is placed over the greater wing of the sphenoid, the middle finger over the pterion, the ring finger behind the ear at the asterion and the little finger over the lateral angle of the occiput. The fingers do not contact merely at the fingertips but along their whole length, giving a greater palpatory contact. The thumbs are placed together as they meet in the midline; they are usually held free of the skull and serve

to form a base for the flexors of the fingers. Initially, for most practitioners, this position is uncomfortable, but with practice and relaxed hands, it becomes second nature. The practitioner's position is most important, seated at the patient's head with the forearms resting on the table. The height of the table is important and should be adjusted specifically for the practitioner to be in a comfortable, relaxed position. This position will create less tension in the hands and body and allow for a freer palpation. The cranial 'vault hold' allows the cranial base to be assessed, i.e. the sphenobasilar synchondrosis. The cranial rhythmic impulse, as mentioned earlier, may be assessed for rate, rhythm, amplitude and quality.

Another method of assessing the cranial rhythmic impulse is to palpate it at the sacrum. The palpating hand is placed under the sacrum of the supine patient and the flexion/extension movement of the sacrum may be assessed as it moves around its transverse or respiratory axis at the level of the second sacral segment. As stated earlier, normal sacral motion is synchronous with that of the occiput via the reciprocal tension membrane. The two ends of the system may be checked together by placing one hand under the sacrum and the other under the occiput. In this manner, one can assess whether or not there is an uninterrupted flow of the cranial rhythmic impulse between the cranium and sacrum.

There are numerous possible 'lesion patterns' that may be found at the sphenobasilar synchondrosis. They include torsion, compression, side-bending/rotation, lateral and vertical strains. These lesion patterns will affect the whole cranium and facial skeleton as well as the sacrum via the reciprocal tension membrane. Conversely, other cranial, facial and sacral lesions can in turn affect the SBS. To expand this theory further, we can add the possibility of a problem in the lower extremity affecting the pelvis, which then, by way of the sacrum and RTM, may create problems with the SBS. It goes without saying that the upper extremity and pectoral girdle will feed into the system in the same manner.

Techniques have been devised for the testing and treatment of all the individual bones of the skull, either directly or indirectly. Furthermore, there are techniques aimed at working on the fluid characteristics of the cranial system including the CSF and vascular systems. It is beyond the bounds of this text to describe each technique in detail. A list of recommended texts may be found at the end of this chapter.

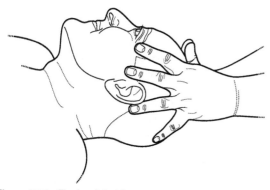

Figure 13.7 The 'vault hold'.

Sutherland considered that the body, including the head, works as a functional totality, and thus should be treated as a whole. As with all modes of osteopathic treatment, the balance of structure and function, when optimal, creates the best defence to 'dis-ease'.

RESEARCH IN THE FIELD OF CRANIAL OSTEOPATHY

Much research has been carried out in the field of cranial osteopathy and it can largely be divided into two distinct areas; that of treatment and that of the origin of craniosacral motion. Both are valid research fields in their own right. Anyone who has experienced, either first hand or in a friend or relative, the beneficial effects of treatment using the involuntary mechanism will undoubtedly agree that it does work, and in some cases remarkably so. In most undergraduate educational programmes, students are required to carry out a research project as part of their studies and many have chosen to study the effects of cranial treatment in clinical practice. There is a wide variety of validity of these research projects; some are quite strictly controlled using double blind or randomized control trials whilst others would not stand up to the weakest scrutiny. Research into the origin of the craniosacral motion, or even its existence, comes under severe critical review from the medical profession and sometimes also from within the osteopathic profession itself. Nevertheless the research continues and it is becoming stronger as experimental design and methods of measurement improve.

The earliest research in the cranial field was carried out by Sutherland himself, on himself! He reputedly inflicted 'cranial lesions' upon himself by various mechanical means and noted the effects. He then proceeded to 'correct' those lesions in order to prove his theory that not only does the phenomenon exist but that it can be affected by treatment.

Much of the early research was aimed at recording sutural motion in the skull and in the 1950s Lippincott and Hewitt[12] made measurements in the frontozygomatic sutures in humans. Unfortunately, the results were inconclusive since the movement measured could easily be due to some other physiological motion rather than from the bones themselves. However, it paved the way for further research under more exacting conditions and in 1992

Adams and co-workers quantitatively measured cranial bone mobility in the anaesthetized cat.[13]

A great deal of work in the cranial field has been produced by the Russian researcher Yuri Moskalenko who, with numerous co-workers, has devoted decades to the study of cranial motion. He suggests that it is the interactions between the volumes and pressures of the blood and CSF that are responsible for the motion of the cranial bones and that of brain tissue.[14]

Many researchers have noted that there seems to be a similarity between the palapatory findings of the cranial rhythm and the Traube–Hering (TH) waves or oscillations. These were first noticed by Traube in 1865 and were described as fluctuations in the pulse pressure that varied synchronously with respiration. The interesting finding was that they persisted even if breathing was temporarily halted. As is always the way in scientific research it requires the same finding by an independent research team to give credence to the first researcher's findings. This confirmation was made 4 years later by Hering and so the oscillations became known as Traube–Hering waves. That was, until 1876, when Mayer noticed another oscillation that was similar in nature but occurred at a much slower rate. And so the whole phenomenon is now sometimes referred to as the Traube–Hering–Mayer oscillation (THM). Nelson[15] notes that 'components of the THM have been measured in association with blood pressure, heart rate, cardiac contractility, pulmonary blood flow, cerebral blood flow and movement of the cerebrospinal fluid and peripheral blood flow including venous volume and body temperature regulation'. Since these physiological reactions are largely under the control of the autonomic nervous system and hence the balance of sympathetic and parasympathetic actions and its effects on the cardiovascular system, they are related to the homeostatic mechanisms of the body. So how does this fit in with the cranial rhythmic impulse? It was stated earlier that the rate of the impulse was considered by Sutherland to be between 10 and 14 cycles per minute. However, as always, there seems to be a certain amount of disagreement on this and numerous studies have put the rate at anything from as low as 3 cycles per minute. These rates have been calculated from studies on both humans and animals. In fact Becker[16] states that there are two rates, one at 8–12 cycles per minute and a far slower one at about 0.6 cycles per minute; he names these 'fast' and 'slow tides' respectively. Other well-known researchers in the cranial field have found diverse findings; Frymann,[17] in addition to the accepted rate, measured long slow cycles of 50 to 60 seconds whilst Upledger[18] measured 9–11 cycles per minute and a slow frequency of 1–2 cycles per minute. Nelson and co-workers[19] used laser-Doppler blood velocity flowmetry and concluded that the 'Traube–Hering component of the oscillation is simultaneous with the fast tide of the CRI'. This fast tide wave is the rate proposed by Sutherland, whilst the slow tide wave as proposed by Becker[15] seems to correlate to the Mayer oscillation. So it seems that there is evidence to support some of the ideas proposed by Sutherland and his followers that the cranial rhythmic impulse does exist – but still the question arises: how does it work?

Nelson[15] has attempted to explain this by looking at the fluctuation of the CSF and the inherent motility of the CNS, two of the five phenomena proposed originally by Sutherland. He cites the works of Feinberg[20] and Enzmann[21] that show motion of the brain and the CSF as 'demonstrated utilizing magnetic resonance velocity imaging'. In short, during the cardiac cycle, in systole, blood flow into the brain creates an increase in its volume which causes the central portion of the brain and the brain stem to move caudally. This creates a net movement of the CSF from the lateral ventricles towards the third ventricle, on to the fourth ventricle and thence to the cranial and spinal subarachnoid spaces. This in turn creates a rise in the pressure of the spinal dural sac. The reverse action takes place during diastole, due to the dural sac's action as a capacitor. Ultrasound studies have shown that blood flow velocity and pressure correlate to the Traube–Hering oscillation.[22] Nelson[23] concludes that this movement is 'synchronous with, and, at least partially because of the THM oscillation, the CSF may well be described as "ebbing and flowing"'. As stated earlier, the THM oscillation has also been associated with peripheral blood flow and venous volume, and Nelson has tried to explain the significance of the THM with respect to lymphatic return. He states that although the lymphatic system does have contractile properties, the sections between two sets of valves, the lymphangion, may contract randomly.[24] However, their efficiency is enhanced when they contract synchronously, which they achieve readily. He feels that it is the Traube–Hering oscillation that facilitates this synchrony by entrainment. He describes entrainment as occurring when 'two systems are oscillating at close frequency … the dominant frequency will force the second oscillation to assume, in synchrony, the same frequency as the dominant input'.[25]

Based on the above discussion it is feasible that a cranial osteopath may be able to palpate and treat from any site on the body. The THM oscillation seems to be reflected throughout the entire body via the nervous and cardiovascular systems and possibly the lymphatics and thus with it are some of the palpable aspects of the cranial rhythmic impulse.

Is the above a case of fitting the research to the needs of the cranial osteopath? Sceptics will undoubtedly feel so, but it seems unlikely. The evidence is becoming stronger and although it may not be the full explanation, it leads the way forwards for further research.

If it can be accepted that the above is strong evidence for the relationship between the Traube–Hering wave and the cranial rhythmic impulse then one would expect to find a change of sorts after cranial treatment. Surgueef and co-workers[25] (incidentally, Nelson was one of them) found exactly that. In a study of only two subjects, a distinct change of the TH wave was found following cranial treatment as measured by laser-Doppler blood flow velocity recording. Prior to treatment, both individuals demonstrated an absence of the normal TH wave and concurrent decreased CRI amplitude. Following cranial treatment both subjects showed a prominent low frequency oscillation waveform characteristic of a normal TH wave. In such a small study, it is easy to criticize the results as merely due to the placebo effect, but it indicates that a much larger study needs to be performed, from which we eagerly await the results.

In the 'Letters to the Editor' section of the Spring 2003 edition of the AAO Journal, Kenneth E Nelson[26] has written a very interesting letter highlighting the similarities between his article 'The Primary Respiratory Mechanism' (AAO Journal, Winter 2002) and an article written by JM Littlejohn[27] 100 years earlier, entitled 'The Physiological Basis of the Therapeutic Law'. Littlejohn was aware that there existed 'brain movements' and that they corresponded to cardiac contractions, respiration and vascular variations of vasomotion. Nelson feels that the latter refers to the THM oscillation. Littlejohn states:

All life and life forms vibrate and pulsate in cycles.
The arterial blood builds up and develops to function
the nervous system, but the nervous system furnishes
stimulus and even nutrition to the artery in order that

it may pulsate in harmony with the master tissue of the body in the supply of food to the entire organ.

He goes on to state:

the brain generates impulses that pass out to all parts of the organism through the nervous system to maintain the tonic, rhythmic, peristaltic or vibratile condition of tissues and organs. This mobility, which is the characteristic of every tissue and organ is maintained by the perpetual stream of vibratile impulses from the brain towards every part of the body. Here we get the vibratility of the vital force.

It is interesting to note that Littlejohn was a student of Andrew Taylor Still at the American School of Osteopathy at the same time as William Garner Sutherland and that although a student, Littlejohn was often responsible for the teaching of physiology. One can only wonder how influential Littlejohn's ideas may have been on Sutherland, especially with respect to the origins of the cranial rhythmic impulse.

METHODS OF TREATMENT

As stated earlier, there are techniques for all the bones of the cranium and their associated structures. It is not the aim of this text to give detailed accounts of these techniques but to try to indicate the ways in which the techniques may be applied and how they achieve their effects.

The aim of the treatment in cranial osteopathy is the same for any aspect of osteopathy: it is to correct structure and thus improve function. Magoun[28] states the specific aims of cranial treatment as to:

1. normalize nerve function
2. counteract stress producing factors
3. eliminate circulatory stasis
4. normalize CSF fluctuation
5. release membranous tension
6. correct cranial articular lesions
7. modify gross structural patterns.

He recognizes that in order to make an effective cranial treatment, it may be necessary to begin by removing certain 'hindrances': myofascial strains from elsewhere in the body, local or generalized infections, nutritional deficiencies and organic poisons.

In order to gain optimum efficiency from the primary respiratory mechanism, it may be necessary to instil a state of 'balanced membranous tension'. This is described as 'the most "neutral" position possible under the influence of all the factors responsible for the existing pattern – all attendant tensions having been reduced to the absolute minimum'. This is achieved by working on the dural membranes, the three 'sickles', falx cerebri and tentorium cerebelli (four sickles if we include the falx cerebelli) and their attachments to 'find' this neutral point where the 'inherent force' can work with optimum efficiency. According to Magoun,[29] finding this state of balance may be achieved by the five different methods of (see also Fig. 13.8):

1. exaggeration
2. direct action
3. disengagement
4. opposite physiological motion
5. moulding.

Exaggeration is a form of indirect technique in which the two (or more) components of the lesion are taken further into the direction in which they were lesioned to a point of balance, and allowing the natural recoil of the tissues to do the correction. If there is the risk that exaggeration would further damage the tissues, then a direct technique would be used. This is more commonly used in younger patients and especially so in children. In this technique, there is a simple but gentle direct retracing of the lesion pattern back to its normal position. Disengagement is a type of indirect technique where the two structures are separated. It is particularly important in cases of impaction and may be used to free up the lesion prior to direct or exaggeration techniques. Opposite physiological motion is a complex combination procedure involving a direct technique for one component of the lesion and an indirect technique for the other. It is used mostly in severely traumatic lesions where the normal physiological pattern has been seriously disrupted. It goes without saying that it requires exceptional skill and experience to recognize when and how to use this technique. Finally, moulding techniques use a direct action. These are used

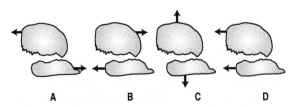

Figure 13.8 Methods for arriving at the point of balanced membranous tension. A – indirect action; B – direct action; C – disengagement; D – opposite physiological motion.

primarily in infants, though they may also be used in adults, in order to normalize the contours of the bones when there are abnormalities due to, for example, intraosseous lesioning from birth trauma.

Once the state of balanced membranous tension has been achieved, some practitioners utilize the patient's breathing in order to further enhance the potency of the inherent motion. Often the patient is instructed to hold the breath at full inspiration for as long as is comfortably possible. However, should the lesion be held into extension or internal rotation, then it is more useful to hold the breath on full expiration.

One of the techniques used in the field of cranial osteopathy is known as the 'compression of the fourth ventricle' (CV4) and amongst the numerous techniques available, this certainly warrants further discussion. It is one of a number of fluid drive or fluid fluctuation techniques which may be local and specific (such as the so-called V-spread) or more global, such as the CV4. The aim of the CV4 technique is to bring the primary respiratory mechanism to a 'still point'. Sutherland described this as a point of balance where there is a brief pause in the rhythm associated with the fluctuation of the CSF. It may be achieved by cupping the hands around the lateral angles and squamous portion of the occiput and gently applying a compression until an 'idling of the motor' is perceived.[30] Its effects are reputedly numerous; enhancing lymphatic drainage, lowering fever, reversing allergic reactions, promoting elimination and hastening detoxification from alcohol and drugs. Furthermore, it can enhance mobility in connective tissue diseases and achieve the correction of somatic dysfunctions that are too painful to be treated by other methods. According to Frymann,[31] it can lower arterial hypertension and it is stated by Magoun[32] that even 'infection in the nares from a pulled hair has responded'!! (our exclamations not his). So how does it achieve this myriad of effects? MacPartland[33] has suggested that entrainment of the CRI and THM oscillation may be the answer. It should be remembered that the nucleus of the tractus solitarius which is responsible for vasomotor activity is to be found in the floor of the fourth ventricle. And it is the neuronal circuits related to this nucleus that coordinate the THM oscillation. This may account for the normalization of the cardiovascular and other homeostatic functions but the nasal hair remains a mystery, although normal homeostatic function will optimize immune function in the case of infection. Magoun,[32] supposedly quoting from some of Sutherland's unpublished works, states 'if you do not know what else to do, compress the fourth ventricle'. It would appear that the CV4 is the 'osteopathic aspirin'.

Alain Gehin,[34] author of the Atlas of Manipulative Techniques for the Cranium and Face, states that of the objectives of the CV4, it is used 'most commonly, to bring about a general relaxation of the patient'. For this reason a cranial treatment will often start with this technique for patients who are 'ill-at-ease'. He goes on to state a second objective 'as a general technique, to enhance the motion of the cranial rhythmic impulse'. With reference to the accepted potency of this particular technique, numerous authors will state it is contraindicated in the case of recent cranial trauma, fracture, haemorrhage and cerebrovascular accidents. Magoun[32] makes the rather bold statement that 'no one is too sick to have this done' and although he recognizes that it should not be used in acute cranial emergencies, he feels that even under these circumstances it may be quite safely carried out from the sacrum.

TREATMENT OF THE NEONATE AND YOUNG CHILDREN

Osteopathy in the cranial field has many important uses due to its gentle nature. One of the most important and frequent applications is in the treatment of babies and young children. Young patients often respond quicker to osteopathic treatment than adults. This may be due to a greater vitality or just because they are much more in touch with their inherent healing mechanisms. Either way, they do respond well and newborns and infants are particularly receptive to cranial treatment.

Although the neonate is not subject to the stresses of everyday life in the same way as an adult, merely arriving in the world is a particularly stressful experience. The adrenal gland in the neonate is much larger proportionally than that of an adult. This is reflected by the massive amount of adrenaline that is required to see the baby through the birth and to begin life in the 'outside world'. The baby has to make the drastic change from relying on its mother for its nutrition, gaseous exchange and elimination through the umbilical attachment to the mother, to that of a relatively self-supporting being. The circulatory system has to become self-sufficient with major changes taking place in the heart, whilst the lungs have to inflate for the first time with life-giving air. The change from the buffering action of a fluid environment to that of a gaseous medium is only part of the trauma. These changes will take place with no rehearsals or pep talks: there is one chance and the baby has to get it right first time. Nowhere else throughout life is so much staked on the normal physiological processes of the body. The baby is subjected to many possible stresses and strains, both in utero and out, but none potentially more traumatic than the birth process itself. However, many babies are born daily throughout the world and most survive. Carreiro[35] states that it is a case that 'the passenger adapts to the passageway' and that in doing so problems may arise.

The baby's head has to undergo a certain amount of compression in order to pass through the birth canal. Its structure is adapted for this function by being much more pliable than that of an adult. The vault of the skull is formed in membrane and the base in cartilage and at birth many of the bones still consist of numerous parts. The sphenoid comprises three parts, the occiput four, each temporal three, frontal, mandible and maxillae two. The osseous components of each bone are held together by cartilage.

At birth the skull is proportionally larger with respect to the rest of the body as compared to that of the adult. However, at birth the facial portion of the cranium is much smaller in proportion to that of the adult; this is due to the underdevelopment of the mandible and maxillae; there are no teeth and the maxillary sinuses have yet to fully develop. Unossified membrane is still present at the angles of many of the developing vault bones, thus forming the fontanelles (Fig. 13.9). The largest is the anterior between the frontal and parietal bones, and a smaller posterior fontanelle is found between the parietals and occipital bone. There are paired lesser fontanelles placed anterolaterally (sphenoidal) and posterolaterally (mastoidal). The fontanelles will close up and ossify as bone growth takes place at various stages; the posterior by about 2 months, the lateral sphenoidal and mastoidal by about 3 months and the anterior within the second year. It is this incompleteness of the bony skull that permits the flat bones of the vault to overlap at the margins and the bones of the cranial base to undergo torsion and compression on passing through the birth canal.

The pliability afforded by the neonatal anatomy allows these events to take place naturally and should also allow the bones to 'spring back' afterwards. In the perfect world, everything would 'pop back' into place and there may be no call for osteopathic intervention. Unfortunately, life is not always

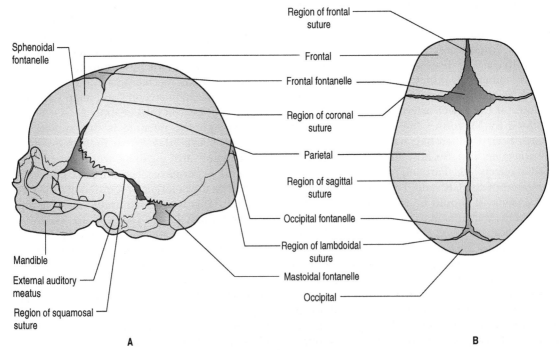

Region of frontal suture

Frontal

Frontal fontanelle

Region of coronal suture

Parietal

Region of sagittal suture

Occipital fontanelle

Region of lambdoidal suture

Mastoidal fontanelle

Occipital

Sphenoidal fontanelle

Mandible

External auditory meatus

Region of squamosal suture

A

B

Figure 13.9   The skull of the newborn baby. **(A)** Lateral view. **(B)** Plan view.

so perfect, not even for the newborn! A prolonged birth or the use of external assistance, such as forceps or suction (ventouse) techniques, may place excessive strains on the baby's head. The mere fact of the mother's anatomy may create complications: a large baby and a small maternal pelvis speaks for itself. Cathie[36] states 'it is the more obscure, the so-called minimal injuries of no apparent clinical significance that too often go undetected and that are so often responsible for problems of development and growth during the periods of infancy, childhood and adolescence'.

Inspection of the baby in the first few days after the birth will make the treatment of any complications much more effective; the sooner the better, and if possible in the first few hours after the birth. Frymann[37] states 'the mobility of the cranial mechanism is much greater at this age than in the adult skull, although the range of motion is of course much smaller'. Delay may permit the lesion patterns to firmly establish themselves, making treatment more difficult. Nevertheless, if treatment is given later it may still be effective but might require more time and effort.

Newborn babies are subject to a completely new environment and it seems that they are only intent on feeding and sleeping (although secretly they are also learning). Some babies seem to cope with these natural functions quite well, but not all. Excessive crying, gastrointestinal upsets such as colic and vomiting are very distressing to both the child and parents. The structural changes such as plagiocephaly, abnormal shape or deformity of the skull, are particularly disturbing for parents and according to Carreiro[38] much help and advice can be given. The success of osteopathically treating babies with these conditions is almost exclusively due to the cranial approach.

As the child grows, other conditions predominate: teething problems, otitis media, pharyngitis and countless others. There seems to be a trend at the current time of 'corrective orthodontic work'. This will naturally place a strain on the cranial mechanism that may be rectified by judicious treatment. It would be better, according to Frymann,[39] to correct any lesions found and create free physiological motion within the mechanism before the orthodontic intervention begins: that way there is no need to force anything but merely to encourage a normal anatomical relationship.

Obviously, cranial treatment does not end with the onset of adulthood. The adult body, too, is subject to the normal stresses, strains and traumas of life and these may be helped by cranial treatment. In fact, cranial treatment may well be the treatment of choice in the elderly or infirm. This does not mean to say that other forms of treatment are excluded, but that the gentle approach afforded by cranial treatment may be more acceptable to some patients and practitioners alike.

References

1. Sutherland WG. With thinking fingers. Missouri: Journal Printing; 1962:12–13.
2. Rosse C, Gaddum-Rosse P. Hollinshead's textbook of anatomy, 5th edn. Philadelphia: Lippincott-Raven; 1997.
3. Williams PL, Warwick R, eds. Gray's anatomy, 36th edn. Edinburgh: Churchill Livingstone; 1980:293–349, 420–429.
4. Lockhart RD, Hamilton GF, Fyfe FW. Anatomy of the human body, 2nd edn. London: Faber and Faber; 1965.
5. Heisey SR, Adams T. Role of cranial bone mobility in cranial compliance. Neurosurgery 1993; 33:869–877.
6. Retzlaff EW, Michael D, Roppel R et al. The structures of cranial bone sutures. J Am Osteopath Assoc 1976; 75:607–608.
7. Sperino G. Anatomia umana, vol 1. Torino: Camilla and Bertolero; 1931:202–203.
8. Magoun HI. Osteopathy in the cranial field. Missouri: Journal Printing; 1966:27.
9. Amonoo-Kuofi HS, El-Badawi MGY. Ligaments related to the intervertebral canal and foramen. In: Giles LGF, Singer KP, eds. Clinical anatomy and management of low back pain, vol 1. Oxford: Butterworth-Heinemann; 1997: 115–116.
10. Still AT. Osteopathy: research and practice. Missouri: Journal Printing; 1898:360.
11. Lockhart RD, Hamilton GF, Fyfe FW. Anatomy of the human body, 2nd edn. London: Faber and Faber; 1965.
12. Lippincott HA, Hewitt WF. Motion at cranial sutures: a method for its mechanical amplification and registration, with preliminary report of frontozygomatic motion in man. J Ost Cran Ass; 1957–1958:51.
13. Adams T, Heisey SR, Smith MC et al. Parietal bone mobility in the anaesthetised cat. J Am Osteopath Assoc 1992; 92:599–622.
14. Moskalenko Y, Frymann V, Kravchenko T et al. Physiological background of the cranial rhythmic impulse and the primary respiratory mechanism. AAO Journal 2003; Summer:21–33.
15. Nelson KE. The primary respiratory mechanism. AAO Journal 2002; Winter:24–33.
16. Becker RE. Motion: the key to diagnosis and treatment. Brooks RE, ed. Life in motion: the osteopathic wisdom of Rollin E Becker, DO. Portland: Rudra Press; 1997.
17. Frymann VM. A study of the rhythmic motions of the living cranium. J Am Osteopath Assoc 1971; 70:928–945.

18. Upledger JE, Karni Z. Mechano-electric patterns during craniosacral osteopathic diagnosis and treatment. J Am Osteopath Assoc 1979; 78:782–791.

19. Nelson KE, Sergueef NS, Lipinski CM et al. The cranial rhythmic impulse related to the Traube–Hering–Mayer oscillation; comparing laser-Döppler flowmetry and palpation. J Am Osteopath Assoc 2001; 101(3):163–173.

20. Feinberg DA, Mark AS. Human brain motion and cerebrospinal fluid circulation demonstrated with MR velocity imaging. Radiology 1987; 163:793–799.

21. Enzmann DR, Pele NJ. Normal flow patterns of intracranial spinal cerebrospinal fluid defined with phase contrast cine MR imaging. Radiology 1991; 178:467–474.

22. Jenkins CO, Campbell JK, White DN. Modulation resembling Traube–Hering waves recorded in the human brain. Euro Neurol 1971; 5:1–6.

23. Nelson KE. The primary respiratory mechanism. AAO Journal 2002; Winter: 24–33. AAO Journal 2003; Summer: 21–33.

24. Olszewski WL, Engeset A. Lymphatic contractions. N Engl J Med; 1979:300–316.

25. Sergueef N, Nelson KE, Glonek T. Changes in the Traube–Hering wave following cranial manipulation. AAO Journal 2001; Spring: 17. AAO Journal 2003; Summer:21–33.

26. Nelson KE. Letters to the Editor. AAO Journal 2003; Spring: 16–19. AAO Journal 2003; Summer:21–33.

27. Littlejohn JM. The physiological basis of the therapeutic law. Journal of the Science of Osteopathy 1902; 3(4).

28. Magoun HI. Osteopathy in the cranial field. Missouri: Journal Printing Company; 1966:94–98.

29. Magoun HI. Osteopathy in the cranial field. Missouri: Journal Printing Company; 1966:100–101.

30. Magoun HI. Osteopathy in the cranial field. Missouri: Journal Printing Company; 1966:110–114.

31. Frymann VM. Cerebrospinal fluid motion. In: Frymann VM. The collected papers of Viola M. Frymann, DO. Indianapolis: AAO; 1998:121–125.

32. Magoun HI. Osteopathy in the cranial field. Missouri: Journal Printing Company; 1966: 114.

33. MacPartland J, Mein EA. Entrainment of the cranial rhythmic impulse. Altern Ther Health Med 1997; 3:40–45.

34. Gehin A. Atlas of manipulative techniques for the cranium and face. Seattle: Eastland Press; 1985:46.

35. Carreiro JE. An osteopathic approach to children. Edinburgh: Churchill Livingstone; 2003: 115.

36. Cathie AG. Growth and nutrition of the body with special reference to the head. AAO Yearbook; 1962:149–153.

37. Frymann VM. The trauma of birth. Osteopathic Annals 1976/5:197–205.

38. Carreiro JE. An osteopathic approach to children. Edinburgh: Churchill Livingstone; 2003:232–235.

39. Frymann VM. Why does the orthodontist need osteopathy in the cranial field? The Cranial Letter 1988; 41:4.

Chapter 14

Balanced ligamentous tension techniques

CHAPTER CONTENTS

INTRODUCTION

It appears that although Sutherland became the 'father of cranial osteopathy' he was often upset by the fact that numerous osteopaths, once skilled in the various cranial techniques, went on to concentrate so much attention on the head that the rest of the body was at times forgotten. To address this issue, he gave classes in an attempt to integrate his ideas for the head with those that Still had used for the rest of the body. Both Alan Becker, who had studied with Sutherland, and his father, Rollin Becker, who had studied under Still, confirmed that Still had actually treated the head along with the rest of the body.[1] Lippincott,[2] a student of Sutherland, followed on in this vein and published an article in 1949 entitled 'The Osteopathic Techniques of Wm G Sutherland' in which he laid the basic foundations for what are today known as balanced ligamentous tension techniques (BLT).

Inherent within Sutherland's approach to the cranial structures is the concept of 'normal alignment' (the bones are maintained by their supporting membranous structures) and that where there is no dysfunction the membranes will be in 'balanced membranous tension'.[3] When dysfunction occurs, the supporting membranes will be affected, and at this point Sutherland would diagnose a membranous strain. Sutherland spoke of membranous tension when referring to the cranial and spinal meningeal tissues, but equally, the same state of balance may be found in articulations outside of the craniospinal complex.[4] All articulations rely on the combination of the shape of the joint surfaces and the muscular and ligamentous tensions acting about that joint in order to maintain stability and articular integrity. Although the techniques have been labelled with the name 'ligamentous techniques' it should be borne in mind that their mode of employment is not limited to those structures known purely as ligaments; it extends to include certain other myofascial connective tissue structures. Nevertheless, the name, rather like 'cranial', seems to have stuck and we will use it throughout this text.

Lippincott reiterated Sutherland's idea that the ligaments working about a joint are in 'a state of balanced reciprocal tension and seldom if ever are they completely relaxed throughout the normal range of movement'.[2] However, an aphysiological range of movement such as trauma, whether micro- or macrotrauma, may result in tissue damage and the end result will be a disturbance in this normal state of balance. Furthermore, it does not necessarily require direct trauma to disturb this delicate balance: dysfunction may result from compensatory changes, infection or inflammation. Whatever the means by which the disturbance is set up, the result will be an osteopathic lesion or somatic dysfunction. The reduced range of motion will be created by the unbalanced tension within the ligaments, with a tendency for easier movement to occur towards the lesion. In other words, should two opposing ligaments become unbalanced, any induced movement will be easier towards that particular ligament that has effectively become 'shortened', the lesion component.

This idea is very simple to see in a joint such as the knee, but the more complex an articulation becomes, the more complex its ligamentous arrangement. In an articulation such as the wrist, the arrangement becomes even further complicated because it is capable of quite a complex series of movements, but there are few direct muscular attachments. During various movements of the wrist the two rows of carpal bones move relative to one another; however, this movement is not achieved by direct muscle pulls onto the carpal bones but, in fact, occurs due to the tensions created within the carpal ligaments. There are numerous small ligaments acting between each of the individual carpal bones, and there are the retinaculae that act over the group of carpal bones; and, in addition, there are the ligaments that attach the carpals proximally and distally. This whole network of ligamentous tissue has a resting tension that can be described as its 'normal' tension. When the wrist is moved into flexion,

the altered positions of the carpal bones will increase tension in some ligaments and decrease it in others, but the sum total of the tensions remains the same, provided the movement remains within the normal physiological range. Take this idea further and apply it to an even more complex articulation such as the foot and ankle and we have to add the extra components of gravity and weight-bearing.

It is the tensegrous nature of the attachments that permits these structures to function under the demands of weight-bearing, which at times can be quite excessive. It is also this tensegrous balance that may become disturbed, causing local problems and widespread knock-on effects.

Since the ligaments are not under voluntary control, Sutherland recommended using the inherent forces, the involuntary forces of the body, to make the change required in order to restore harmony to the unbalanced ligamentous articular mechanism. The main involuntary force used is that of respiration, although it is possible to use fluid mechanics or to treat by altering the posture in certain instances. Respiration is not merely an expansion and contraction of the thorax, it has a mechanical effect that is reflected throughout the body.[5] It is apparent to the naked eye of a lay onlooker that breathing has an effect on the abdomen; not so easy to see is the effect on the vertebral column which flattens slightly on inspiration. This mechanical change will be reflected to a greater or lesser extent throughout the whole body via the connective tissue components of the musculoskeletal system.

The aim of the treatment is to restore the state of balance, and this is achieved by careful palpation and gentle but precise positioning of the affected part. The success of the technique lies in achieving a state of balance in the tissues in which all the forces are at zero, or at least, at a minimal level, a neutral point. When this point is reached, the involuntary inherent forces within the body can be utilized to correct the problem.

If we imagine a normally functioning, pure hinge joint that has only flexion and extension movements, there will be, at a certain point somewhere between those two movements, a point of balance where the ligamentous tension will be at a minimum. Should the joint become injured, by whatever means, a state of dysfunction ensues and the balance point will be moved to a different position. The practitioner will find the point at which the forces are minimal and hold the joint at this point until the inherent forces reset the tensions to the preinjury point.[6] At the moment of resetting, since the neutral point is no longer at the point being maintained by the practitioner, it is possible to sense a slight increase in tension as the joint resets. It is important at this point of resetting that the practitioner allows the change to take place; too firm a hold will prevent it and so the hold should be passively supportive. The very same procedure will be used for any joint of the body but obviously all joints do not possess only flexion and extension movements and so a combined movement will be necessary, adding all the vectors together to find the point of balance.

This approach is considered to utilize indirect techniques, that is to say the practitioner is not forcing the change, but merely helping the body to access its own inherent self-healing mechanisms, mobilizing its forces to enable normalization of the dysfunctional state and thereby restoring homeostasis. This self-healing mechanism is now thought by many to be a consequence of the tensegrous nature of the body. BLT is perhaps one of the best examples of how the concept of tensegrity can be applied in treatment. As discussed in Chapter 4, inherent in the concept of tensegrity is the idea that once the force maintaining the dysfunction is overcome, the tensegrous structure will self-stabilize/normalize. In BLT, the practitioner offers support, be it physical or perhaps some form of energetic support, that matches the restricting forces, thereby enabling the articulation to reestablish its correct tensegrous harmony.

References

1. Speece CA, Crow WT. Ligamentous articular strain. Seattle: Eastland Press; 2001.
2. Lippincott HA. The osteopathic technique of Wm G Sutherland DO. 1949 Yearbook of the Academy of Applied Osteopathy. Indianapolis: AAO; 1949.
3. Sutherland WG. Teachings in the science of osteopathy. Portland: Rudra Press; 1990.
4. Magoun HI. Osteopathy in the cranial field, 3rd edn. Kirksville: Journal Printing; 1976.
5. Carreiro JE. Balanced ligamentous tension techniques. In: Ward R, ed. Foundations for osteopathic medicine. Philadelphia: Lippincott Williams and Wilkins; 2003.
6. Becker RE. Motion: the key to diagnosis and treatment. Brooks RE, ed. Life in motion: the osteopathic wisdom of Rollin E Becker, DO. Portland: Rudra Press; 1997.

Chapter 15

Visceral osteopathy

CHAPTER CONTENTS

INTRODUCTION

Visceral osteopathy has taken its place in the treatment approaches used by osteopaths. Increasingly, the importance of visceral conditions, dysfunctions and thus techniques have crept into the osteopathic repertoire over the last decade or two. Certain names have become synonymous with visceral osteopathy, Jean-Pierre Barral and his many co-workers in France, Caroline Stone in the UK and Franz Buset in Belgium. Each has developed their own ideas and together they have increased the knowledge of the visceral system and integrated it into the osteopathic understanding. However, AT Still was the founder of osteopathy and likewise was also the founder of visceral osteopathy. Still frequently made reference to the visceral system and although the techniques may have changed or been adapted since his time, the underlying principles remain the same. 'The Rule of the Artery is Supreme', the axiom attributed to Still, remains as solid in its message today as ever. The links between innervation, nutrition and drainage are still to be seen in all of the visceral techniques that are used by today's osteopaths.

Simply stated, the visceral system encompasses all the organ systems that lie anatomically within the thorax, abdomen and pelvis. They receive their innervation from the autonomic nervous system, in most cases a dual innervation from both the sympathetic and parasympathetic components. It will include the respiratory, cardiovascular, gastrointestinal and genitourinary systems, the glands associated with these systems, their blood and lymph vessels, the hollow and solid organs. In this case, it may be extended to include the associated structures found in the anterior throat region. As distinct from the musculoskeletal system which provides us with locomotion, the visceral system provides the gaseous supply and exchange, digestion, assimilation and excretion systems (and the procreation) that allows the body to function as it does. It may be argued that without the musculoskeletal system the body could not function by acting as a food gatherer for itself. Nevertheless, this chicken and egg syndrome results in the exquisite systemic interplay of the fully functioning body and any self-respecting osteopath would never neglect this interplay. However, some may choose to exert their effect on this interplay by coming at it from a different direction to others. Most osteopaths who choose to use visceral techniques would also recognize that optimum function cannot be achieved without appropriate work on the musculoskeletal system, thereby recognizing the importance of this interplay.

The link between the visceral and musculoskeletal systems is made by the attachments of the organs and structures involved. A cursory look at the anatomy will remind the practitioner that the organs are not merely contained within the body compartments of the throat, thorax, abdomen and pelvis but many are fixed relatively solidly and uniformly to the surrounding framework (Fig. 15.1). Furthermore, certain organs are attached to one another. The axial portion of the musculoskeletal system not only provides protection to the organs within but also support. It is through the supporting mechanisms that function or dysfunction may arise and it is via the attachments that a number of osteopathic visceral techniques have their mode of employment.

The statement that the viscera are attached to the surrounding framework or to one another may imply that they are immobile. This is certainly not the case, as is seen, for example, with the movement

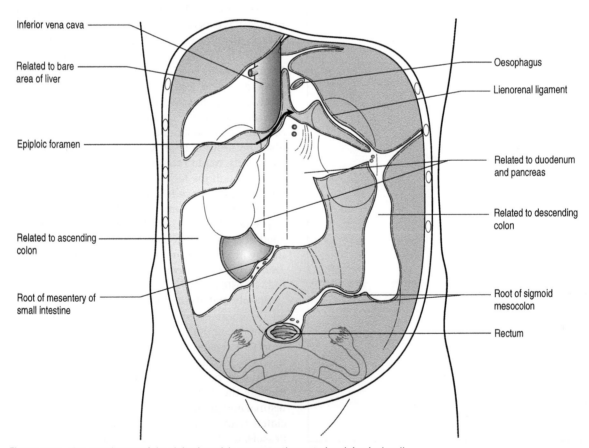

Figure 15.1   The attachment of the abdominopelvic organs to the posterior abdominal wall.

of the liver and other organs during diaphragmatic excursion with respiration. Mobility of the organs is permitted by the serous membranes of the thorax and abdomen and the areolar tissue between fascial compartments of the throat and in the pelvis, which create a number of sliding surfaces. These serous membranes are the thin outermost mesothelial layer of connective tissues that secrete a serous fluid permitting a relatively free movement of the organs over one another and over the internal aspect of the respective body compartment. As such, the serous membranes of the abdomen are to be found on those surfaces of the organs directly adjacent to the peritoneal cavity. Certain surfaces not adjacent to the peritoneal cavity, for example the posterior sur-

faces of the large intestine, are serous free and remain a non-secretory connective tissue. These sliding surfaces are essential to normal everyday physiological processes, deglutition, respiration, defaecation, micturition and parturition. They allow organs to move relatively freely over one another, within the limits of their attachments, permitting expansion and retraction of the hollow organs as in the case of a full/empty stomach, bowel or bladder. In the case of the abdomen it is the peritoneum which is the largest and most complexly arranged serous membrane of the body[1] (Fig. 15.2). In the thorax, the pleurae line the cavity and cover the lungs, leaving the midline space between them free, the mediastinum.

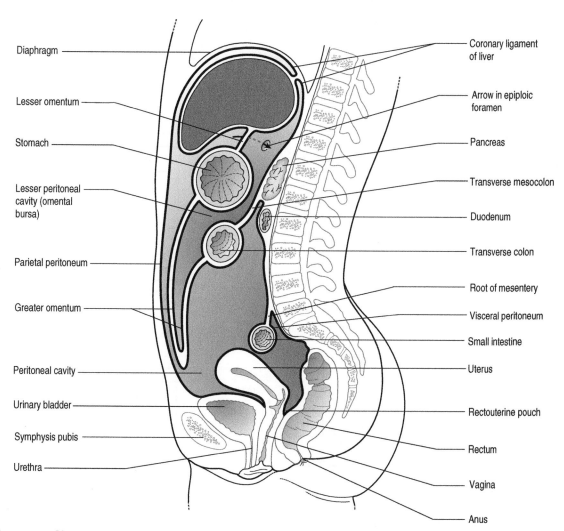

Figure 15.2   Diagrammatic representation of a sagittal section through the abdomen and pelvis to show the peritoneum.

The thorax presents its own kind of problem to treatment in that it has a bony barrier to overcome in order to reach the viscera contained within. It is this inaccessibility that makes this very important area difficult to treat. One approach is as follows: if the thorax is viewed as a series of three cylinders, one either side containing the lungs and a central cylinder containing the mediastinum, the problem becomes surmountable. By extending the idea of the cylinders, it is possible to view the thoracic vertebral column as a relatively hard but nevertheless flexible posterior cylinder that undoubtedly may have an effect on the mobility of the other cylinders. Finally, this series of four cylinders, three soft and one hard, is contained within an all-encompassing larger cylinder, the thoracic cage. By working on the aforementioned sliding surfaces that exist between the structures, the osteopath is able to influence the mobility and motility indirectly. It is conceivable that by gently 'rolling' the cylinders, one against the others, in all possible axes of movement, mobility may be tested and, if restrictions are found, treated using direct or indirect methods (Fig. 15.3). As a result of improved mobility, blood supply, venous and lymphatic drainage and nerve supply would also be improved, resulting in better function of a previously dysfunctioning organ or viscus.

The central cylinder is the mediastinum, which anatomically is divided into superior and inferior parts by a line drawn from the sternal angle anteriorly to the inferior border of the body of the fourth thoracic vertebra posteriorly. The superior mediastinum contains the great vessels, vagus, cardiac and phrenic nerves, trachea and oesophagus, thoracic duct and numerous important lymph nodes. The inferior mediastinum is divided into anterior, middle and posterior portions. The middle mediastinum contains the heart in the pericardium and the great vessels as they enter and exit. Furthermore, it contains the bifurcation of the trachea and the two bronchi, the azygos vein, the deep part of the cardiac plexus and some tracheobronchial lymph nodes. The anterior mediastinum, lying between the sternum and the pericardium, is narrow due to the approximation of the lungs in their pleural sacs anteriorly and may contain the vestiges of the

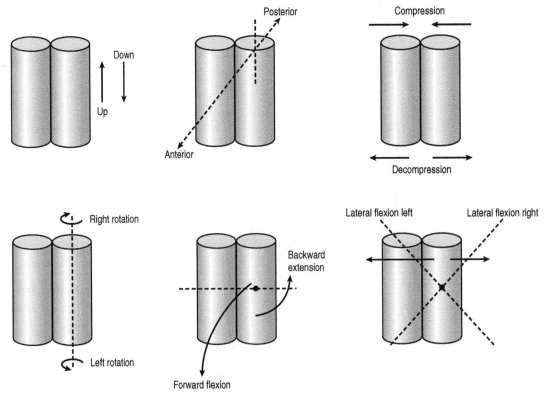

Figure 15.3 Axes of movement of the 'cylinders'. Any of these axes might become restricted, resulting in a restriction of the 'sliding surface' motion. Only two cylinders are shown for clarity.

thymus gland, some lymph nodes and some areolar tissue. The posterior mediastinum contains the thoracic portion of the descending aorta, the azygos and hemiazygos veins, the splanchnic and vagus nerves, oesophagus, thoracic duct and some lymph nodes. With respect to innervation, nutrition and drainage, the mediastinum may be seen as a very important area to the body as a whole and so judicious treatment will be indicated where restriction exists.

Naturally, the lungs as essential organs of respiration can only benefit from a full and unhindered range of movement, and so to address the lungs in their pulmonary pleura separated from the internal aspect of the thoracic wall by the parietal pleura should not be overlooked. Restrictions in mobility may arise from any number of causes: principally, primary lung or pleural disease, thoracic trauma, pneumothorax or as a result of thoracic surgery.

The posterior cylinder, vertebral column and the surrounding thoracic cage will obviously need to be addressed in any treatment of the internal cylinders. This highlights the importance of the attachments of the viscera with the bony thorax, the sternopericardial and the vertebropericardial ligaments. In addition, the suspensory apparatus of the pleura in the region of the thoracic inlet and the pericardial attachments to the diaphragm become important.

Finally, the attachments of the diaphragm to the sternum, lower six ribs and costal cartilages, and the upper three or four lumbar vertebrae should also be considered, as should the attachments inferior to the diaphragm.

The idea described above of the thorax as a series of cylinders may be equally applied to the abdomen, pelvis and neck regions.

The neck may be viewed as two large cylinders, a posterior one containing the cervical vertebral column with its associated muscles and ligaments and an anterior cylinder containing the anterior throat (Fig. 15.4). It is possible to view these as a relatively hard bony cylinder posteriorly, which although mobile may be restricted by its vertebral articulations or the soft tissues attaching to it. Anteriorly, the cylinder is composed largely of soft tissues with the hyoid bone, thyroid, cricoid and tracheal cartilages interposed within it.

In the upper neck, this anterior cylinder houses the pharynx which is suspended from the base of the skull by the superior constrictor muscle of the pharynx and the pharyngobasilar fascia. Inferiorly, it separates into two distinct cylinders as the oesophagus posteriorly and trachea anteriorly. Lying anterior to the trachea is the isthmus of the thyroid gland with its two lobes extending superi-

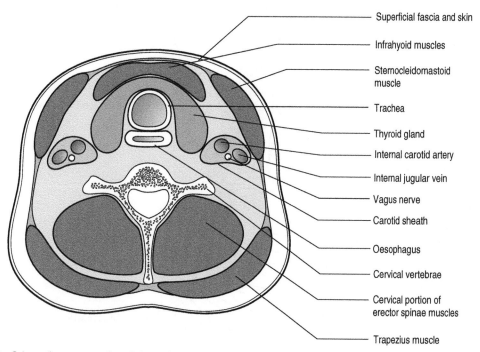

Superficial fascia and skin

Infrahyoid muscles

Sternocleidomastoid muscle

Trachea

Thyroid gland

Internal carotid artery

Internal jugular vein

Vagus nerve

Carotid sheath

Oesophagus

Cervical vertebrae

Cervical portion of erector spinae muscles

Trapezius muscle

Figure 15.4   Schematic representation of the neck as two cylinders.

orly and inferiorly from it enclosed in the pretracheal fascia. Lying just posterolaterally to these are the bilateral cylinders of the carotid sheath containing the common carotid artery (internal carotid artery superiorly), the internal jugular vein and the vagus nerve. This group of anterior cylinders is separated from the posterior cylinder by the prevertebral fascia and the whole series of cylinders are surrounded by the investing fascia of the neck. These fascial layers permit movement of the sliding surfaces in order to facilitate in deglutition, phonation and movements of the head and neck. This region is a prime example of the relationship between the visceral and musculoskeletal systems. Surrounding the whole series of internal cylinders is a relatively mobile muscular tube anteriorly comprising the superficial anterior throat musculature, including the supra- and infrahyoid muscles, sternocleidomastoid and platysma. This connects the anterior throat to the skull above and the pectoral girdle below and is closely linked with the stomatognathic system (Fig. 15.5). The stomatognathic system refers to the interrelationship between the head, neck, jaw,

hyoid and pectoral girdle and it has been proposed that this system has a direct influence via proprioceptive feedback pathways on the comportment of the whole body.[2] In the above discussion, we have brushed aside the all too obvious direct connection of the cervical spine and the posterior compartment of muscles. It may be seen that by overlooking this 'visceral' aspect of treatment, the osteopath may be neglecting a major component of treating the patient 'structurally'. And so, osteopaths who consider themselves 'structural' workers and who baulk at the thought of treating 'viscerally', are most likely going to have an effect viscerally whether they like it or not!

The viscera of the abdomen may also be viewed in a similar 'cylinder' fashion although due to the gross derangements of position during embryological development, the pattern is not so easily seen and tends to change rather more dramatically throughout its length than in the thorax.

A transverse section made through the upper abdomen at the level of the twelfth thoracic vertebra reveals a large cylinder composed of the abdomi-

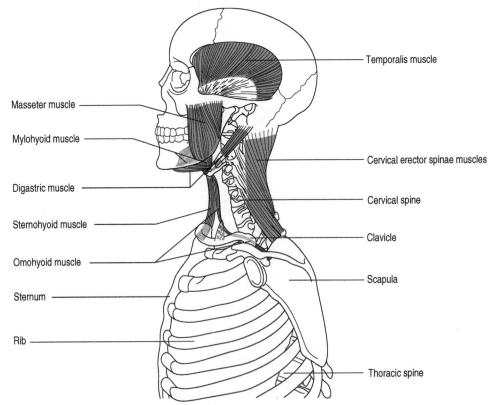

Temporalis muscle

Masseter muscle

Mylohyoid muscle

Digastric muscle

Sternohyoid muscle

Omohyoid muscle

Sternum

Rib

Cervical erector spinae muscles

Cervical spine

Clavicle

Scapula

Thoracic spine

Figure 15.5 The linkage system from the head to the neck and thence to the pectoral girdle, as part of the stomatognathic system.

nal wall lined internally with a serous membrane, the peritoneum (Fig. 15.6). Posteriorly lies the vertebral column and lying either side of this are the two kidneys ensheathed in the renal fascia and a varying amount of fat. At this level, it is possible to see two solid organs, the liver on the right side and the spleen on the left, with a 'hollow organ', the stomach, lying between them. The main neurovascular bundle of the abdomen, containing the abdominal aorta, the inferior vena cava and the paravertebral ganglionic chains of the sympathetic nervous system, lie just anterior to the vertebral column. They are situated retroperitoneally behind the posterior wall of the omental bursa. The parasympathetic part of the autonomic nervous system is largely represented in the abdomen by the vagus nerve which has followed the oesophagus through the diaphragm as the anterior and posterior vagal trunks. The vagal component supplies the gastrointestinal tract as far as the splenic flexure. The vagal trunks will form the gastric plexus and then continue into the coeliac, superior and inferior mesenteric ganglia with the sympathetic components of the autonomic supply to the viscera.

A transverse section made lower down at the level between the second and third lumbar verte-brae reveals a loss of the solid organs and a predominance of the hollow organs. However, depending on the individual examined, it may still be possible to view the lower border of the right lobe of the liver wedged between the greater omentum and the ascending colon. The presence of the psoas major muscle, forming its bulk on the sides of the lumbar vertebral column, has pushed the two kidneys laterally although at this level only the very ends of the lower poles may be visible. The right kidney extends further inferiorly than the left due to the presence of the liver on the right side and so it may still be visible. Lying anterior to the vertebral column is the neurovascular bundle, still lying retroperitoneally. The main features seen at this level are the ascending and descending colons with the descending colon lying slightly more posteriorly than the ascending portion. At this level, both the ascending and descending colons are in a retroperitoneal position and on either side of them are the paracolic gutters or sulci. A confusion to the vertical cylinder idea arises at this level: it is possible to see two horizontal cylinders, anteriorly is the transverse colon and posteriorly, the duodenum. Lying between these two horizontal cylinders are the coils of the small intestine: the jejunum and ileum which

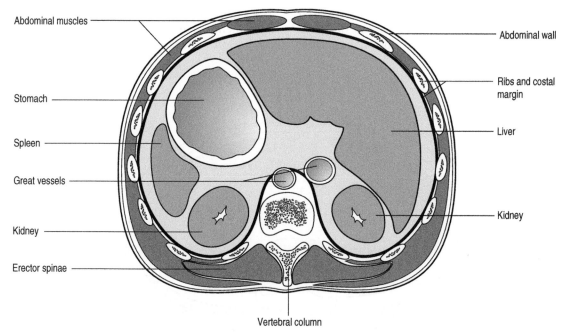

Figure 15.6 Transverse section through the body at about the twelfth thoracic vertebral level. Some of the sliding surfaces between the cylinders formed by the viscera at this level may be seen.

are attached to the vertebral cylinder by the root of the mesentery. The major part of the anterior and lateral portions of the peritoneal cavity is filled by the greater omentum.

Finally, the pelvis may be viewed in the same manner. In the upper pelvis, the sigmoid colon is found on the left side, whilst lower down it continues more centrally and posteriorly as the rectum (Fig. 15.7). In the female pelvis, lying anterior to the rectum is the uterus and more inferiorly the vagina; further anteriorly lies the bladder. In the male, the arrangement is similar with the exception that the uterus is replaced by the seminal vesicles whilst the bladder sits on the prostate gland. The contents of the pelvis in both male and female lie inferior to the peritoneum and a number of blind-ending, peritoneal-lined pouches or recesses may be seen. Lying between the rectum and uterus in the female is the rectouterine Pouch of Douglas whilst anterior to the uterus is the vesicouterine pouch separating the body of the uterus from the bladder. In the male, the absence of the uterus creates a rectovesical recess. The pelvis is lined internally by an endopelvic fascia and the contents are further lined by fascial sheets named correspondingly to their adjacent structures.

This simplified version of viewing the body compartments as a series of cylinders enables treatment to be applied with respect to the mobility of the viscera by moving a particular cylinder on its neighbour or neighbours, or within a larger cylinder. However, it does not consider individually all of the numerous attachments of the various structures contained within. Major attachments such as the mesentery of the small intestine have been mentioned but many more, smaller but nevertheless important ligaments and fascial condensations have been omitted. Any osteopath working with visceral techniques would need to be familiar with these attachments that are far too numerous to be described in a text such as this.

In addition to the supporting system, there is another aspect to visceral osteopathic techniques that uses the inherent motility of the organs. In a similar way to which the involuntary mechanism has been applied to the craniosacral system, it has been proposed that the visceral organs also possess a 'motility'. Motility differs from mobility in that the latter is a measurable extrinsic motion of a structure, whereas motility is an inherent motion. In the case of the liver, a visible motion is afforded by the diaphragm which when raising and lowering in the normal course of respiration, causes the liver to ascend and descend with it. In addition to this mobility, the liver also possesses an innate motion independent to the mobility. Barral[3] describes this intrinsic motion as a 'low frequency and low amplitude movement that is invisible to the naked eye'. He believes that it is not dependent on the primary respiratory motion but arises as a result of 'cellular memory of embryological movements'. He proposes that it 'represents an oscillation between accentuation of the embry-

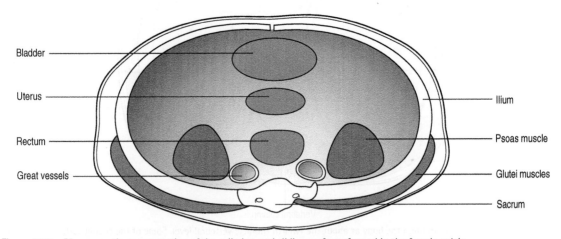

Figure 15.7   Diagrammatic representation of the cylinders and sliding surfaces formed in the female pelvis.

ological movement and a return to the original position'. Barral and Mercier state that visceral motility has a frequency of approximately 7 cycles per minute as opposed to the 10–14 cycles per minute frequency seen in the 'primary respiratory motion' proposed by Sutherland.[4] By way of differentiating it from the extrinsic mobility created by diaphragmatic excursion, Barral and Mercier describe the motility as 'expir' when the organ moves closer to the median axis and 'inspir' as it moves away (Fig. 15.8). To describe motility of organs on the median axis, they describe 'expir' as an anterior movement and 'inspir' as a posterior movement.

Passive palpation of the motility of the viscera is known as 'listening' and allows the osteopath to assess whether the movement is normal or abnormal. The rate, amplitude and symmetry are assessed and if it is decided that there is an abnormality, then treatment may be applied directly to the organ affected. In order to localize areas of dysfunction, a 'general listening' technique is performed (Fig. 15.9). This is usually performed with the patient in the sitting position and involves the practitioner placing one hand over the posterior aspect of the skull and the other over the sacrum. An indication of laterality, level and sense of position in the sagittal plane is obtained by the involuntary movement of the body towards the restriction. Therefore, for example, a lateral flexion to the right with an associated amount of flexion in the sagittal plane may indicate a restriction at the level of the

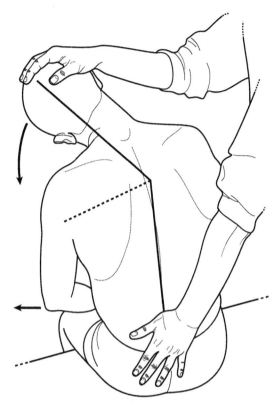

Figure 15.9   General listening.

liver. In order to verify the position of the restriction, 'local listening' is performed which involves placing a hand over the organ or region where a restriction is suspected, thus homing in on the restricted element (Fig. 15.10). Finally, the motility of the individual organ must be tested and, once again, this requires additional knowledge beyond the scope of this book. Each individual organ possesses its own axis of movement and in order to assess this fully, a working knowledge of the whole system of visceral motility is essential. In order to treat dysfunctions of motility an 'induction' technique is used which basically 'induces' normality by directly accentuating the more normal part of the cycle until either a release is felt or normal motility is restored. The release may or may not be accompanied by a still point. As with all osteopathic techniques for palpation and treatment an enormous amount of practice is required in order to reach perfection.

With respect to treatment, osteopaths may choose to work with the mobility, the motility or both. It is likely that one will affect the other and that considering only one aspect will still result in a

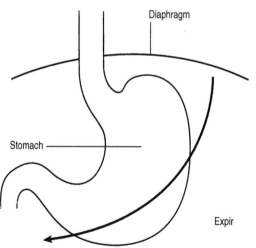

Figure 15.8   'Expir' motion of the stomach as described by Barral and Mercier.

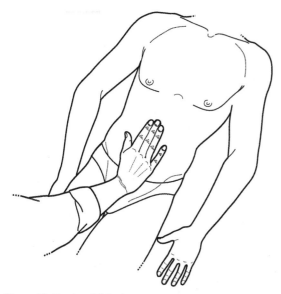

Figure 15.10 Local listening.

change with the other, although the extent of the effect remains a controversial point between osteopaths. Some practitioners will insist on working with the motility as a deeper form of treatment; others feel they may be too inexperienced or lack the palpatory skill required to work with such a fine movement.

Barral[5] states that he often uses a technique that appears to be a mixture between an induction and a mobilization technique. Once again, this is a controversial remark: some may feel that the mixing of techniques is sacrilege whilst others, it would appear Barral included, feel that this is fine. A moot point for anyone embarking on this form of 'technique mixing' would be not to mix functional techniques with structural tests or vice versa. Use of a structural technique first requires diagnosis by a structural test. Mixing the two may confuse the novice and most certainly make their treatment at least ineffective, and at worst dangerous.

References

1. Williams PL, Warwick R, eds. Gray's anatomy, 36th edn. Edinburgh: Churchill Livingstone; 1980: 1321–1333.
2. Walther DS. Applied kinesiology, vol II. Head, neck and jaw pain and dysfunction – the stomatognathic system. Colorado: Systems DC; 1983.
3. Barral JP, Mercier P. Visceral manipulation. Seattle: Eastland Press; 1988: 5–29.
4. Sutherland WG. With thinking fingers. Missouri: Journal Printing Company; 1962.
5. Barral JP. Visceral manipulation II. Seattle: Eastland Press; 1988.

Recommended reading

A series of books have been written by JP Barral and published by Eastland Press, on various visceral regions and techniques.

Caroline Stone has written two books on visceral approach published by Tigger Publishing, Maidstone.

Chapter 16

Indirect approach technique: myofascial

INTRODUCTION

Osteopaths have often used the fascia as a means of examination, diagnosis and treatment, but it is only recently that we have really begun to understand the true functioning of the fascial system. This development in our understanding has helped explain the effectiveness of this valuable osteopathic tool. It has become clear that the fascia is very closely associated with the muscular system both structurally and functionally. It is for this reason that the term 'fascial techniques' is today being replaced by the term 'myofascial techniques'. This false separation into two separate systems was misleading. Still[1] was more than aware of the importance of the fascia and wrote:

> If we are to have anything like a clear overview of soft tissue dysfunction it is necessary to add into the equation the influence of fascia which invests, supports, divides, enwraps, gives cohesion to and is an integral part of every aspect of soft tissue structure and function throughout the body and which represents a single structural entity, from the inside of the skull to the soles of the feet.[1]

In order to truly appreciate the continuity of the myofascial system we need to remind ourselves of some basic anatomy.

The holistic approach adopted by the osteopath will of necessity have a respect for integration of the whole body anatomy and physiology. In its simplest form, anatomy, especially that of the musculoskeletal system, is a continuum. The public at one time regarded osteopaths as 'dealing with the joints' and it is true that we do have a great deal of interest in joint function. The articular integrity of a joint is dependent on three major factors (Fig. 16.1):

1. The shape of the articular surfaces and hence the congruity of the joint.
2. The tension of the ligaments acting about that joint.
3. The tension of the muscles acting about that joint.

What is so important to the osteopath is how a particular joint functions with respect to others, and one of the major factors in linking joint function together is the muscular system.

Any anatomy text book will give us the origins and insertions of skeletal muscles. Their attachments bind muscles at each end to various bony points and possibly other soft tissue structures, but in numerous anatomy texts their continuity is often neglected.

If we take a simple example, the upper extremity is attached to the bony axial skeleton at the sternoclavicular joint and is afforded its great mobility by the structure and nature of this joint and that of the scapulothoracic articulation. At this point, many anatomy texts will then describe the muscles attaching the humerus to the scapula and clavicle under the heading of the upper extremity muscles. They will then describe serratus anterior, trapezius, rhomboids and levator scapulae as axial muscles attached to the scapula (and clavicle in the case of trapezius).

Let us take a closer look at trapezius. It is attached from the superior nuchal line of the occiput, to the ligamentum nuchae, supraspinous ligament and spinous processes down as far as the dorsolumbar junction. We would, then, agree that it might be axial in 'origin' but that it has a major role to play in the stabilization and mobilization of the scapula and hence will have an influence on upper extremity function. By virtue of its vertebral attachments, any restriction of mobility in the dorsal or cervical spine may have an effect on scapula mobility and thus on upper extremity function. It would be rational to suggest that any dysfunction of upper extremity mobility may have an effect on vertebral function.

We know from basic anatomy that the rhomboids, major and minor, and the levator scapulae also attach to the spine in the cervical and upper dorsal regions, and also to the scapula, thus reinforcing the possibility of an interaction of vertebral-upper extremity dysfunction. Now consider serratus anterior with its attachments to the ribs and we further compound the idea by the possible compromise of rib mobility. Pectoralis major with its sternoclavicular and humeral attachments further complicates the picture, as do pectoralis minor and coracobrachialis with their attachments to the coracoid process of the scapula, the humerus, the ribs and the costal cartilages.

Although at this stage we have not discussed the rest of the muscles of the upper extremity we can picture that the muscular links are extended right down to the fingertips. Most of us are aware that even a minor problem such as a sprained wrist or elbow affects the way we hold our arm and so we can imagine the repercussions that may take place more proximally at the shoulder and so on.

We could propose that a simple shoulder dysfunction could compromise rib function, or vice versa. We are aware that a major function of ribs is the act of breathing but if we explore the anatomical relations of the costal articulations we develop a broader picture. Posteriorly, the ribs possess costovertebral and costotransverse articulations and lying in close proximity to the internal aspects of these articulations is the sympathetic ganglionic chain. It is these ganglia that are responsible for the

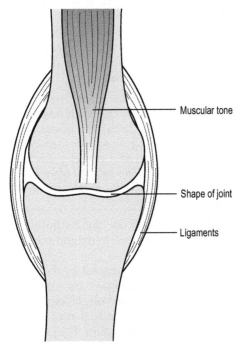

Figure 16.1   Articular integrity = shape + muscle tone + ligamentous tension. Congruity may be increased by cartilage, e.g. menisci, labrum.

Muscular tone

Shape of joint

Ligaments

transmission of the sympathetic impulses supplying the thoracoabdominal-pelvic viscera, their importance having been discussed in Chapter 6. To complete our holistic picture of the musculoskeletal system we need to add the lower extremity and the head.

Most anatomical texts, when referring to the hip joint of the lower extremity, would list the hamstrings, adductors, lateral rotators and glutei muscle groups. They would also make mention of iliopsoas as a hip flexor and the actions of sartorius and rectus femoris of the anterior compartment group of muscles. The anatomical integrational aspect neglected by many texts may be demonstrated by exploring the relationship between the paravertebral muscles and the gluteus maximus. The multifidus portion of the paravertebral muscles group attaches to the sacrum and extends throughout the whole vertebral column. In its lower part it is enclosed by the external and intermediate layers of the thoracolumbar fascia which itself is anchored to the sacrum and the iliac crest of the innominate bone. Gluteus maximus forms a raphe with multifidus on the sacrum and with its iliac fibres then passes to the gluteal tuberosity of the femur and the fascia lata. In addition to this we should note that piriformis passes from the anterior aspect of the sacrum to the greater trochanter of the femur whilst the psoas portion of iliopsoas passes from the lumbar spine to the lesser trochanter of the femur.

In a similar fashion to the upper extremity, we have a direct connection between the vertebral column and the lower extremity. With these connections in mind, we could then propose the idea of a dysfunction interaction working between the lower extremity and the axial skeleton.

Likewise, with the upper extremity we have not discussed the more distal muscle links but again it is not difficult to imagine the interactions taking place between the distal and proximal muscle groups, and if we add to this the effect of weight-bearing we can easily imagine the repercussions that may take place.

The muscle latissimus dorsi arises from the iliac crest, thoracolumbar fascia and lumbar spine and passes upwards, taking slips from some of the ribs and the inferior angle of the scapula before attaching in the floor of the bicipital groove of the humerus, linking the pelvic girdle and the upper extremity.

We may assume that structural problems of either upper or lower extremities may create dysfunction in the spine or vice versa and thus compromise the body's ability to perform as a functional entity. If there was no interrelationship between the upper and lower extremity function they would not be necessary for coordinated movements and we would be able to run marathons quite comfortably with our hands in our pockets!

The head is balanced precariously on the cervical spine and is prevented from toppling by an intricate system of muscles that are attached on all sides. We have already mentioned the attachments of trapezius to the superior nuchal line of the occiput and we made a brief mention of the paravertebral muscles that run the length of the vertebral column from the sacrum to the skull. The longus colli and longus capitis muscles run on the anterior and lateral aspects of the cervical spine and again attach to the base of the skull. On the lateral aspect of the cervical column we have the scalene muscles which attach to the first and second ribs and the sternocleidomastoid muscle which passes from the skull to the sternum and clavicle. So this intricate arrangement of muscles from the skull and cervical spine also links to the thoracic spine, the ribs and the pectoral girdle – and so in the same way that we have seen the possibility of dysfunction interactions elsewhere, we can now see the same possibility for the head and neck. Furthermore, we have an even more intricate arrangement of muscles that connect the occiput and the upper two cervical vertebrae, the rectus capitis and obliquus capitis muscles. Finally, we have a set of muscles that lie superficial to the structures of the anterior throat and connect the skull, mandible, hyoid bone, sternum and the scapula, forming part of the stomatognathic system.

We have not given any deep anatomical detail as yet but already we can see that there is a muscular linkage system that extends throughout the whole body. This is no great revelation in the world of anatomy but the consequences of dysfunction are frequently overlooked by many within the healthcare professions. To many, a 'muscle strain' is just a 'muscle strain' and no further thought is given to the possible repercussions throughout the system as a whole. Osteopaths will use this linkage system as a means to establish an overall picture as to how the body functions as a unit and not as a series of disconnected segments. The muscular links of the body are only part of the picture; we now need to look at the fascial links.

The conventional viewpoint of fascia has recognized its continuity but often dismissed it as a kind of 'extra connective tissue'. *Butterworths Medical Dictionary*[2] defines fascia as 'a layer or sheet of connective tissue separating or enclosing groups of muscles or other organs; the connective-tissue sheath of an organ'. *Gray's Anatomy*[3] states that 'fascia is a term so wide and elastic in usage that it signifies little more than a collection of connective tissue large enough to be described by the unaided eye'.

The structure of fascia is highly variable and depends on its location and function. Anatomists do not always agree on nomenclature, dividing it into a number of layers and locations.

Superficial fascia lies deep to the dermal layer of the skin and is composed of a loose areolar tissue that is both fibrous and elastic. It contains branches from the subcutaneous nerves, vessels and lymphatics, fat and some superficial skin muscles, though the latter are more predominant in other mammals than in humans. Its loose nature allows the skin to move quite freely on the underlying tissues and its fat content creates an insulating layer. In colder climates the proportion of fat is higher than in warmer regions. There is also a difference in the proportion and distribution of the fat between the sexes. Superficial fascia is dense in the scalp, soles of the feet and palms of the hands, but thinner in the dorsums of the hands and feet. Other areas requiring freedom of movement, including the face, sides of the neck, anus, penis and scrotum are again proportionally thinner. The superficial fascia is a potential space for pooling of excess fluids and metabolites which allows us as osteopaths to palpate for tissue texture changes.

Deep fascia is composed largely of collagen fibres but they are denser and more regular than superficial fascia in their arrangement. The deep fascia is the compartment-forming fascia, enclosing single muscles and groups of muscles. It may act as an anchor point for muscles and in these cases is termed an 'intermuscular septum'. In certain areas the structure of the deep fascia is modified to perform specific functions, as in the retinacula of the wrists and ankles and the fibrous sheaths of the digits.

The internal fascia is the name usually given to the endothoracic, endoabdominal and endopelvic fascias. They fix the parietal layer of the pleura in the thorax and the peritoneum in the abdomen and the pelvis to the inner aspect of the body wall. In certain regions, the internal fascia is well defined and usually takes the name of the adjacent structures, e.g. psoas fascia.

A fourth category of fascia is sometimes referred to as the 'subserous fascia'. It lines the individual viscera. In places this has become organized into structurally more independent bands which somewhat confusingly are then called ligaments. In fact, the term ligament means 'to bind together' and so naming these fascial bands as ligaments is not as strange as it may at first appear.

These visceral ligaments are many and diverse, and may be named after the person who first 'discovered' them or by the structures that they bind together. They are also diverse in structure, some being merely connective tissue bands whilst others are fibromuscular in nature with varying amounts of fibrous and smooth muscle tissue contained within them.

Some texts state that 'true' visceral ligaments must contain smooth muscle and those that do not are 'false' ligaments, but there seems to be no strict ruling as to how much or how little smooth muscle needs to be present in order to prevent the ligament from being termed a muscle!

Nevertheless, whether these structures are termed ligaments, muscles, fascia or otherwise there seems to be a unanimous decision that this connective tissue is somewhat continuous throughout the whole body.

Osteopaths have recognized for many years that there appears to be an inherent motility in fascia and that this motility may be employed in order to assist us in examination, diagnosis and treatment of patients. As is often seen in osteopathy, until recently there was never a plausible scientific explanation for this motility. However, as is the case already seen with cranial osteopathy, recent research may begin to interpret these findings and pave the way to a clearer, if only partial, explanation.

It was considered for many years that it was the mechanical properties of fascia that could explain its effective usage in osteopathic treatment. Fascia was considered a continuous medium that could undergo physical change by the use of manual manipulation. It is well accepted that collagenous tissue when placed under a constant load will undergo elongation. Once its maximal elongation is reached, if the load is sustained for a prolonged period of time, then a subsequent further subtle elongation occurs that is known as 'creep'.[4] On releasing the applied load, the tissue will return towards its original length but at a different rate to that at which it lengthened. The difference between the rate of change of length in loading and unloading is known as 'hysteresis'.[4] Moreover, it may not return to its original length, the difference being known as a 'set'.[4] It was these properties of fascia and other connective tissues that osteopaths and other practitioners such as massage therapists thought responsible for the efficacy of treatment of the fascia. One such therapist, Ida Rolf,[5] published a book in 1977 on her own method of treatment utilizing the fascia, which she called 'Rolfing'. It involves a form of pressure type massage in order to change the physical properties of the fascia. Rolf's explanation was that the fascia underwent a change from the 'gel' to the 'sol' state, making it more pliable. This increase of pliability in the fascia reduced tensions and as such resulted in reduced pain. Although these changes from gel to sol do occur when the fascia is subjected to heat or mechanical application, this is not the full story in the sense of the osteopathic usage. The gel to sol or 'thixotropic change'[6] is acceptable as an explanation for short-term effects but the changes reputedly experienced by osteopaths require further explanation.

Osteopaths have always felt that they can sense a 'release' in the fascia when working on it. So what does this mean and how is it experienced? There are numerous approaches to working fascially; there are the more gentle indirect approaches that allow the tissue to do the guiding until a release point is achieved, and there are the more direct techniques which are more confrontational in nature. The latter techniques employ the use of more, and sometimes a great deal more, force, than the indirect techniques. Practitioners of both techniques will report similar findings at the point when the technique has its effect: there is 'release of the tissues'. This is a term bandied about quite frequently in osteopathy and it basically refers to a palpable change in the tensions of the tissues being worked upon; there is a 'melting' or 'giving way' of the restrictive components of the structure being treated. As can be demonstrated with the thixotropic changes there are measurable changes that take place in the fascia but this requires a great deal more force than that normally used by an osteopath; moreover, it requires more time than that usually available in a standard treatment session.[7] So if osteopaths really do feel something releasing, it is probably not the thixotropic change.

Another explanation proposed was the 'piezo-electric effect' in which a small electrical charge is produced as an effect of the treatment and this then stimulates fibroclastic activity (and possibly inhibits fibroblastic activity). Although this has been shown to be an effective process in certain cases of bone repair after fractures and in some aspects of wound healing,[8] it is the time factor that prevents this from being the explanation in osteopathic fascial techniques.

Fascia is quite heavily supplied by the nervous system and a very high number of its sensory nerves come from a variety of mechanoreceptors. Since fascia is the all-enveloping and attaching structure that medical science accepts it to be, it is quite normal for it to have some kind of biomechanical role and as such, it requires not only a feedback system, to itself, but also a 'feed forward' system, to other structures. It makes sense that the mechanoreceptors found in the fascia can report back to the central nervous system on the state of tissue tensions throughout the body. It has been shown that stimulation of the mechanoreceptors does, in fact, create measurable effects in skeletal muscles.[9] The effect seen is much greater in the gamma motor neurones than in the alpha, thus implying that the fascia is having primarily a direct proprioceptive effect but, in addition, a secondary effect on skeletal muscle tonus. If we divide the mechanoreceptors found in fascia into their separate types, we can see that the responses to stimulation are not just limited to muscular effects. Schleip[10] notes that in addition to decreasing tonus in striated muscles and proprioceptive feedback, these responses are responsible for inhibition of sympathetic activity, vasodilatory changes and plasma extravasation (see Table 16.1 for details).

Much work has been performed on the viscoelastic properties of fascia and Schleip cites the work of Yahia and co-workers[11] and Staubesand[12] who carried out two related but independent studies. Yahia found that some connective tissues when subjected to an isometric tension actually began to

Table 16.1   Receptor types and their effects (After Schleip R. Fascial plasticity – a new neurobiological explanation, Part 1. Journal of Bodywork and Movement Therapies 2003; 7(1):11–19)

Receptor type	Effects
Golgi type Ib	Decreased tone in associated skeletal muscle
Pacini type II	Proprioception
Ruffini type II	Inhibition of sympathetic activity
Interstitial type III and IV	Vasodilatory changes Plasma extravasation

increase the tension. She concluded by proposing the possibility of muscular action taking place within the fascia and suggested a histological study. Staubesand published his work 3 years later, to show that there were indeed smooth muscle cells interspersed with collagen fibres in the fascia cruris. Schleip states that 'it seems justified to say that both studies taken together show that there are smooth muscle cells embedded in the fascia, and that it is highly probable that they are involved in the regulation of an intrafascial pretension'.[10] Staubesand also found the presence of both myelinated and unmyelinated nerve fibres in the fascia and although unable to categorically state their functions, he proposed that it seems likely that the myelinated fibres are sensory in nature whilst the unmyelinated fibres are autonomic efferents to the smooth muscle or perform some other autonomic function. Finally, Staubesand also noted the presence of perforations in the superficial fascia at points where the perforating branches of nerve, artery and veins (the neurovascular bundle) gained access to the muscular compartments. Studies[13] have shown that these perforations are often associated with a thickened band of collagen fibres around the nerves and vessels in patients suffering from chronic shoulder or neck pain. Furthermore, microsurgical intervention to 'release' unusually thickened bands resulted in significant pain reduction.

The recent progress in research into understanding the fascial system may help us as osteopaths to explain what is actually occurring under our hands as we work. The presence of smooth muscle fibres in the fascia may account for the inherent motion that we feel we are able to palpate. The release that we feel when we are treating could be accounted for by a relaxation of these muscle fibres due to proprioceptive feedback. The positioning of the patient in certain procedures could place the fascial system at a point of reduced sensory input. Naturally there will still be some afferent activity but it is quite conceivable that there will be a reduction in any abnormal activity from a dysfunctioning, overstimulated point. This reduction or normalization of proprioceptive feedback may create its effect by two possible routes: directly, creating an inhibition of the smooth muscle activity, or indirectly, by reducing abberant skeletal muscle activity. It seems quite likely that the two are working concurrently and that the proprioceptive balance achieved is responsible for the lasting effects. Up until now, the presence of smooth muscle fibres has only been reported in larger flat sheets of fascia which are responsible for postural changes and thus require a good proprioceptive mechanism. However, osteopaths feel that the same palpatory findings can be made in visceral ligaments which are much less likely to be involved in a postural mechanism. In this case it is more likely that the effect is felt due to relaxation of striated or unstriated muscle fibres in associated structures. It is possible that there could also be a feedback loop to the organ itself and that physiological changes may be provoked in the function of the particular viscus, creating a sensation of change. Many osteopaths will describe a feeling of local warmth at the site of a release; this may well be explained as the vasodilatory changes that are mediated by the interstitial type III and IV mechanoreceptors found in fascia, whilst the increased vasomotor activity may well reinforce this effect.

'Fascial listening' is a term used by osteopaths to describe the process of using the fascia to aid in the examination and diagnosis or assessment of the patient. Some practitioners will place their hands gently on the body in places known as the 'fascial listening posts' (Fig. 16.2). With the patient lying comfortably on their back, commonly used fascial listening posts are the feet, the thighs, over the pelvic region, the lower thoracic cage and the upper thoracic cage or shoulders. There may be a sensation of pulling towards a particular region, indicating the possibility of dysfunction. For example, a pulling up from the feet associated with a pulling down from the thighs may indicate a problem at the knee. However, if there is further pulling up from the thighs and pelvis but a pulling down from the lower thorax, this may indicate a problem in the abdomen. If this is the case, the laterality will be decided by which side is pulling more; a symmetrical pulling would indicate a problem centrally. From there, an idea of depth may be gained by making an anteroposterior (AP) contact, one hand beneath the patient, one hand on top. There may be a sense of rotatory movement in the hands and if, for example, the sensation in the upper hand is stronger or moves more with respect to the lower hand, then the problem is deemed to be more posterior. It has been described as a spiral type movement that is felt with the narrow end of the spiral closest to the problem (Fig. 16.3). The use of the word 'problem' is deliberate: this particular method of diagnosis is used in order to locate dysfunction and not necessarily to define the structure that is dysfunctioning. It will give an approximate location

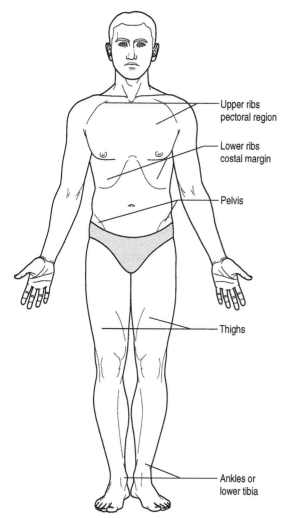

Figure 16.2   Fascial listening posts.

and the knowledge of anatomy will then indicate the structure affected. However, with experience, some practitioners feel confident to name the structure and to state the exact nature of the dysfunction

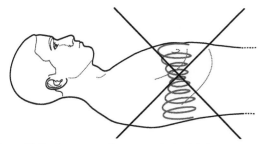

Figure 16.3   Anteroposterior contact in fascial diagnosis helps to reveal the depth of the structure or structures involved.

by using these methods. Barral[14] has often been quoted for his analogy to the wine connoisseur: he states 'the osteopath is a mechanic in the noblest sense of the word – really a micromechanic ... No one argues with the wine taster who, by using his palate, can tell us the characteristics of a wine – its region, its vineyard or even its vintage. The education of touch can go at least as far'.

Another method of using the fascia to aid in location of dysfunction is to use the standing and sitting listening tests. The patient is instructed to stand relaxed, and the practitioner places a hand on the head of the patient. The patient is then instructed to close their eyes, at which point a sense of pulling or falling either forwards or backwards may be experienced. This is said to indicate if the dysfunction is vertebral or visceral in nature, forward pulling indicating visceral dysfunction and backwards, vertebral. The same test may be performed with the patient in the sitting position in order to localize problems in the trunk. An asymmetrical pulling to one side or the other will indicate the laterality of the problem. Paoletti[15] uses an 'induction' or indirect method of treating the fascia after using the listening tests. It involves following the tension found in the fascia in its particular axis, of which there may be two or three, and, once these axes are found, waiting for the aforementioned 'release of the tissues'. He stresses that if any axis of tension is left untreated, the technique will not be successful.

A method of treatment known as 'fascial unwinding' may be employed in order to release the structure concerned. It may be performed as a local technique to the region concerned or more globally as part of the so-called 'total body unwinding' technique. This involves 'following' the dysfunctioning part into its pattern of movement until a point of balance is achieved and a release is felt. The practitioner supports and facilitates the unwinding process but does not instigate it. However, it may be necessary to firmly resist any avoidance movements; that is to say, with experience it may be possible to detect that the unwinding process is avoiding a particular point in the sequence of movements. This avoidance manoeuvre is often seen in traumatic injuries, either physical or emotional, where unwinding may provoke unsettling memories of the trauma. It has been described as a 'walling off' or encapsulation of a problem that the body has decided to 'overlook'. It requires a great deal of experience on the part of the practitioner to recognize this, and even more to confront it.

Dealing with emotional trauma takes a lot of time and is something that once started is not easily, and sometimes not safely, stopped once the process is under way. It may also be necessary to advise the patient to seek professional help in the form of psychological counselling.

The fascia is seen as the continuous, all-enveloping and compartmentalizing connective tissue structure of the body. The explanations for the osteopathic treatment of the fascia and of using the fascia to treat the person are becoming a little clearer as our knowledge of this tissue becomes clearer. It must be borne in mind that the continuity of the fascia as connective tissue means that whether the osteopaths' chosen method of technique is GOT or MET, or any other for that matter, there will have to be some effect on the fascia and vice versa. Myers[16] states that 'a tensegrity model of the body – unavailable at the time of their pioneering work – is closer to the original vision of both Dr Andrew Taylor Still and Dr Ida Rolf'.

References

1. Still AT. Philosophy of osteopathy. Missouri: Academy of Osteopathy; 1899.
2. Butterworths Medical Dictionary, 2nd edn. London: Butterworths; 1978.
3. Williams PL, Warwick R, eds. Gray's anatomy, 36th edn. Edinburgh: Churchill Livingstone; 1980:523.
4. Bogduk N. Clinical anatomy of the lumbar spine and sacrum, 3rd edn. Edinburgh: Churchill Livingstone; 1997: 71–76.
5. Rolf IP. Rolfing: The integration of human structures. Santa Monica, CA: Dennis Landman; 1977.
6. Twomey L, Taylor J. Flexion, creep dysfunction and hysteresis in the lumbar vertebral column. Spine 1982; 7(2):116–122.
7. Threlkeld AS. The effects of manual therapy on connective tissue. Phys Ther 1992; 72(12):893–901.
8. Oshman JL Energy medicine. Edinburgh: Churchill Livingstone; 2000.
9. Johansson H, Sjolander P, Sojka P. Receptors in the knee joint ligaments and their role in the biomechanics of the joint. Crit Rev Biomed Eng 1991; 18(5):341–368.
10. Schleip R. Fascial plasticity – a new neurobiological explanation: Part 2. JBMT 2003; 7(2):104–116.
11. Yahia LH, Pigeon P, DesRosiers EA. Viscoelastic properties of the human lumbodorsal fascia. J Biomed Eng 1993; 15(5):425–429.
12. Staubesand J, Li Y. Zum Peinbau der Fascia cruris mit besonderer Berücksichtigung epi- und intrafaszialer Nerven. Manuelle Medizin 1996; 34:196–200.
13. Bauer J, Heine H. Akupunkturpunkte und Fibromyalgie – Moglichkeiten chirugischer Intervention. Biologische Medizin 1998; 6:257–261.
14. Barral JP, Mercier P. Visceral manipulation. Seattle: Eastland Press; 1988:29.
15. Paoletti S. Les Fascias: Rôle des Tissus dans la Mécanique Humaine. Vannes: Sully; 1998:254–256.
16. Myers TW. Anatomy trains: Myofascial meridians for manual and movement therapists. Edinburgh: Churchill Livingstone; 2001:46.

Chapter 17

Functional technique

CHAPTER CONTENTS

INTRODUCTION

Functional technique, as practised by most osteopaths, is classed as an indirect technique. These are defined as methods of treatment in which the restrictive barrier to motion is disengaged; in other words the dysfunctional part is moved in a direction away from the restriction. Much of the credit for functional technique is given to three American osteopaths: Charles Bowles, Harold Hoover and William Johnston. During the period from 1952 to 1957 there was a series of study sessions of the New England Academy of Osteopathy that went under the heading of 'a functional approach to specific osteopathic manipulative problems' and the name functional appears to have had its origins from that time. Bowles[1] said, 'This is not the birth of a new entity in osteopathy, but simply a new type of measuring stick for evaluating the Still lesion as a process of aberrated function'. Bowles[2] later stated that the term functional technique was 'somewhat of a misnomer since all osteopathic manual technique is primarily structural and treats structural dysfunctions'. Sutherland[3] was also aware of the possibility of releasing cranial sutures by disengagement and so though the credit may go in part to Bowles, Hoover and Johnston, they may well have been adapting an already recognized, but unnamed, technique. Hoover[4] described functional technique as using 'the perceived activity of the body', whilst Bowles[1] wrote of it as 'constantly guided by the tissue need and the tissue response'.

However, in differentiating between structural and functional techniques, it has been suggested that structural relates more to the *quantity* of movement of a joint whereas functional relates more to the *quality* of the movement. An example of a structural approach to treatment would be to take the dysfunctional articulation to its motion barrier and to then apply a thrust or another form of technique that 'moves' the motion barrier and creates a greater range of motion, a direct technique. Conversely, in functional technique the overall aim is to avoid confrontation with any barriers and to remain within the range of motion available, allowing the inherent reflexes to effect the change, an indirect technique.

When working with functional technique, for example on the vertebral column, the practitioner will place one hand directly over the segment to be worked on in order to palpate; this is termed the 'listening hand'. The other hand is the 'motor hand' and is responsible for guiding the movements that will take place during the technique, the so-called 'motion demands'. Motion demands are fine movements where the practitioner is 'asking' the tissues if they will allow movement in a certain direction. It is essential that the roles of the hands remain separate, the 'listening hand really has to listen', and the early pioneers of functional technique stated that 'you can't talk and listen at the same time'.[1] The listening hand is palpating for the quality of the movement. Poor quality movement that is resistant to smooth mobility is termed as 'bind'; it is an active opposition of a muscle to a motion demand. An easy smooth movement where there is compliance or cooperation of a muscle in response to a motion demand is termed 'ease'. The basic principle behind functional technique is to avoid any movements that create bind and to follow the ease (Fig. 17.1).

In a form of functional technique sometimes described as 'dynamic functional',[5] 'the listening hand monitors the response to motion by the motor hand and directs the motion demand along the path of increasing ease'. The aim is to restore the previously dysfunctional articulation to its normal movement patterns by avoiding excessive inappropriate neural feedback. It is the muscle spindle that is responsible for the moment to moment control of joint behaviour. It is thought that by avoiding the bind the practitioner is reducing the afferent proprioceptive input to the reflex mechanism that is maintaining the dysfunction. As the technique follows further along the path of ease, the afferent feedback is reduced further, allowing a greater range of motion by reducing the gamma efferent

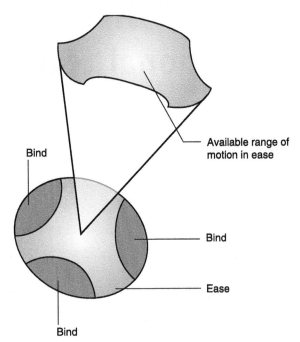

Figure 17.1   Functional technique works within the ease and avoids the bind.

activity. This cycle repeated will eventually allow the control mechanisms to return to normal and restore symmetrical movement. However, as was seen in the cases of fascial and muscle energy technique, the muscle spindle theory may not be the complete explanation and it may be the mechanoreceptors in the fascia that are giving the reduction in afferent input to the spinal cord that results in the inhibition of the reflex. When the fascia is put in a position of ease, there will also be a better exchange of fluids, blood and lymph which gives the subjective feeling of warmth and release to patient and practitioner alike.

In the above technique, the practitioner partly relies on the inherent motion to guide the movement, although it is the motor hand that is actively following the path of ease in the procedure. A variation known as 'balance and hold'[5] involves the stacking up of movements until a release is achieved. Quite simply, using the example of a vertebral segment, there are six different directions of 'pure movement' possible, two about each of the x, y and z axes (Fig. 17.2). Flexion and extension take place about the x axis, right and left rotation about the y axis and right and left side-bending about the z axis. By working about each axis one at a time, the point of ease is found for each separate axis and

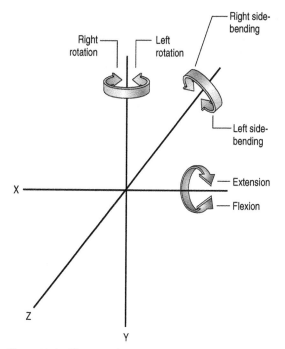

Figure 17.2   The axes of pure movement.

is sequentially stacked upon the next. The next stage of the treatment is to do the same with the possible translation movements, both left and right and anterior and posterior. Then some compression and distraction will be added, always to the direction of ease, and finally a respiratory movement. Again, as with the vertebral movements, the phase of respiration that creates the most ease, expiration or inspiration, will be maintained. Usually the patient is instructed to hold the breath in the desired phase for as long as is comfortable before slowly returning the breathing pattern to normal again. This whole sequence of events may be repeated a number of times until the practitioner is satisfied that there is an acceptable level of change. The dynamic functional technique may involve combining movements, for example side-bending with rotation or flexion, whereas the balance and hold technique keeps the movements pure. Nevertheless, it is the stacking up of these pure movement patterns that eventually finds the same vector of ease achieved by combining them dynamically that will allow a resetting of the normal neural feedback mechanisms. Stacking or combining of the vectors is important because a return to neutral before making a different motion demand may alter the position from the ease

already gained to a point of relative bind. So there should be a new direction added to the last movement made, not further into the same direction where bind may be felt, and likewise not a retracing of steps. It is not of great importance in which order the stacking is carried out but it must be sufficient to maintain the ease. Once an ease response has been elicited in several directions, it tends to occur in response to all normal motion demands at the concerned joint and this indicates that there has been a spontaneous release of the holding pattern.

Functional technique when performed on vertebral restrictions is not aimed at the positional elements of the lesion but more at the behaviour or functional activity of the lesion; this is made up of the vertebrae, the associated paravertebral soft tissue structures and their related neural reflexes.[6]

Though the techniques have been described here with respect to the vertebral column, they can be performed on any articulation. Obviously, the symmetry will be altered in asymmetrical joints such as the wrist or knee but it is always the quality of the movement being monitored that is more important in functional technique.

Functional technique does have some advantages over structural technique in the treatment of acute patients, elderly, infirm or postoperative patients and may well be the preferred choice of technique by both patient and practitioner. In the patient with an acute low back, treatment may be given in any position, sitting, standing or lying. The gentle nature of the technique combined with minimal movements may be applied throughout the whole spine, not just to the acutely lesioned segment. A screening procedure performed before commencement of treatment will indicate the primary problem and any other secondary compensations. The cumulative effect of making numerous small releases throughout the whole body will certainly be appreciated by the patient as a return towards normal functioning.

In elderly or infirm patients with low vitality, the functional approach may well be a good alternative to the more dynamic structural type techniques. It can be performed with a minimum of traumatic input and may be repeated frequently without causing reactions. Since functional technique is not merely addressing faulty joint position but is also aimed at rebalancing of the neural mechanisms, it will also be useful in problems of a more chronic nature.

References

1. Bowles CH. A functional orientation to technic. AOA: 1955 Yearbook; 177–191.

2. Bowles CH. Functional technique: A modern perspective. J Am Osteopath Assoc 1981; 80:5.

3. Lippincott HA. The osteopathic technique of WG Sutherland DO. In: Northup TL. 1949 AAO Yearbook of Osteopathy. Michigan: Edward Bros; 1949:1–24.

4. Hoover HV. Functional technic. AOA: 1958 Yearbook; 47–56.

5. Greenman PE. Principles of manual medicine. Baltimore: Williams and Wilkins; 1996:105–108.

6. Haycock W. The techniques of Dr CH Bowles DO and Dr HV Hoover DO. Functional technique. In: White RJ, ed. Osteopathy principles and practice, vol. 2 Maidstone: Institute of Classical Osteopathy; 2000:60–72.

Chapter 18

Jones technique

INTRODUCTION

In 1964 Lawrence H Jones[1,2] took up the cause of the indirect functional approach in his article in *The D.O.* 'Spontaneous Release by Positioning', introducing the concepts that have now become known as strain and counterstrain (SCS) and which were further developed in 1981 in his book of the same name. In the book he considers how dysfunction may arise and how it may be treated using an indirect approach, taking patients into the point of ease, and monitoring this process by means of assessing tender points.

As with many of the different approaches to osteopathic treatment, his approach has been modified by subsequent practitioners; Chaitow, D'Ambrogio and Roth, Deig and Schiowitz to name but a few.[3-6] However, in this chapter we will try to give the ideas and principles as proposed by Jones.

Jones relates that he discovered the two principal features of SCS by chance. Firstly, in attempting to treat an individual who was too acute to employ any of his usual manipulative techniques, in desperation he placed the patient in a position that could at least offer some comfort, and then left him there for 20 minutes. After this time, to his great surprise, the patient appeared to have improved generally. The second important and serendipitous discovery was that on the anterior aspect of the body, there appeared to be small areas of dense tissue that, though tender to palpation, were not themselves painful. These appeared often to be in the area opposite to that 'strained', and when the position of ease was obtained the tenderness diminished.

Jones[1] offered two definitions of the SCS approach:

- *Relieving spinal or other joint pain by passively putting the joint into its position of greatest comfort.*
- *Relieving pain by reduction and arrest of the continuing inappropriate proprioceptor activity. This is achieved by markedly shortening the muscle that contains the malfunctioning muscle spindle by applying mild strain to its antagonist. In other words, the inappropriate strain reflex is inhibited by application of a counterstrain.*

To understand these definitions it is necessary to look at how Jones considered somatic dysfunction to arise. He realized that, excluding obvious trauma, the time of onset of a problem was often the time of returning to neutral position. Thus, if an individual has been flexed for a long time and then attempts to rapidly stand upright again, it is at the moment that they begin to extend that the pain begins.

Jones explained this with regard to the muscles. Thus if an individual has remained flexed for a protracted period, the posterior musculature is lengthened and anterior musculature shortened. If they return slowly to the upright position, the body will reestablish balance between the two sets of muscles and no problems will arise. However, if the return is done too quickly, the shortened anterior muscle is unable to respond fast enough and becomes 'strained'. The dysfunction will be found in the asymptomatic shortened antagonist anterior muscles, evidenced by the individual being able to flex, but extension is limited by the anterior muscles and so the pain is experienced posteriorly. Thus, the time of onset of the joint dysfunction is not the moment of the strain itself, it is the body's reaction to the strain, an overactive panic reaction to too rapid an attempt to return to the neutral position.

It has long been observed that the body often exhibits tender points in relation to dysfunction (acupuncture points, Chapman's reflex points and Travell's myofascial trigger points to name but a few), and Jones found these to be of particular diagnostic value.[7,8] He described his own findings as small areas, usually about 1 cm across, of oedematous and tense muscle or fascia that are tender to palpation. They may be singular or multiple and Jones found that there was a repeatable pattern of distribution of these points and somatic dysfunction. These occasionally parallel, but do not exactly reproduce, Travell's myofascial trigger points and

Chapman's reflex points. Jones charted his points, approximately half of these being located posteriorly in the paravertebral muscles. They tend to be closely related to the spinal somatic dysfunction and the patient is usually aware of them being painful as well as tender to palpation. The other half are to be found on the anterior aspect of the body; however, unlike the posterior points, these are tender on direct palpation, but the patient is usually unaware of their presence until they are probed by the practitioner. This pattern of distribution is also repeated in the limbs, with tender points being found in the pain-free aspect, opposite to the site of pain and weakness. The prevalence of the tender points in the muscles opposite to the previously considered strained muscle further supports the hypothesis that the site of dysfunction is in the anterior shortened muscles.

Jones found that by palpating the tender point and asking the patient for feedback regarding the level of tenderness as he sought the position of ease, he could accurately localize the exact position of ease as the tenderness disappeared. This is different to many approaches where the tender points are treated by direct pressure, needling or injecting. In effect, Jones' use of the tender points is truly as a functional indirect approach whereby the tender points are used only to aid the practitioner in finding the optimum position of ease, whereas Chapman and Travell utilize their points as an aid to treatment by working directly on the points themselves. Nevertheless, in all three methods, the practitioner also noted a palpable loss of tension in the tender point being worked on or monitored.

Treatment consists of taking the patient back into the point of ease, which is the direct opposite of the point of pain, and by finding the 'mobile point' which is described as the point where there is maximal relaxation and increase in joint mobility. This is thought to be the point at which the strain occurred. At this point the previously painful tender point should become pain free. The patient is then held in this position for about 90 seconds, and then very slowly returned back to the upright position. Although Jones' initial chance treatment lasted 20 minutes, by experimentation he found that 90 seconds was the optimum time required for an effect to take place. One of the key elements is that it is essential that the return to neutral is done slowly, particularly the first few degrees of movement (Jones recommended the first 15°). If it is not performed slowly it may lead to a recurrence of the original problem by a reinstallation of the aberrant reflex. It would appear that in the long term, a somatic dysfunction creates a sensitization of the reflex neural circuits and so even after restoration of normal function, this 'memory' of the dysfunction remains especially susceptible to insult and may result in a resensitization.[9] It is for this reason that Jones found by experience that the return to the normal position had to be very gentle and that it was good practice to advise the patient to take it easy for a day or so following the treatment. If the actual cause of the problem is known, perhaps after bending over for a prolonged period whilst gardening, for example, then this action especially should be avoided for a couple of days in order to prevent resensitization.

The indications for using SCS methods are immediately apparent, and the fact that a principle of the technique is to find the most comfortable position for the patient makes it extremely useful in the acute patient. In the case of chronic problems, more applications may be required but then that is the case for most approaches to treatment.

References

1. Jones LH. Spontaneous release by positioning. The DO Jan 1964:109–116.
2. Jones LH. Strain and counterstrain. Colorado: AAO; 1981.
3. Chaitow L. Positional release techniques: advanced soft tissue techniques. New York: Churchill Livingstone; 1996.
4. D'Ambrogio KJ, Roth GB. Positional release therapy: assessment and treatment of musculoskeletal dysfunction. St Louis: Mosby; 1997.
5. Deig D. Positional release technique: from a dynamic systems perspective. Butterworth-Heinemann: Boston; 2001.
6. Schiowitz S, DiGiovanna EL, Dowling DJ. Facilitated positional release. In: Ward, RC, ed. Foundations for osteopathic medicine. Philadelphia: Lippincott Williams and Wilkins; 2003:1017–1025.
7. Owen C. An endocrine interpretation of Chapman's reflexes. Carmel: American Academy of Osteopathy; 1932.
8. Travell JG, Simons DG. Myofascial pain and dysfunction: the trigger point manual. Baltimore: Williams and Wilkins; 1983.
9. Patterson MM. Neural mechanisms of the strain-counterstrain technique. L'Osteopathie 2002; Winter 8:5–9.

Chapter 19

Trigger points

CHAPTER CONTENTS

INTRODUCTION

Many different authors have documented and mapped the presence of trigger points in a variety of tissues. The best known and most important contribution of work in this field is without a doubt that provided by Travell and Simons.

A trigger point[1] is described as *a focus of hyperirritability in a tissue that, when compressed, is locally tender and, if sufficiently hypersensitive, gives rise to referred pain and tenderness, and sometimes to referred autonomic phenomena and distortion of proprioception.* They are usually found in a taut band of skeletal muscle or fascia though they may also be found in other structures.

There are two types of trigger points palpable: active and latent. Active trigger points are tender, may be already referring pain at rest, or may refer pain on palpation or muscular contraction, and resist muscle lengthening. Latent trigger points require a probing pressure on them to elicit a response and otherwise remain clinically quiescent. It is because of the quiescence of these latent trigger points that unless a full examination is performed, they may not be noticed, leading to a misdiagnosis and thus unsuccessful treatment.[2]

Myofascial trigger points possess all the requirements of a somatic dysfunction: increased sensitivity, tissue texture changes, asymmetry and a reduced range of motion.[3] As such, they may be utilized in the differential diagnosis and treatment of a number of clinical presentations that may not only be muscle related; they could include pain syndromes and disability and disrupted visceral function.[2]

Of the many trigger points mapped by Travell and Simons, the most common sites are in the upper trapezius and quadratus lumborum muscles. There are certain factors that are known to perpetuate new and existing trigger points, including mechanical disturbances, certain metabolic and endocrine disorders, nutritional deficiencies, psychological stress, allergies, infection and prolonged immobility.[1,4] So, for example, a compensatory pattern set up from the pelvis may initiate a reflex from the quadratus lumborum muscle which may sensitize the interneurones at the spinal cord levels associated with the muscle. This in turn may increase the tension in the muscle creating a taut band which when compressed is painful: a trigger point. If there is visceral dysfunction, facilitation in the spinal cord from the viscera may well perpetuate the trigger point; likewise, the trigger point may be able to set up visceral dysfunction. It has been noted by Travell and Simons that 61% of patients with cardiac disease were found to have trigger points in the thoracic region. Trigger points may give rise to symptoms other than pain.[4] Numerous autonomic effects have been noted: vasoconstriction, alterations in local temperature control (usually colder skin), piloerection and sweating.[1,4] Other symptoms noted include dysmenorrhoea, diarrhoea, dizziness and vasoconstrictive headache.[2]

Treatment of trigger points requires their deactivation, which may be achieved by a number of methods but the success will be permanent only if any other perpetuating factors are also resolved, for example any other compensatory dysfunctional patterns. A manual method for deactivation of trigger points involves the application of firm digital pressure which may be a combination of alternating pressure and release for up to 2 minutes. There are many and varied approaches to using digital pressure and each individual has a preferred method. The pressure is thought to create a local ischaemia which inhibits the neural activity maintaining the reflex, causing the associated taut band to release. Another technique is the cryotherapeutic approach or the so-called 'spray and stretch' which involves spraying a coolant onto the trigger point and then manually stretching the taut band. Other approaches include dry needling or wet needling with local anaesthetic, ultrasound or microcurrent applications. Within the osteopathic approaches, trigger points may be treated by using muscle energy technique, myofascial release and combined techniques.

There seems to be a certain amount of overlap between various trigger points and tender points along with those of Chapman's and the lesser known Jarricot's points.

References

1. Travell JG, Simons DG. Myofascial pain and dysfunction: the trigger point manual, vol 2. Baltimore: Williams and Wilkins; 1992.
2. Kuchera M, McPartland JM. Myofascial trigger points as somatic dysfunction. In: Ward R, ed. Foundations for osteopathic medicine. Philadelphia: Lippincott Williams and Wilkins; 2003: 1034–1050.
3. Chaitow L. Modern neuromuscular techniques. Edinburgh: Churchill Livingstone; 2003: 39–68.
4. Travell JG, Simons DG. Myofascial pain and dysfunction: the trigger point manual, vol 1. Baltimore: Williams and Wilkins; 1999.

Chapter 20

Chapman's reflexes

INTRODUCTION

This system of reflex points, originally used by Frank Chapman DO, was described by Charles Owens DO. These reflexes present as predictable anterior and posterior fascial tissue texture abnormalities assumed to be reflections of visceral dysfunction or pathology (viscerosomatic reflexes). A given reflex is consistently associated with the same viscus; Chapman's reflexes are manifested by palpatory findings of plaque-like changes of stringiness of the involved tissues.[1]

Frank Chapman was an osteopathic physician who worked in the USA in the 1920s. Although Chapman never documented his work, it was collected and published by Charles Owens, Ada Hinkley Chapman and WF Link in 1932.[2] Very little research has been directed at Chapman's reflexes and as such, it still remains a system based purely on empirical values. The true value of Chapman's reflexes in current osteopathic practice seems to be more as a diagnostic tool or as an aid to differential diagnosis. However, a number of osteopaths use it as a system of both diagnosis and treatment.

Chapman found a series of reflex points located throughout the body that he proposed as reflections of visceral dysfunctions. These reflex points are characterized by a small, firm, palpable nodule of about 2–3 mm in diameter. They are located in the deep fascia or periosteum and as such lie deep to the skin and superficial subcutaneous tissues. On gentle but firm palpation, a distinct, sharp, distressing but non-radiating pain is reported by the patient. All attempts at histological examination by biopsy have proved fruitless; nevertheless, they are repeatable and consistent in their anatomical location. Chapman is reported as mapping two sets of reflex points for each viscus, one on the anterior aspect of the body and the other posterior.

It has been proposed that the anterior reflex points were originally used for diagnosis, whilst the posterior points could be used for treatment. Diagnosis using the anterior reflex points needs to be confirmed by locating a sensitive corresponding posterior point. Treatment is effected by a deep, circular massage of the point by the fingertip as if to 'dissipate the local swelling of the nodule'. This massage is generally maintained for between 20–30 seconds but some osteopaths will 'treat' for up to 90 seconds – or as long as either the patient or practitioner can tolerate! It appears that the anterior points are often too tender to treat in this manner, hence the use of the posterior points principally for the treatment. It has been argued that the posterior points are often 'inadvertently treated' by soft tissue work to the paraspinal musculature by osteopaths with no working knowledge of Chapman's points.

Whether Chapman's points are used purely as a means of diagnosis or as a system of diagnosis and treatment together, correlation with the case history examination and physical findings is still necessary. Furthermore, examination of the points should be performed prior to any other form of osteopathic treatment in order to prevent modification of results.[3] Critics highlight the non-holistic nature of this push-button system of treatment; however, Chapman emphasized the importance of treating by this method only after any pelvic function had been addressed.[4] Although 'correction' of the pelvis is part way towards a holistic viewpoint, it is hardly 'true holism' as osteopathic principles define it. As an attempt to incorporate Chapman's reflexes into a holistic approach, it is possible to use them in conjunction with other treatment modalities. On examining all the anterior points, it may be found that there is a predominance of points that correspond to one particular system of the body, for example, the urogenital or respiratory systems. The osteopath may then decide to treat this system using a series of direct visceral techniques. Naturally, testing of the specific viscera beforehand will be required in order to dictate which specific techniques are required. Then, as a means of confirmation, re-testing of the previously diagnosed reflex points should reveal the desired change. Conversely, the osteopath may find the dysfunctions in accordance with the case history by using standard visceral osteopathic testing, confirm this by Chapman's testing and treat the posterior points. Re-testing of the specific viscera afterwards should confirm the desired change from the treatment using the reflex points.

References

1. Chapman's Reflex. Glossary of osteopathic technology. Glossary review committee. In: Ward RC, ed. Foundations for osteopathic medicine. Baltimore: Williams and Wilkins; 1997: 1127–1140.
2. Owens C. An endocrine interpretation of Chapman's reflexes. California: AAO; 1932.
3. Kuchera ML, Kuchera WA. Osteopathic considerations in systemic dysfunction, 2nd edn. Ohio: Greyden Press; 1994: 200–201.
4. Patriquin DA. Viscerosomatic reflexes. In: Patterson MM, Howel JN, eds. The central connection: somaticovisceral–viscerosomatic interactions. Ohio: University Classics; 1992: 4–18.

Chapter 21

Soft tissue techniques

INTRODUCTION

There are two reasons for treating the soft tissues: firstly, as part of treating the whole body and secondly, in treating a real local soft tissue problem. In osteopathic thinking, the former should be the *only* reason for working on the soft tissues, as part of a global treatment aimed at restoring balance to the body. However, in reality, there may be times when the osteopath is called upon to perform a 'first aid' type treatment to relieve a particular soft tissue injury. As we have already seen, the interconnections of all the connective tissues of the body, soft and hard, mean that even in the latter case of working directly on the soft tissues for a certain intrinsic problem, there will automatically be some kind of secondary effect on the other tissues.

Osteopaths have 'borrowed' soft tissue techniques from other disciplines, sometimes adapting these techniques to fit in with the osteopathic principles, and in certain cases have invented their own techniques. The techniques used are many and varied but their aims are much the same: to restore homeostatic mechanisms, whether they are neural, fluid, immune or other in nature, and probably to relax the tissues, though some soft tissue techniques are performed to stimulate the tissues. Osteopathically, the removal of somatic dysfunction may be possible by soft tissue techniques alone, or it may help to prepare the dysfunction for removal by other methods. The changes that take place when a somatic dysfunction has been removed may be aided by soft tissue techniques and thus prevent reinstatement of previous compensatory lesion patterns.[1]

One of the basic soft tissue applications used by osteopaths is that of massage. Therapeutic massage has been known for thousands of years and although seemingly first documented in early Egyptian times, it does not need a wild imagination to think that it first appeared when the first person to walk the earth stubbed a toe! Rubbing a site of minor injury is an action that aims to reduce pain and improve circulation. Even animals will patiently lick an injured paw and so it appears that self massage, at least, is actually an instinctive reflex.

Massage techniques may be divided into three generally used 'strokes': effleurage, petrissage and friction.[2] Effleurage is the most commonly used massage technique and may be used in preparation of the tissues for other techniques. It consists of a gliding movement over the skin that requires a firm and even pressure, and allows the operator to explore the tissues for areas of increased muscle tonicity. It is performed from the superficial layers towards the deeper layers with sensitive hands monitoring the change through the layers. The superficial stroking used to begin effleurage will help to warm and prepare the tissues for the deeper work and other techniques. Petrissage is a type of kneading of the tissues, it involves lifting and gentle squeezing of the tissues. It will aid the venous and lymphatic return and free up minor adhesions. Friction massage allows penetration to the deeper tissue layers; it involves small circular movements that move the deeper tissues but not the skin. A fourth massage technique not used so often in osteopathic practice is tapotement. It requires much practice to reach perfection and may well best be left for the professional massage therapist. It is used when stimulation is required and involves tapping the body with a series of brisk blows using various parts of the hands and various hand positions. Commonly used tapotement techniques include hacking, cupping, slapping and tapping.

Although the above described techniques may be at times useful to the osteopath, should the patient be in need of a 'real' massage then obviously a professional should be sought. A close working relationship with a massage therapist may prove useful to both parties.

INHIBITION

Inhibition, or functional inhibition technique as it is sometimes known, is used on specific regions of increased tonus or spasm in muscles. It consists of a very gentle manual pressure that is usually applied perpendicular to the direction of the muscle fibres. Where the fibre orientation makes a perpendicular action difficult, the same principles may be applied by stretching along the line of the fibres.

It appears that Still, whilst a young boy, was the 'inventor' of this technique.[3] He relieved his headaches by lying on his back with his upper neck resting in a rope sling and whilst sleeping for a while in this position reduced the tension in the suboccipital muscles. This reduction in tension produces an increase in fluid exchange and a decrease in reflex activity. The same principles are applied today in the technique known as 'suboccipital inhibition' whereby the practitioner's fingertips replace Stills' rope. With the patient lying supine and the osteopath cupping the occiput, a gentle pressure is applied into the suboccipital region in order to release the tension within the muscles. As the tension releases, the slack is taken up by the fingers, creating a longitudinal stretch on the muscles.

An example of perpendicular stretching would be in the long muscles of the back. If there is a region of hypertonicity in the erector spinae muscles of the mid-thoracic region, the patient will lie comfortably in the prone position with the practitioner seated beside them. Contact is made just beside the hypertonic region, usually with the thumb; this is the sensory contact and monitors the state of the tissues being worked upon. The other hand is used as the motor hand and supplies the active force across the muscle fibres. This use of sensory and motor hands is the reason that this technique has come to be known as 'functional' inhibition. The force applied across the direction of the muscle fibres results in a lengthening of the muscle that is constantly being monitored by the sensory hand. Should the application of the force be too great or too rapid then the muscle spindle reflex will create more tension in the muscle as a result of the stretch reflex. The applied pressure is very gentle to begin with but may increase as the technique progresses; as more relaxation takes place it requires the taking up of more slack in the tissues. In most cases, the greater the tonicity, the slower the release and the whole procedure of taking up the slack may take a few minutes. The slack in the tissues is taken up until no further release is felt and the hypertonicity is resolved. At this point, the tension created by the motor hand must be released in a very slow and controlled manner in order to prevent the recurrence of the same aberrant reflex.

Functional inhibition techniques are very useful in acute cases such as muscle spasm of the back following lifting, but may be used anywhere in the body. Excessive pressure may result in irritation of the tissues, especially in the acute case, and so a constant feedback from the sensory hand and good palpatory skills are required.

NEUROMUSCULAR TECHNIQUE

This particular technique was developed by Stanley Lief and his cousin Boris Chaitow who between them had a mixture of chiropractic, naturopathic and osteopathic backgrounds.[4]

Originally, neuromuscular technique (NMT) was used as a way of diagnosing and treating soft tissue lesions which may have been the complete treatment or, more often, as part of a treatment.

Lief[5] associated certain phenomena with the soft tissue lesion that has become known as a 'neuromuscular lesion': congestion with a related acid-base disturbance, adhesions and chronic changes in muscle tonicity. Possible causative factors include trauma, postural compromise, nutritional deficiencies, fatigue and psychosomatic causes.

Lief believed that the application of deep pressure on muscle or some other connective tissue structure will lead to a reduction of the symptoms and an improvement of the general function. As pressure is applied to tissues, a transient relative ischaemia in the area being treated occurs, due to the interference of the normal blood flow, this being reversed as soon as the pressure is released and possibly creating a period of increased blood flow which may have the effect of flushing the tissues and removing the metabolites. Constant pressure in this manner acts as a counterirritant by overloading mechanoreceptor stimulation, which may result in neurological inhibition via the gate control mechanism and thus lead to a decrease in nociceptive information reaching conscious levels.[6,7] As the reticular formation screens and filters information of body contact awareness, it may require the spinal cord to 'turn down' this awareness when it becomes overloaded. An everyday example of this is the wearing of clothes or sitting on a chair: the body screens out this information so that we are not consciously aware of these inputs. In addition, there may also be a local or general release of endorphins, the body's naturally produced painkillers.

NMT can be applied to any connective tissue of the body as either a global or local treatment; the application is similar for both approaches. In order to apply the pressure to the tissue, the thumb is most commonly used, but knuckles or elbow may also be utilized. A firm, constant contact is required, and the use of a lubricant is recommended. The technique consists of gliding along the muscle desired, using two strokes, the first one being mainly diagnosis, and the second one treatment. If areas of fibrosis are found, three or four strokes may be needed to achieve persistent changes.

The pressure applied should vary depending on the states of the tissues and their reaction: lighter pressure for healthy tissues and stronger pressure for contracted or fibrosed tissues. Release of the superficial tissue should be performed before that of the deep, and in order to aid efficient lymphatic drainage, it is best to work first on the proximal segment to decongest and open up the lymph channels there before proceeding to the more distal segments.

NMT may be applied locally to the site of fibrosed tissue, congestion, trigger points and Chapman's reflex points. In the case of a muscle tear or ligament sprain, the technique must be adapted to the degree of chronicity. If the tissue is still in the acute stage, it may be better to wait, or at least to drastically modify the technique to a very low level of pressure. Lief used a type of general treatment approach which involved a procedure for working on all areas of the vertebral column and adjacent tissues.[4] He completed his treatment with an abdominal technique. This approach at first may seem like a 'massage with a difference' but he used it successfully throughout his career, adding articulation and springing techniques as necessary. By applying an osteopathic understanding to the body, the global NMT becomes quite a specific treatment. During the treatment, emphasis may be made of areas of particular dysfunction. For example, a liver dysfunction may require special attention around the paraspinal structures of T6 to T10 and the lower ribs on the right covering the liver. It is recommended that the back should be treated first, so that the neurological reflex may predominate.

Age is not a limiting factor for the application of NMT, although as with any technique it may need to be adapted for the individual patient with respect to vitality of the patient and chronicity of the lesion. With respect to contraindications, common sense should prevail: pressure applied directly over the site of infection, acute inflammation or broken skin should be avoided because of possible dangerous consequences.

References

1. Kuchera WA, Kuchera ML. Osteopathic principles in practice, 2nd edn, Colombus: Greyden Press; 1992.
2. Tappan FM. Healing massage techniques: holistic, classic and emerging methods, 2nd edn. Norwalk: Appleton and Lange; 1988.
3. Still AS. Autobiography of AT Still. Revised edn. Kirksville: Still; 1908.
4. Chaitow L. Soft tissue manipulation: a practitioner's guide to the diagnosis and treatment of soft tissue dysfunction and reflex activity. Rochester: Healing Arts Press; 1988.
5. Leif P. The neuromuscular lesion. British Naturopathic Journal 1963; 5:10.
6. Wall PD, Melzack R, eds. Textbook of pain. Edinburgh: Churchill Livingstone; 1984.
7. Kandel ER, Schwartz JH, Jessell TM. Principles of neural science, 4th edn. New York: McGraw-Hill; 2000: 482–488.

SECTION 4

Clinical conditions

In this section, we will look at a number of commonly presenting case scenarios. It was decided by the authors NOT to give case histories and treatment details from their own individual patient lists, as is often seen in text books. The main reasons for not doing so are, firstly, because we do not wish to promote the idea that the methods given are the *only* ways in which to treat a person with such a presenting condition, and, secondly, because the theme throughout this book is that treatment should be individually tailored for the person in front of us. If a certain series of techniques helped a particular patient with their constipation, it certainly does not follow that the same set of techniques, performed in the same order and manner, will work for another patient with constipation. However, in practice there is likely to be a certain amount of overlap and in some circumstances, treatments may appear identical to the casual observer – but the different nuances between them may have been overlooked and obviously cannot be described in a text such as this.

Finally, although we have covered a number of common presentations, it must be remembered at all times that there is no osteopathic technique for constipation, and that osteopaths do not treat dysmenorrhoea. However, osteopaths do treat *patients* with dysmenorrhoea and they may use a technique that in another patient might help in the relief of their constipation. The difference is subtle, but nevertheless important. Osteopathy is about treating patients as a whole and not their individual conditions: if we lose sight of this concept we also lose sight of the true philosophy of osteopathy.

The aim of this section is to give an idea as to how an osteopath might approach a patient suffering from any of the conditions covered in the chapters in this section. Firstly, we will give an overview of the disease, its presentation, what are considered to be the pathological processes, its progression and possible outcomes. Osteopaths should always be aware of the so-called 'red flags' and these considerations will, within reason, be discussed. Finally, we will highlight points of particular importance that an osteopath may consider during his or her treatment approach.

Chapter 22

Dysmenorrhoea

CHAPTER CONTENTS

INTRODUCTION

Dysmenorrhoea is the medical term used to describe painful menstruation. It is a relatively common condition; it is estimated that in excess of 50% of postpubescent women experience painful periods. It may be incapacitating enough for the sufferer to take time off work and as such it is the greatest single cause of lost working hours amongst young women.[1]

Menstrual abnormalities may be subdivided into the following categories:

- premenstrual syndrome
- primary dysmenorrhoea
- secondary dysmenorrhoea
- amenorrhoea
- menopausal.

In this section we will look at the first three: premenstrual syndrome, and primary and secondary dysmenorrhoea.

Premenstrual syndrome (PMS) can be defined as a condition characterized by nervous tension and emotional instability, frequently with irritability, anxiety and depression. Associated with it may be headaches, swelling of the abdomen and/or breasts with or without pain, and fatigue. In fact the list of symptoms is almost endless since other complaints that the woman suffers may be exacerbated during this period. It usually occurs somewhere between 7–10 days before the onset of the menses and is usually relieved by the arrival of the menses. However, the picture of relief may become obscured by the onset of dysmenorrhoea. The pattern of symptoms may vary greatly between different women and within the same woman but during different cycles. Some women have significant but not overly disturbing symptoms whilst others are quite markedly disturbed by their symptoms. Orthodox medical treatment tends to be directed at relief of the symptoms with which the individual presents, hormonal manipulation, counselling to help with coping strategies and in some cases tranquillizers for psychological management.

Primary dysmenorrhoea is described as cyclic pain associated with the menstrual cycle in the absence of demonstrable lesions of the reproductive system. It is sometimes known as functional dysmenorrhoea and is thought to occur as a result of uterine contractions and ischaemia. It is estimated that primary dysmenorrhoea is the most common menstrual disorder and affects 30–50% of young women, including teenagers, resulting, once again, in much lost working and school time.[1] The severity of the condition is directly related to the duration and volume of menstrual flow. The pain is located in the lower abdomen, particularly anteriorly, but may radiate to the thighs and/or lower back. It may be associated with headache, nausea, tiredness, dizziness and possibly an alteration of the bowel habits.

Although secondary dysmenorrhoea (sometimes known as acquired dysmenorrhoea) has a similar pain presentation to primary dysmenorrhoea, it is distinguished from it in that in secondary dysmenorrhoea there is a demonstrable lesion, and so a thorough pelvic examination must be performed in order to exclude pelvic pathology. Examples would include pain resulting from fibroids, infections, endometriosis or even tumours. It may be associated with other symptoms such as abnormal discharge, infertility or dyspareunia.

Dysmenorrhoea that begins early after the menarche, within the first 2–3 years, is most likely to be primary dysmenorrhoea, whereas secondary dysmenorrhoea is most likely to begin much later.[2]

In the case of menstrual irregularities, numerous causes may be considered, and the presentation will guide the differential diagnosis, but 'red flags' would include vaginal discharge other than blood, excessive bleeding and complications of pregnancy.

PATHOPHYSIOLOGY

Dysmenorrhoea seems to be due to an increased production of prostaglandins from the endometrium.

It has been shown that prostaglandin F (PGF_{2a}) may be produced in quantities as high as 10 times that in asymptomatic women.[3] The result of the increased levels of these hormones is a greater than normal contraction of the myometrium, coupled with vasoconstriction of the endometrial vessels. The overall result is ischaemia, bleeding and pain. The pain appears to peak during the first 2 days, when the prostaglandin production is at its greatest level. Once the prostaglandins and their metabolites enter the systemic circulation there may be other systemic symptoms, such as nausea, headache or vomiting. Normally, as the prostaglandin levels diminish so do the symptoms. Oral contraception may also relieve the symptoms, as do prostaglandin inhibitors.

OSTEOPATHIC CONSIDERATIONS

Many women consider that pain associated with menses is normal and should simply be accepted, and so they make no great complaints. It is often the case that the osteopath is the first practitioner to discuss the problem with the patient, in that it is the time devoted by the osteopath to case history taking that may reveal the problem. If this is so, then it is important that any possible pathology should be ruled out before treatment proceeds. Contact with, and/or referral to the patient's gynaecologist may be necessary. Once the 'all clear' has been given, the treatment may then proceed with the osteopath considering the following points.

During the case history examination the true 'cause' of the problem may be revealed. For example, it could be that the patient developed dysmenorrhoea 9 months before and that it coincided with a fall, or after starting a course of orthodontic treatment, or following a change of circumstances such as moving house or a relationship break-up. Often the patient will not have been aware of these connections and it is only the time and care taken in the case history examination that reveals them. The osteopathic physical examination will need to be structured with these findings in mind, looking closely at the involuntary mechanism in the case of orthodontic work or structural imbalance due to the fall. Occasionally, the cause will be revealed retrospectively: on finding the somatic dysfunction or lesion pattern, the osteopath may pose questions that remind the patient of a previously forgotten fall.

The innervation of the uterus and female genital tract should not be overlooked with respect to outflow levels and routes of the nerves (Fig. 22.3). Afferents from the uterus pass via the uterovaginal and pelvic plexuses and thence via the hypogastric nerves back to the aortic plexus. Since the sympathetic supply to the uterus is responsible for smooth muscle contractions it may be implicated in dysmenorrhoea, especially in the case of somatic dysfunction or facilitated segment at its outflow levels of T10–L2. The parasympathetic supply to the uterus, although not responsible for muscle contraction but more so for glandular secretions, comes via the pelvic splanchnic nerves from the S2–4 levels. However, the parasympathetics will have an effect of inhibition on the sympathetics when controlling uterine contraction, and on vasomotor activity. Afferent pain fibres from the upper vagina and cervix pass via the pelvic splanchnics whilst those from the lower vagina and perineum pass in the pudendal nerve. Although these pathways should not truly be involved in dysmenorrhoea it would be worth investigating the possibility of their compromise as a possible exacerbating factor.

Naturally, the osteopath should look very closely at the pelvis for dysfunction of the articulations and the muscles working around it. Since the accepted pathophysiology recognizes that there is ischaemia in the uterine tissues, then improved circulation and drainage will be of paramount importance and naturally, this goes hand-in-hand with normal pelvic mobility. Kuchera and Kuchera[4] advocate the use of a technique of 'firm, continuous pressure over the sacral base'. By working with the involuntary mechanism from the sacrum it is possible to effect a type

of sacral CV4 technique. This is one method which will be effective in relieving tissue congestion and normalizing any disturbance of the parasympathetic outflow from this level.

Self-help exercises may be of use to calm the cramps and to aid pelvic decongestion. One such exercise often recommended by healthcare practitioners is that of adopting the kneeling position, with the upper body resting on the floor. In this position the pelvis is held higher than the upper body and this relieves pressure from the viscera in the pelvic bowl and facilitates drainage.

A technique often used by general osteopathic treatment (GOT) practitioners known as 'oscillations' or 'oscillatory technique' has been seen to be particularly helpful in dysmenorrhoea.[5] It involves a gentle side-to-side rocking of the body in the prone position. One hand drives the movement from the sacrum whilst the other hand works up the vertebral column encouraging normal movement and inhibiting abnormal muscle tensions.

The osteopath conversant with visceral techniques may choose to work directly on the structures of the pelvis if indicated. Naturally, an important place to begin looking for dysfunction would be the uterus itself. Is it in its normal position? Is it anteverted, retroverted or laterally flexed? (Fig. 22.1). Both mobility and motility should be checked and then the numerous ligamentous attachments (Fig. 22.2). The cardinal or Mackenrodt's ligament (lateral cervical ligament) carries the uterine vessels from the internal iliac vessels on the inner aspect of the pelvis. There is a quite dense venous plexus within the pelvis and associated with it is the lymphatic system. Both may benefit from judicious pumping techniques. The pelvis is not solely there for the benefit of the genital system; the lower gastrointestinal tract passes through as does the urinary system. These three systems are separated from one another in the pelvis by different layers of fascia and this creates the perineopelvic spaces, an absolute playground for fascial techniques.

Interestingly, in premenstrual syndrome, dietary factors seem to play quite a role. It has been suggested that eating six small meals a day, increasing complex carbohydrates, fibre and water intake whilst decreasing that of caffeine, alcohol, animal fat and sugar appears to be beneficial. Vitamin B6 supplements seem to help with the associated depression and irritability.[6,7]

Lack of exercise is a known exacerbating factor, as is that famous 20th century disease, stress! This is

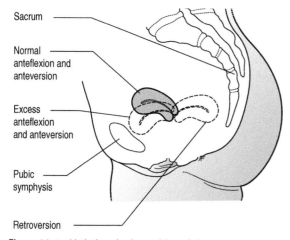

Sacrum

Normal anteflexion and anteversion

Excess anteflexion and anteversion

Pubic symphysis

Retroversion

Figure 22.1 Variations in the position of the uterus.

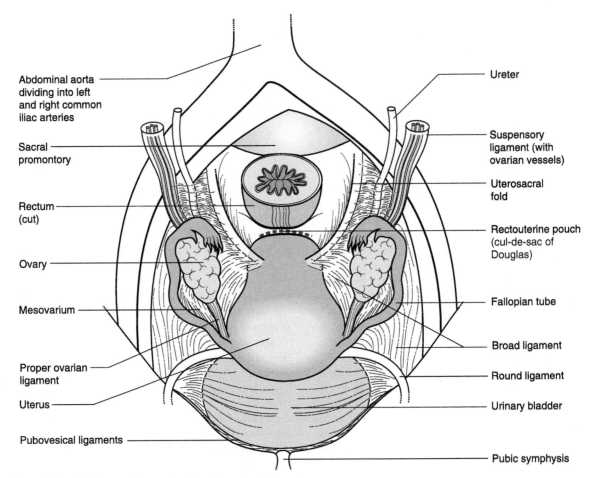

Figure 22.2 Relations and ligaments of the uterus viewed from above.

Abdominal aorta dividing into left and right common iliac arteries

Sacral promontory

Rectum (cut)

Ovary

Mesovarium

Proper ovarian ligament

Uterus

Pubovesical ligaments

Ureter

Suspensory ligament (with ovarian vessels)

Uterosacral fold

Rectouterine pouch (cul-de-sac of Douglas)

Fallopian tube

Broad ligament

Round ligament

Urinary bladder

Pubic symphysis

an occasion when the osteopath has to wear two hats, those of counsellor and therapist. Emotional stress and, in this case in particular, low self-esteem and possible interpersonal relationship problems will benefit from time and a sympathetic ear, both of which the osteopath can provide. At the same time, treating this particular patient as a whole may help their body to eradicate a number of minor problems

that are contributing factors to the overall picture. It is quite common to find that underlying physical or even psychological problems may become aggravated with premenstrual syndrome (or dysmenorrhoea); this then becomes a vicious circle which further exacerbates the symptoms. By taking an holistic approach, the vicious circle may be broken or at least brought under control.

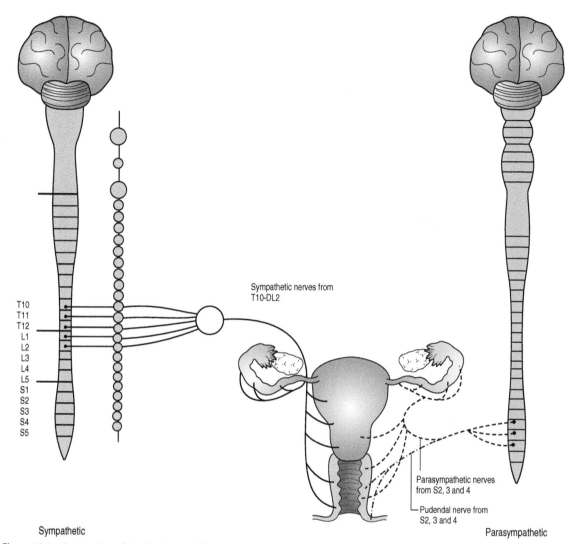

Figure 22.3   Innervation of the female genital system.

References

1. Fauci AS, Braunwald E, Isselbacher KJ et al. Harrison's principles of internal medicine, 14th edn. New York: McGraw-Hill; 1998.
2. Seller RH. Differential diagnosis of common complaints. Philadelphia: WB Saunders; 1996: 200–227.
3. Pickles VR, Hall WS, Best FA. Prostaglandins in endometrium and menstrual fluid from normal and dysmenorrhoeic subjects. B J Obstet Gynaecol 1965; 72:185.
4. Kuchera ML, Kuchera WA. Osteopathic considerations in systemic dysfunction. Colombus: Greyden Press; 1994: 139–142.
5. Campbell C. The anatomical, physiological and mechanical basis of the Maidstone oscillatory technique. Unpublished. Maidstone College of Osteopathy.
6. Wurtman JJ, Brzezinski A, Wurtman RJ, Laferrère B. Effect of nutrient intake on premenstrual depression. Am J Obstet Gynecol 1989; 161:1228–1234.
7. McCance KL, Heuther SE. Pathophysiology: the biologic basis for disease in adults and children. Missouri: Mosby; 1998: 753.

Chapter 23

Irritable bowel syndrome

CHAPTER CONTENTS

INTRODUCTION

Irritable bowel syndrome (IBS) is possibly the most common gastrointestinal disorder to present in clinical medical practices. Though not a life-threatening disease, it is, nevertheless, very distressing for the patient and quite frustrating for the medical practitioner in that, currently, there seems to be no good solution for treatment. It is characterized by altered bowel function, including constipation, diarrhoea, or alternating bouts of both; it is usually accompanied by abdominal discomfort and possible distension. The symptoms are often intermittent and are usually present for 3 months before a diagnosis of IBS is given.[1] The diagnosis is mainly made on account of the presenting symptoms in the absence of structural, biochemical or infectious aetiologies. As such, it is often considered a 'functional' disorder. Its prevalence is estimated at 10–22% of the adult population, with a female predominance twice that of males.[1]

Medical considerations in the differential diagnosis procedure are varied. They include:

- intestinal malabsorption or infection
- inflammatory bowel disorders (Crohn's disease or ulcerative colitis)
- neoplasm
- endometriosis
- depression
- obstructive disorders.

'Red flags' to indicate sinister causes which require referral include blood in the stools, weight loss, fever and pain or diarrhoea that awakens the patient from sleep. The physical examination should be unremarkable.

As aforementioned, IBS is considered a functional disorder of gastrointestinal motility and as such may, at times, be considered to be stress related. Although there is little evidence to support stress as a cause, it is often implicated as an exacerbating factor.[2]

Passage of the contents of the digestive system is achieved by a delicate balance of muscular contractions termed 'motility', which is controlled by the enteric nervous system. The term 'motility' is used here in the medical context, that is to say not in the osteopathic sense of the word. The enteric nervous system consists of the Auerbach's and Meissner's plexuses found throughout the wall of the gastrointestinal system. Auerbach's plexus is found between the muscular walls of the gastrointestinal tract and controls the muscular contractions and relaxations that propel the contents along. It is sometimes known as the myenteric plexus. Meissner's plexus, otherwise known as the submucosal plexus, lies, as the name suggests, in the submucosal lining of the gastrointestinal tract (GIT). It is responsible for the glandular secretions that cause digestion and mucous production, thus contributing to motility. In effect, the GIT is quite capable of functioning independently of the rest of the nervous system by using the connections of the enteric nervous system; however, it may be greatly influenced by the autonomic component of the nervous system. Quite simply, sympathetic influence tends to slow or shut down enteric activity whilst parasympathetic influence restores it. This would make sense in that when we are in a state of sympathetic hyperactivity (as in the case of the fight or flight response), we do not need to waste energy and blood supply on digestion or intestinal motility. After the 'stressor' has passed, we can restore our homeostatic balance and continue the everyday activity of digestion, reabsorption and elimination. It is this autonomic influence that is thought to be responsible for the stress-related part of IBS. A series of stressors followed by stress-free periods could end up disorganizing the coordinated balance of the enteric and autonomic nervous systems to the point of producing the symptoms of IBS, or if a patient is already predisposed to IBS, it is very likely that stress will then worsen the situation. A study of gastrointestinal motility[3] showed that there is a response of motility to external stressors, for example, placing a subject's hand in cold water or participating in a pressured interview. It seems that those subjects with a greater tendency to diarrhoea have a response in the large

intestine, whilst those who are prone to constipation showed a response in the small intestine. So it would seem that the response is quite specific, targeting nerves that are most likely already facilitated. Furthermore, if a stressor such as temperature or psychological pressure can create such a response it would not be implausible to consider that the same may occur with a mechanical stressor, especially if it were connected in some way or another to the neural levels influencing those organs. In other words, it is possible that mechanical disturbance in the thoracic or upper lumbar regions could influence sympathetic outflow from those levels and, thus, influence the supply to the small or large intestines.

From the above discussion we are able to see that stress influences IBS to a greater or lesser extent but there are other possible factors to consider. Undoubtedly diet will be an important factor in the patient's condition and any necessary improvements should be made. Other considerations will include occupation, sport and exercise and pregnancy. A sedentary occupation and social life is quite capable of creating reduced gastrointestinal motility whilst an excess of sport is capable of the reverse. This seems to be contrary to the accepted ideas on autonomic control of the GIT, but hyperactivity of the sympathetic system not only turns down digestive activity but promotes voiding of the lower colon. This voiding takes place before the necessary reabsorption of water has occurred, resulting in loose, liquid stools.

Kuchera and Kuchera[4] discuss a number of different types of contractions that are found in normal bowel function. There are two slow wave frequencies associated with normal function and these may be disturbed in a patient suffering from IBS. There are two normal slow wave frequencies, one at 6 cycles per minute and the other at 3 cycles per minute. They state that there is a balance of 90% of the 6 cycles per minute and 10% of the 3 cycles per minute in the normally functioning bowel. However, in the IBS sufferer the ratio changes from 90 : 10 to 60 : 40, resulting in a dysfunction of the normal flow of bowel contents. It is normal for the bowel to have 'mass movements'; they usually occur within the first hour or so after eating a meal. They are partly caused by the gastrocolic and duodenal reflexes and are mediated in part by the myenteric plexus, although the hormone gastrin released from the mucosa of the antrum of the stomach also plays a role. It appears that in IBS sufferers (and in other irritative conditions of the bowel) there is a much higher frequency of mass movements and in certain cases they may occur almost constantly.[5]

OSTEOPATHIC CONSIDERATIONS

The first approach to treatment that the osteopath can offer is one of support. IBS is a very distressing problem and the mere fact that there is contact with someone who understands is a positive first step. It is estimated that only 15–50% of IBS sufferers seek medical help.[1]

Nutritional advice will be given where necessary, although in the majority of cases the patient will have tried most things already, or altered their diet and lifestyle to cope better. The osteopath's main input to treatment will be their efforts at restoring homeostatic balance within the body.

Particular attention will undoubtedly be paid to the areas most important in the autonomic influence of the GIT (Fig. 23.1). These areas will include the sympathetic outflow to the intestines from D7 to the L2 region. Conversely, the parasympathetic outflow via the vagus and the pelvic splanchnics will be important: the region of the subocciput, carotid sheath and mediastinum for the vagus and the S2–4 levels, sacroiliacs and thus pelvic function for the pelvic splanchnics. Direct techniques would involve articulation of the relevant vertebral levels and ribs,

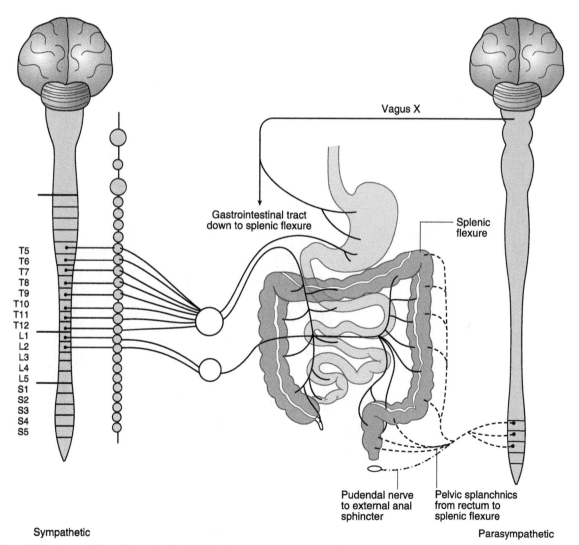

Figure 23.1   Innervation of the gastrointestinal system.

suboccipital traction, and soft tissue rolling of the cervical region. Application of the knowledge of Littlejohn's mechanics of the spine may highlight any significant areas which would then be treated with respect to their dysfunction.

Obviously, there are endless possibilities of visceral dysfunction in this case, but certain lesion patterns may be more likely than others. It has been mentioned that a major part of the symptoms of IBS is linked to the large intestine and so it would be prudent to test and rectify any problems of the colon. This may include working in the paracolic gutters, the colic flexures or the ileocaecal valve. Since the blood supply and nerve supply to the GIT follow much the same root, the innervation, nutrition and drainage rule of osteopathic principles will remain of utmost importance. Treating the root of the mesentery, the coils of the small intestine and the possibility of intestinal adhesions by gentle direct visceral techniques may be of some use. Using structural techniques to the spine, articulation or HVTs, at the levels of the attachment of the

Figure 23.2 The lymphatic system.

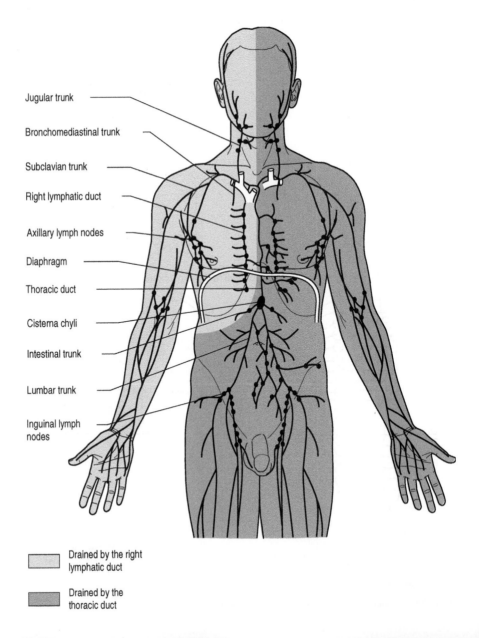

Jugular trunk

Bronchomediastinal trunk

Subclavian trunk

Right lymphatic duct

Axillary lymph nodes

Diaphragm

Thoracic duct

Cisterna chyli

Intestinal trunk

Lumbar trunk

Inguinal lymph nodes

Drained by the right lymphatic duct

Drained by the thoracic duct

mesentery may well be indicated and augment the direct work on the mesentery itself. The importance of the autonomic plexuses, namely the coeliac, superior and inferior mesenteric plexuses and the superior and inferior hypogastric plexuses, should not be overlooked, primarily because of their role in influencing the enteric system.

Autonomic function is under the control of the central nervous system and important areas include the hypothalamus and limbic system. The limbic system seems to be involved with just about every area of the brain but the hypothalamus, arranged on either side of the third ventricle, will be easier to 'contact' osteopathically by using the involuntary mechanism techniques. For the vagal outflow, the relationship of the occiput and hence the jugular foramen are considered important. Link this with the sacral parasympathetic outflow and the harmonious balance between the occiput and sacrum should then be tested and treated accordingly.

Lymphatic and venous congestion should be a major consideration in the treatment of patients with IBS (Fig. 23.2). Since the lymph channels ulti-mately find their way back into the venous system these two systems are closely linked. The lymph from the large intestine drains to the lumbar lymph nodes and via the lymph vessels back to the thoracic duct. On passing from the abdomen to the thorax the lymph passes through the cisterna chyli group of lymph nodes, located at around the level of the thoracolumbar junction. The vessels pass beneath the crura of the diaphragm and so close attention should be paid to all the attachments of the diaphragm. A technique known as 'doming of the diaphragm' has been reported by many osteopaths to be of some aid in return of venous blood and lymph from the abdomen to the thorax.

Chapman's reflex points have been used by many osteopaths in the treatment of IBS and other similar visceral disturbances.

All of the above considerations should be made in order to ease the discomfort and maintaining factors of this functional disorder. The aim is not just to give symptomatic relief at the time of treatment but, in addition, to change the intrinsic mechanisms that perpetuate the problem.

References

1. Lynn RB, Friedman LS. Irritable bowel syndrome. In: Fauci AS, Braunwald E, Isselbacher KJ et al, eds. Harrison's principles of internal medicine, 14th edn. New York: McGraw-Hill; 1998.
2. Sapolsky R. Why zebras don't get ulcers: an updated guide to stress, stress-related diseases, and coping. New York: WH Freeman; 1998: 73–74.
3. Wangle A, Deller D. Intestinal motility in man. Gastroenterology 1965; 48:69.
4. Kuchera ML, Kuchera WA. Osteopathic considerations in systemic dysfunction. Columbus: Greyden Press; 1994: 109–122.
5. Guyton AC, Hall JE. Textbook of medical physiology, 10th edn. Philadelphia: WB Saunders; 2000: 496–497.

Chapter 24

Asthma

INTRODUCTION

Asthma is a chronic relapsing inflammatory disorder characterised by hyperreactive airways, leading to episodic, reversible bronchoconstriction, owing to increased responsiveness of the tracheobronchial tree to various stimuli.[1]

It has been described as a complex disorder involving biochemical, autonomic, immunologic, infectious, endocrine and psychologic factors in varying degrees in different individuals.[2]

It is divided into two main types, extrinsic or allergic and intrinsic or non-allergic asthma.[3] In allergic asthma, there is usually a family history of asthma or related diseases such as eczema, and there are increased levels of immunoglobulin E (IgE) in the serum. In non-allergic asthma, there appears to be no family history of related diseases and no increased IgE level. However, a strict distinction is often difficult to make, with some patients falling into a 'grey area' between the two groups. A common feature of both types is inflammation, resulting in an increased irritability of the airways; this creates a bronchial spasm due to the release of inflammatory mediators. Further reduced diameter of the airways then ensues secondary to vascular congestion, oedema and excess mucus production. The patient complains of chest tightness, wheezing and dyspnoea. During an attack there may be a non-productive cough which later, as severity increases, progresses to the production of a stringy mucus. It is a highly distressing problem for the individual as the feeling of an inability to breathe may create panic, which only serves to exacerbate the problem. Status asthmaticus is severe asthma which may become life threatening and requires immediate emergency intervention. Normal treatment is ineffective and the patient has an incapacitating cough, dyspnoea and airway obstruction. Intensive care is required.

Precipitating factors are many and varied. Environmental factors include the climate: a rapid change of temperature or humidity may be sufficient to provoke an attack, such as coming out of a warm office or school into cold damp air. Air pollution is increasingly implicated in urban areas and busy cities. Occupational factors such as the workplace are obviously a consideration, exposure to certain chemicals and dust being the most obvious issues. For children developing asthma, household pets and dust should also be considered, and the parents' habits, such as smoking, need to be taken into account. Certain drugs can provoke attacks, notably aspirin and some food additives such as colourings. Even certain foods are enough to provoke attacks in some individuals: nuts, certain grains and some forms of seafood are the most commonly reported culprits. Exercise-induced asthma is often seen but on closer inspection it may be the temperature or humidity changes mentioned earlier that are the true causes. For example, a person who exercises by jogging may experience a problem in winter but not in summer, or a person may find that jogging provokes attacks all year round, but swimming in a heated indoor pool causes no ill effect whatsoever. Respiratory infections seem to provoke a large number of attacks, especially so in the case of viral infections. As always, our old nemesis emotional stress also takes its share of the blame – some reports suggest in up to 50% of cases![2,3]

Standard medical treatment is the use of inhaled (nebulized) drugs that effect dilation of the airways and/or prevent inflammation. If this is unsuccessful or inadequate then steroids may be prescribed, either inhaled or taken orally.

An interesting study by Balon and co-workers[4] published in *The New England Journal of Medicine* in 1998 compared active and stimulated chiropractic treatment as an adjunctive treatment for childhood asthma. Although both sets of treatments produced positive effects the researchers concluded that there was no significant difference between them. The active chiropractic treatment consisted of high velocity spinal manipulation. Sadly, what was not pointed out by the chiropractors who performed the study was that the simulated treatment that they described

as 'soft tissue manipulation and gentle palpation to the spine, paraspinal muscles and shoulders' is exactly what many an osteopath will use as a basis for the treatment of asthma. Furthermore, the treatment was 'simulated' by using low-amplitude, low-velocity impulses to other areas of the body that the researchers considered insignificant in the treatment of asthma, notably the head and occipital region. To an osteopath, these areas are of great significance in the treatment of asthma due, amongst other reasons, to the course of the vagus. It is hardly surprising that there was 'no significant difference', as they are both valid treatments in their own right! Any number of classical osteopathic texts will have described a treatment for asthma that consisted of precisely these types of manoeuvres.

OSTEOPATHIC CONSIDERATIONS

There is a difference between treating an asthmatic during an attack and treatment between attacks. The treatment needs to be modified for the situation but the structures addressed will be similar in both cases. Naturally, techniques used during an attack should be generally inhibitory in nature. Having stated that, there are some osteopaths who feel that stimulation during an attack will increase sympathetic activity and thus create bronchodilation.[5] There is a fine line for an asthmatic between feeling in control and losing control during an attack and so stimulatory treatment is probably best left for those with considerable experience.

Most osteopaths recognize the importance of working on the thorax in the case of asthmatic patients. They are interested not only in the intervertebral articulations but also in the costovertebral and costotransverse articulations. These articulations are involved in thoracic mechanics and hence any restrictions will limit the ability for a full respiratory motion. In addition, the sympathetic ganglionic chain is lying very close to these articulations and it is thought that any possible dysfunction of these articulations could affect the nerves and hence their targets. It is the upper five or six thoracic spinal levels that supply the sympathetic outflow to the lungs and bronchi and so these levels should undoubtedly be checked.

Breathing is not merely a movement of the ribs. In asthma the diaphragm will be important and so the sternal, costal and vertebral attachments will need to be considered (Fig. 24.1). In addition, the

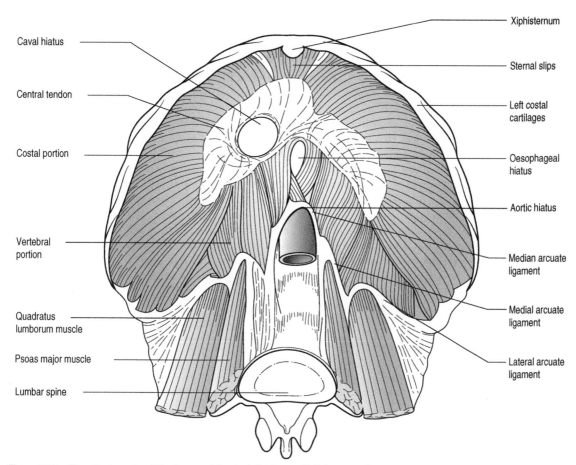

Figure 24.1 The attachments of the thoracoabdominal diaphragm (inferior aspect).

motor supply to the diaphragm comes via the phrenic nerve which has its origins at the C3–5 levels and so any somatic dysfunction at these levels should be addressed.

The constricting feeling that accompanies an asthma attack may be relieved by working into the mediastinum. This is the space between the two pleural sacs. In theory it is anatomically subdivided, but it is the mediastinum as a whole that houses the trachea and bronchi, the roots of the lungs and their associated vessels. It contains the heart in the pericardium and the great vessels. The heart and lungs have their cardiac and pulmonary plexuses respectively, which are made up of a mixture of sympathetics from the upper thoracic region (T1–6) and parasympathetics from the vagus. It is the autonomic nerves that control the smooth muscle of the airways and hence their diameter. Furthermore, the drainage vessels from the lungs, both venous and lymphatic, have to traverse the mediastinum in order to reach their respective major conduits, the superior vena cava and the thoracic and lymphatic ducts. Since a major part of the pathogenesis of asthma is congestion, any aids to reduction of congestion would be welcome. It would be prudent for any osteopath treating a patient suffering from asthma to look closely at the mediastinum and to release any tensions found therein. Gentle pumping techniques to the thorax may be of help, but it is stressed that they should be kept to a minimum in order to avoid overstimulation. It is relatively easy to provoke an attack by using too forceful a compression to the thorax.

Since respiration is controlled by the respiratory centre which is located in the upper medulla lower pontine region of the brain stem, it makes sense to examine this region using cranial techniques and to work on anything indicated. The relationship of the occiput to the cervical fascia and thus the continuity to the mediastinum, especially with the vagus nerve contained within, should not be forgotten. The imbalance of the autonomic nervous system in asthma is accepted as an overactivity of the vagus creating bronchospasm and an underactivity, at least initially, of the sympathetics. It is for this reason that during an attack a CV4 technique may help to restore autonomic balance. This may be the treatment of choice in an anxious patient having an attack rather than trying to inhibit the parasympathetics and stimulate the sympathetics. It is quite likely that in the case of an anxious patient, the sympathetic system is already working overtime and although the action is to bronchodilate, there may well be an excess of mucus that is obstructing airflow. Restoring a harmonious balance to the autonomics may be the way to calm the attack but it should be borne in mind that most asthmatics, during the course of an attack, will not be happy to, or benefit from, lying down and so the technique may need to be performed sitting. In fact Still stated that he sometimes treated asthmatic patients 'while they are standing up'.[6] Still wrote in his book *Osteopathy – Research and Practice*[6] that his treatment for asthma included treating all the ribs and muscles of the thorax until he was satisfied that 'this part of the work is absolutely normal'. He then advised practitioners to 'keep your hands off the patient for at least one week'; this is quite sound advice since it is relatively easy to provoke an asthmatic attack in some patients by overzealous handling or overadministration of treatment. 'Find it, fix it, and leave it alone.'

References

1. Busse W, Holgate S. Asthma and rhinitis. Boston: Blackwell Scientific; 1995.
2. McCance KL, Huether SE. Pathophysiology. Missouri: Mosby; 1998: 1176–1178.
3. McFadden Jr ER. Diseases of the respiratory system: asthma. In: Fauci AS, Braunwald E, Isselbacher KJ et al, eds. Harrison's principles of internal medicine, 14th edn. New York: McGraw-Hill; 1998: 1419–1426.
4. Balon J, Aker PD, Crowther ER et al. A comparison of active and simulated chiropractic manipulation as adjunctive treatment for childhood asthma. N Engl J Med 1998; 339:1013–1020.
5. Umanzio CB. The allergic response. In: Hoag JM, Cole WV, Bradford SG, eds. Osteopathic medicine. New York: McGraw-Hill; 1969: 685–708.
6. Still AT. Osteopathy – research and practice. Kirksville: Still; 1910: 174–177.

Chapter 25

Low back pain

CHAPTER CONTENTS

INTRODUCTION

Osteopaths in the UK and in many other countries throughout the world have earned the label of being fairly good at treating back problems. Even if our patients do present with a number of different problems it is quite likely that at some stage we would be called upon to treat a 'bad back'. Back pain and, in particular, low back pain is one of the major reasons that patients consult their preferred healthcare professional. It accounts for an enormous amount of public funds in terms of loss of work, insurance payments and medical costs, pharmacologically or otherwise, and one would expect that much research has been performed in solving this worldwide problem. Indeed, much work has been done, but unfortunately, the medical profession as a whole (which includes the osteopathic profession) has a poor knowledge of what is actually going on with the average bad back and worse still, what to do with one![1] This does not mean that advances have not been made in our understanding of back pain but merely that, at the end of the day, there does not seem to be an agreed 'cure'.

Low back pain is probably one of the most controversial areas of medicine with respect to any form of agreement on what is best for the patient. Fortunately for healthcare practitioners and patients alike, the ideas are changing. Sydenham[1] recognized the importance of mobility in arthritic and rheumatic patients as early as 1734. Seriously ill people had taken to the sick bed as a consequence of the disease and not as a form of treatment. Then along came Hunter[1] in 1794 and Hilton[1] in 1887, two surgeons dealing with surgical disease who wholeheartedly recommended rest as an essential part of recovery. This idea then became adopted right across the field of medicine and so it became fashionable that bed rest was advised as the first line of attack in overcoming back pain. However, this was not always the case; there were a number of black sheep who disagreed.[2,3,4] 'Rest or activity' has been the cause of considerable research.[5–8] Others have been more pointed in their research, directing it towards the harmful effects of rest.[9,10]

But it was in the mid-1980s that the question of how long the duration of bed rest should be was posed. Once again, wide-ranging ideas and much disagreement seemed to be the outcome. Finally, in 1997, Waddel and co-workers[11] made a systematic literature search for all randomized controlled trials of advice for bed rest and that of staying active. The overall conclusion was that activity is far more useful than inactivity. With so much disagreement as to whether rest or activity is more important, it comes as no surprise to learn that those who do agree that activity is more important then disagree as to how much and by what methods!

Sadly or gladly, depending on your viewpoint, recent research has shown that 80–90% of patients with acute low back pain will 'recover' within 12 weeks regardless of the type of treatment administered.[12,13] In these particular research studies, recovery was seen as 'no longer seeking medical advice' and so numerous patients may have returned to work and, as such, were no longer seeking medical advice. It appears that the longer someone is off work with back pain, the lower their chances are of returning to work, especially if the injury occurred in the workplace.[14,15] However, when pain is used as a measure, the outcome looks different: fewer than 50% are pain-free after 1 month, after 3 months more than 40% are still experiencing discomfort, and 60% will have recurrence within 1 year.[16–20] This could change our viewpoint on low back pain; should it 'really be regarded as not simply an acute disease but (often) a recurrent disease that has symptom free periods interspersed with frequent exacerbations?'.[21] With this in mind, our approach to treatment may need rethinking.

So how does the osteopathic approach differ from other modalities? Before answering this question, we should consider a number of points. Firstly, we have already seen that across the medical profession there is considerable disagreement on how

best to achieve good results. In addition, the thinking has changed with time. Osteopathy is no different. Two different osteopaths may have two different ideas on how the same patient should be treated. However, most osteopaths would agree that every patient is a different individual and thus treatment should be individualized too.

PATIENT + DISEASE = ILLNESS

The only constant factor in this equation is that of the disease; it may be exposure to the cold virus that affects two separate patients. These two patients are different; they may have different ages, occupations, genders, past medical histories, etc. And as they represent the variables in the equation, they will thus vary the manifestation of the illness. One may have a cold that leaves them feeling dreadful and laid up for a week whilst the other has a sore throat for a day. It may be argued that this is merely a differing response due to the efficiency or inefficiency of their immune systems and that this cannot be applied to low back pain. Let us apply the equation to a musculoskeletal condition.

If we consider only the vertebral column for a moment, we may see it as a team, for example a football (soccer) team. Like any team, it is composed of a number of players and in order for it to give its best performance, all members of the team must pull together. Each member of the team plays an important part in the match although their roles differ. We need speedy forwards that can flit about looking for any opportunity to slot in a goal, the cervicals. The defence (lumbars) needs to be solid enough to repel the opposition whilst the midfield (thoracics) has to be flexible enough to link the two but at the same time lend solidity to the defence. The vertebral column, composed of its vertebrae and interposed discs, provides the individual members of the team but it is the connecting tissue between them that completes the action of teamwork. Take this analogy a step further and we see the nervous system as the manager. Naturally enough, some members of the team are more important than others – as highlighted by Littlejohn's views of pivots and pivotal roles – but to a greater or lesser extent all members of the team have a role to play. The problems arise when a member of the team is shown the red card or becomes injured. This places an extra strain on the other members of the team and may create the undesirable situation of a member of the team having to perform a role to which he is not really suited.

This will create a weakness in the team's performance and, furthermore, may highlight previously unnoticed weaknesses elsewhere within the team. A player who is under some strain due to a niggling problem now has to give 110% to make up for his sent-off team mate, and in doing so his weakness becomes apparent. This analogy may be applied to the vertebral column. A segment of the column may be under strain, due to, for example, a knee problem, but the column as a whole compensates and continues to function, albeit not to its best ability. Bring along another strain, which may be relatively innocuous, and the previously compromised compensatory system begins to falter. Previously unnoticed weaknesses become apparent: in other words, the subclinical problems now show symptoms. This could be what is happening in the asymptomatic patient who has developed low back pain for 'no apparent reason'.

Any of the members of the above team that receive an innervation may be responsible for the nociceptive input felt by the patient as low back pain. These structures include muscles, ligaments, fascia, articulations or discs of the lumbar spine. Obviously there are a number of other structures that could refer pain to the low back, for example the urogenital structures and lower intestinal viscera, but in this discussion we will look solely at the lumbar spine structures. Of these, the intervertebral disc has received much attention for many years and the commonly made diagnosis of 'slipped disc' was fashionable for some time. In fact, for some practitioners and patients alike, it is still used quite freely.

The intervertebral disc comprises an outer portion, the annulus fibrosus, and an inner nucleus pulposus. Structurally, the annulus fibrosus is composed of 10–20 closely packed concentric layers of collagen known as lamellae.[22] It is this portion of the disc that can withstand considerable compressive forces. The nucleus pulposus is a hydrated gel that when under compressive force pushes radially out towards the annulus. It is the resistance of the annulus against the gel of the nucleus that creates the combination of strength and pliability so characteristic of the intervertebral discs. In addition to the above described portions of the intervertebral disc, the superior and inferior surfaces are covered with cartilage plates known as vertebral end plates, which bind the discs firmly to adjacent vertebral bodies.[22] One of the numerous problems that can occur is disruption of the annulus portion, with displacement of both nuclear and annular material beyond the normal perimeter of the disc; this is known as a disc prolapse. The true problem for the patient arises when it begins to press upon pain-sensitive structures such as the posterior longitudinal ligament, spinal nerves or their roots, or worse still, the spinal cord itself. Pressure on the pain-sensitive structures will result in a change from an asymptomatic to a symptomatic condition, for example, pain in the back or sciatica.

Numerous studies have shown that disc abnormalities such as dehydration, bulging and herniation may be demonstrated by magnetic resonance imaging (MRI) in up to 50% of asymptomatic subjects, and studies have shown similar results using computer-assisted tomography (CAT) and X-ray investigations.[23–26] If there are so many of us walking around with 'undiscovered' back problems it is no wonder that we see so many patients who have no real idea as to how their back problem began. Could it be that the others, those that can give a reason, are merely doing so because it is easy to 'find' a reason retrospectively?

Since Nobel Prize winners Bloch and Purcell first reported the phenomenon of magnetic resonance in 1946 and Damadian and Lauterbur put these principles to the first clinical uses, many patients have benefited. Conversely, it could be argued that a great number of patients have been dealt a disservice by it! Consider the scenario of a patient presenting with back pain of 1 month's duration. On MRI a disc herniation is revealed. Where does the treatment regimen take the patient? One hopes for a conservative approach, but in many cases surgical intervention may be the outcome. Would it not be better to consider that if we had performed an MRI on this patient 1 month *and 1 day* ago, the chances, according to the previously mentioned studies, are 50:50 that they will have shown a disc herniation but no symptoms? If this is the case, would it not be better to try to find out what has taken place to create the new situation, and to try to reverse it without the need for surgery? Could it be that we are now looking for the player who has received the red card and who, in doing so, has placed extra strain on the team, highlighting his team-mate's weakness? Imaging by magnetic resonance was a major medical breakthrough but also a potential disaster as it is too easy, in some cases, possibly up to 50% of cases, to make the 'false' diagnosis of disc herniation as the 'true' cause of the patient's distress.

OSTEOPATHIC CONSIDERATIONS

A study published in 1999 compared treatment of chronic and subchronic back pain by osteopathy with that of standard medical care.[27] The conclusion was that both had similar clinical results; however, there was a far greater financial cost with standard medical care and obviously a much higher use of medication. Furthermore, two major publications in the UK[28] and the USA[29] provided guidelines for the management of back pain conditions. Both agreed that it is important to avoid passive approaches and resort to the 'positive' approach of return to normal activity as soon as possible. This, in the majority of cases, is also the wish of the patient. The studies stressed that it was important to address the psychosocial aspect of the problem as well as the physical aspect. In this respect, the osteopath has a distinct advantage over the classic allopathic approach: most osteopathic treatment sessions provide ample time for patient–practitioner interaction. During the course of a treatment, the osteopath has the opportunity to give positive corrective advice with respect to posture, ergonomics of work station and relevant exercises.

With respect to the 'real hands-on treatment', as we have already stated, osteopaths will differ in their beliefs and methods and thus their approaches. However, we shall try to give an outline as to how the osteopath approaches low back pain. It will be a mixture of numerous ideas!

Let us first consider a patient who consults with acute low back pain. Naturally, the patient may be in considerable pain, and a primary requirement of the osteopath is to reduce that level of pain. Associated with acute pain is the concept of fear. Fear that any movement is going to produce more pain but, in addition, fear that some irreparable damage has been done. And so a calm, reassuring but positive attitude on behalf of the osteopath will be required. In this case the history will be of utmost importance: the onset and reason for onset must be considered. By far the most common reason for onset of acute lumbar pain is lifting, either lifting an object that is too heavy, or lifting in an awkward position. Having stated that, a number of patients present with acute pain without having actually lifted the intended object, or having lifted an object that was quite light. Either way, it is possible that the patient may actually have done significant damage to certain structures and so the questions posed will need to ascertain other possible symptoms such as neurological deficit. In this case, 'red flags' would include saddle anaesthesia, impaired sphincter control or progressive motor weakness: these would alert the osteopath to serious damage and require urgent referral. Other neurological symptoms such as paraesthesia or pain radiating into the lower extremity would be assessed in the physical examination by motor, sensory and reflex testing and then by using other indicated specific tests such as Lasegue's or Bragard's.

In the case of acute lumbar strain, aggravating factors would include anything that provokes brisk movements such as coughing or sneezing, though commonly this may be misread as a 'false positive' indication of raised intraabdominal pressure creating the pain. In most cases this can be ruled out by asking the patient to perform a controlled Valsalva's manoeuvre. Should the pain still be present then thecal involvement must be considered and investigated. In the majority of cases, the patient will admit to immobility as an ameliorating factor and this should be apparent by their body language.

Consideration must be given to the patient's age. In a 25-year-old, bending to lift a light box may produce an acute lumbar strain that is exquisitely painful – but the same action in a 75-year-old osteoporotic woman may produce the same strain plus a pathological stress fracture!

Once the history and physical examination have ruled out serious injury or pathology then treatment may proceed. As mentioned earlier, most acute presentations will feel better with the avoidance of movement and so treatment may be best provided by using techniques that are gentle. However, in certain cases a high velocity low amplitude thrust technique may be indicated; this will depend on the individual osteopath and patient. An experienced practitioner, with the patient's clear understanding and consent, may choose to perform a thrust technique as a rapid means of 'unblocking' the patient's back. In fact, some patients will consult an osteopath with that outcome in mind: 'a quick crack and back to work'! A study comparing osteopathic manipulation with chemonucleolysis for sciatica concluded that 1 year after the treatments the clinical outcomes were not significantly different.[30] However, the study did show that the manipulation produced a quicker improvement in both back pain and disability. Nevertheless, some patients and osteopaths alike will shy away from manipulative methods under these circumstances and turn to the more 'gentle' indirect approaches. Regardless of the technique used, the true depth of the osteopath's mastery will become apparent after the unblocking has taken place. Many of us have been called upon to perform wonders on acute backs but what we are doing is merely first aid; the true reason for the breakdown in the normal spinal and hence body mechanics should be sought. It may be that a good working knowledge of the biomechanics of the spine and an understanding of the Littlejohn mechanics will provide the route to untwining the complex stacking of lesion patterns, uncovering the root of the problem and enabling the osteopath to restore mechanical harmony, and helping to prevent further recurrence of the 'locked back syndrome'. With reference to the earlier analogy of the workings of the spine and body as a team, as the various team members become compromised and compensations are set up, 'reading' of the lesion patterns will enable a treatment programme to progress without further exacerbations of pain. This requires experience built upon empirical values rather than a prescriptive treatment regimen. It is important for the osteopath to realize that an unchecked acute problem may progress to a chronic problem and that this may then trigger further complications, mechanically, psychosocially and possibly even pathologically.

Chronic pain is quite different from acute pain, in that pathological change may occur in the tissues, both locally and in distant tissues. Locally, fibrotic infiltration of the soft tissue structures of the lumbar spine may occur and if compensations are set up due to adaptation of a slowly progressing chronic problem then other areas of the spine or other articulations may become involved. It has been shown by histological examination of the multifidus muscle in patients with low back pain that metaplasia, fibrosis and atrophy may occur.[31–34] The multifidus muscle plays an important role in the self-bracing mechanism of the pelvis and thus in the transfer of energy from the upper body to the lower extremities[35,36] (Fig. 25.1). This mechanism involves the multifidus increasing tension in the thoracolumbar fascia, sacroiliac ligaments and sacrotuberous ligaments and so the anatomical connections are clearly at risk of compromise in failure of this system due to chronic low back pain. Add to this the continuation of the connective tissue structures, the ligamentous stocking of the lumbar spine and sacroiliac joints with their connections to the muscles, both prime movers and stabilizers, and we form an integrated structure that encompasses both the hard

and soft tissues of the low back.[37] It is this integrated system that combines mobility and stability. It is a combination of the shape of the bony components and the tension of the connective tissue structures that creates a balance of what are known as 'force' and 'form' closure[34] (Fig. 25.2). If there is failure in the balance of any of the components of this system, it is likely that pain will ensue as a result of this dysfunction.

The osteopath recognizes these connections and in the global view of the body will assess not only how each of these structures functions, but also how their functions interact. The osteopath should then extrapolate these connections to take in the whole body picture of the individual patient before him; this includes the mind-body-spirit connections discussed earlier in the book.

Clearly, looking at a case scenario as 'simple and straightforward' as low back pain becomes ever more complicated when other factors are considered. It was mentioned earlier that on case history examination and potential hypothesis making, age may play a part in distinguishing between a simple strain and something far more traumatic. But another factor that may alter our total body picture is past surgical intervention. If we consider two patients of the same age presenting with exactly the same type of low back pain, where one has no past history of surgery and the other has had an appendectomy, inguinal hernia repair and two Caesarean sections, it is likely that our management plan of treatment will differ between the two. The abdominal wall musculature plays a critical role in stabilization of the low back and pelvis, especially on forward flexion.[38] In the case of our patient with a history of extensive abdominal surgery, her compromised anterior abdominal wall may have been responsible for creating her low back pain and so this will need addressing as part of her treatment. However, it does not necessarily require surgery in order to weaken the abdominal wall and thus the low back; postpartum hypotonia is seen quite commonly, and abdominal hypotonia is not confined to women!

Furthermore, abdominal surgery may result in adhesions which could further destabilize the lower back and pelvis by altering the ability to contract the abdominal muscles or, indeed, by altering the posture. This in turn may become an important factor in the management of a patient who simply presents with low back pain. It may not be sufficient to treat the patient without the use of some

Figure 25.1 The self-bracing mechanism and the transfer of energy from the upper body to the lower extremities through the thoracolumbar fascia.

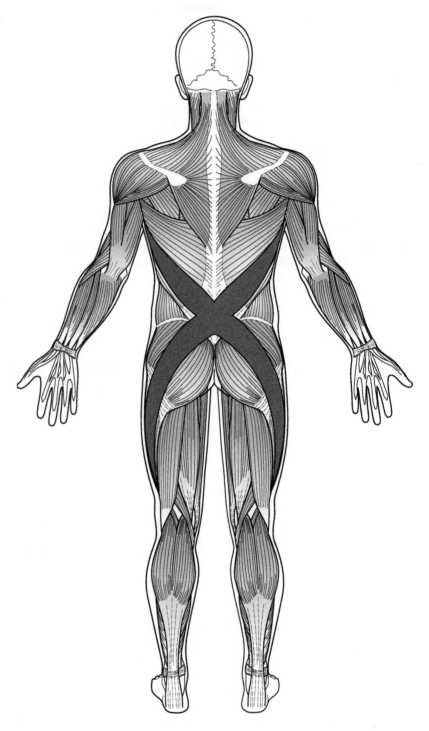

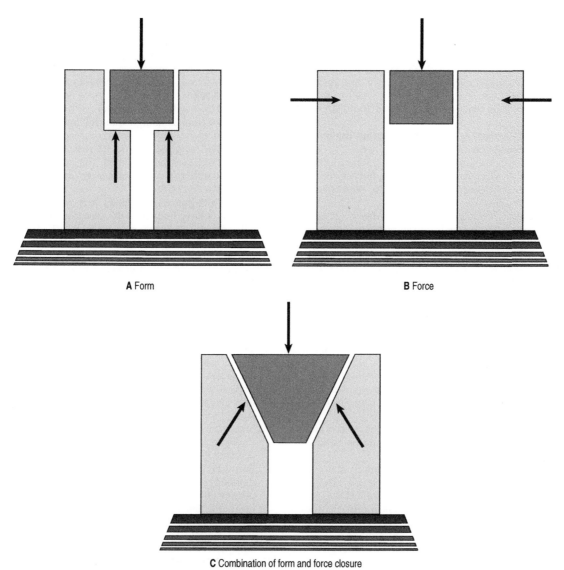

A Form

B Force

C Combination of form and force closure

Figure 25.2 Form and force closure. **(A)** The shape creates the stability but at the cost of reduced mobility. **(B)** Force applied through a tight band creates stability with mobility. **(C)** A combination of form and force closure is seen in the human pelvis, creating a balance of stability with mobility. (Reproduced with permission from Snijders et al.[35])

visceral work, or at best, it may just result in a series of oscillations between relapses and remissions, the oft-seen cyclic recurring back problem. It is the consideration of these factors that distinguishes osteopathic treatment of patients presenting with low back pain from some other forms of treatment.

In summary a quotation from Radin[39] will suffice:

functional analysis, be it biological, mechanical or both, of a single tissue will fail to give a realistic functional analysis as, in all complex constructs, the interaction between the various components is a critical part of their behaviour.

This is the rule that osteopaths should apply to every patient, no matter what the presenting complaint.

References

1. Waddell G. The back pain revolution. Edinburgh: Churchill Livingstone; 1998.

2. Johnson G. A lecture on backache and the diagnosis of its various causes with hints on treatment. BMJ 1881; 1:221–224.

3. Asher RAJ. The dangers of going to bed. BMJ 1947; 967–968.

4. Cyriax J. Textbook of orthopaedic medicine. Baltimore: Williams and Wilkins; 1969: 460–462.

5. Cherkin DC, MacCornack FA, Berg AO. Managing low back pain – a comparison of the beliefs and behaviours of family practitioners and chiropractors. West J Med 1988; 149:475–480.

6. Battie MC, Cherkin DC, Dunn R et al. Managing low back pain: attitudes and treatment preferences of physical therapists. Phys Ther 1994; 74:219–226.

7. von Korff M, Barlow W, Cherkin D et al. Effects of practice style in managing back pain. Ann Intern Med 1994; 121:187–195.

8. Svensson H, Andersson G. The relationship of low back pain, work history, work environment and stress. A retrospective cross–sectional study of 38 to 64 year old women. Spine 1989; 14:517–522.

9. Bortz WM. The disuse syndrome. West J Med 1984; 141:691–694.

10. Hides JA, Stokes MJ, Saide M et al. Evidence of lumbar multifidus muscle wasting ipsilateral to symptoms in patients with acute/subacute low back pain. Spine 1994; 19:165–172.

11. Waddell G, Feder G, Lewis M. Systematic reviews of bedrest and advice to stay active for acute low back pain. Br J Gen Pract 1997; 47:647–652.

12. Andersson GB. Epidemiology of low back pain. Acta Orthop Scand Suppl 1998; 281:28–31.

13. Coste J, Delecoeuillerie G, Cohen de Lara A et al. Clinical course and prognostic factors in acute low back pain: an inception cohort study in primary care. BMJ 1994; 308:577–580.

14. McGill CM. Industrial back problems: a control program. J Occup Med 1968; 10:174–178.

15. Abenhaim L, Rossignol M, Gobielle D et al. The prognostic consequences in the making of the initial medical diagnosis of work-related injuries. Spine 1995; 20:791–795.

16. Chavannes AW, Gubbels J, Post D et al. Acute low back pain: patients' perceptions of pain four weeks after initial diagnosis and treatment in general practice. J R Coll Gen Pract 1986; 36:271–293.

17. Cherkin D. Proceedings of the First International Forum for Primary Care Research on low back pain, Seattle, October 1995. Spine 1996; 21(4):2819–2929.

18. Croft PR, Macfarlane GJ, Papageorgiou AC et al. Outcome of low back pain in general practice: a prospective study. BMJ 1998; 316:1356–1359.

19. von Korff M, Deyo RA, Cherkin D et al. Back pain in primary care: outcomes at one year. Spine 1993; 18:855–862.

20. von Korff M, Saunders K. The course of back pain in primary care. Spine 1996; 21:2833–2839.

21. Lively MW. Prevalence of pre-existing recurrent low back pain in college athletes. W V Med J 2002; 98(5):202–204.

22. Adams MA, Bogduk N, Burton K et al. The biomechanics of back pain. Edinburgh: Churchill Livingstone; 2002: 64–78.

23. Wiesel SW, Tsourmas N, Feffer HL et al. A study of computer-assisted tomography: 1. The incidence of positive CAT scans in an asymptomatic group of patients. Spine 1984; 9:549–551.

24. Witt I, Vestergaard A, Rosenklink A. A comparative analysis of X-ray findings of the lumbar spine in patients with and without lumbar pain. Spine 1984; 9:298–300.

25. Boden SD, Davis DO, Dina TS et al. Abnormal magnetic-resonance scans of the lumbar spine in asymptomatic subjects. A prospective investigation. J Bone Joint Surg Am 1990; 72:403–408.

26. Jensen MC, Brant-Zawadzki MN, Obuchowski N et al. Magnetic resonance imaging of the lumbar spine in people without back pain. N Engl J Med 1994; 331:69–73.

27. Andersson GB, Lucente T, Davis AM et al. A comparison of osteopathic spinal manipulation with standard care for patients with low back pain. N Engl J Med 1999; 341:1426–1431.

28. Clinical Standards Advisory Group. Management guidelines for back pain. London: HMSO; 1994.

29. Agency for Health Care Policy and Research. Management guidelines for acute low back pain. Rockville: US Department of Health and Human Services; 1994.

30. Burton K, Tillotson KM, Cleary J. Single-blind randomised controlled trial of chemonucleolysis and manipulation in the treatment of symptomatic lumbar disc herniation. Eur Spine J 2000; 9:202–207.

31. Hadar H, Gadoth N, Heifetz M. Fatty replacement of the lower paraspinal muscles: normal and neuromuscular disorders. Am J Roentgenol 1983; 5:895–898.

32. Lehto M, Hurme M, Alaranta H et al. Connective tissue changes of the multifidus muscle in patients with lumbar disc herniation. An immunohistologic study of collagen types I and III and fibronectin. Spine 1989; 14:302–309.

33. Mattila M, Hurne M, Alaranta H et al. The multifidus muscle in patients with lumbar disc herniation. A histochemical and morphometric analysis of intraoperative biopsies. Spine 1986; 11:732–738.

34. Parkkola R, Rytokoski U, Kormano M. Magnetic resonance imaging of the discs and trunk muscles in patients with chronic low back pain and healthy subjects. Spine 1993; 18:830–836.

35. Snijders CJ, Vleeming A, Stoeckart R. Transfer of the lumbosacral load to iliac bones and legs. Part 1: Biomechanics of self-bracing of the sacroiliac joints and its significance for treatment and exercise. Clin Biomech 1993; 8:285–294.

36. Vleeming A, Pool-Goudzwaard Al, Stoeckart R et al. The posterior layer of the thoracolumbar fascia: its function in load transfer from spine to legs. Spine 1995; 20:753–758.

37. Willard FH. The lumbosacral connection: the ligamentous structure of the low back and its relation to back pain. In: Vleeming A, Mooney V, Dorman T et al, eds. Second Interdisciplinary World Congress on Low Back Pain: The Integrated Function of the Lumbar Spine and Sacroiliac Joint. Rotterdam: ECO; 1995: 29–58.

38. Don Tigny RL. Dysfunction of the sacroiliac joint and its treatment. J Orthop Sports Phys Ther 1979; 1:23–35.

39. Radin EL. The joint as an organ: physiology and biomechanics. First World Congress on Biomechanics, La Jolla, September 1990; Volume 2:1 Abstracts.

Chapter 26

Headache

INTRODUCTION

There are probably very few people lucky enough never to experience a headache at some time in their lives. It is such a common occurrence; estimates are made that at least 40% of individuals worldwide experience severe disabling headaches annually.[1]

It is a vast subject to try and cover in a small chapter like this and so we will give just the salient points. Headaches can come as a result of anything from psychoemotional stress to tumours. However, although many individuals who suffer a severe disabling headache are inclined to fear the worst, most headaches are of a benign origin. It is estimated that only 5% of patients presenting to the emergency departments of hospitals are found to be suffering from a serious underlying neurological disorder.[1] Having stated that, it is important to be able to differentiate between those headaches of benign origin and those of a more sinister nature.

The International Headache Society (IHS)[2] uses a classification system that separates headaches into 13 different categories (Box 26.1).

It is interesting to note that there is a category (4) for miscellaneous headaches that are not associated with structural lesions (they are obviously not referring to structural lesions in the osteopathic sense) and a further category (13) for 'not classifiable' headaches. These are the *'well I really can't give a definite diagnosis so I guess you have a category 13 headache'* headaches! Even with this ambiguity, by far the commonest type of headache is the migrainous type.[1]

Box 26.1   International Headache Society classification of headache (After Olesen J. Headache Classification Committee of the International Headache Society: Classification and diagnostic criteria for headache disorders, cranial neuralgia and facial pain. Cephalalgia 1988; 8(7):1. Reproduced with permission)

1. Migraine
2. Tension-type headache
3. Cluster headache and chronic paroxysmal hemicrania
4. Miscellaneous headache not associated with structural lesion
5. Headache associated with head trauma
6. Headache associated with vascular disorders
7. Headache associated with non-vascular intracranial disorder
8. Headache associated with substances or their withdrawal
9. Headache associated with non-cephalic infection
10. Headache associated with metabolic disorder
11. Headache or facial pain associated with disorder of facial or cranial structures
12. Cranial neuralgias, nerve trunk pain, and deafferentation pain
13. Not classifiable headache

Box 26.2   Symptoms associated with headache that may suggest a sinister origin – 'red flags'

First severe headache ever
Subacute worsening over days or weeks
Disturbs sleep or is present immediately upon awakening
Abnormal neurological examination
Fever or other unexplained systemic signs
Vomiting precedes headache
Induced by bending, lifting or cough
Known systemic illness (e.g. cancer, collagen vascular disease)
Onset at age 55 or older

A study[3] performed using the IHS classification system found that many patients actually needed two or three, and sometimes four, different classifications for the same headache. Although it was found that migraine was indeed the most common type, only 25% of subjects had migraine as their sole diagnosis, and 75% of those diagnosed with migraine also had either a chronic tension type headache or drug-induced headache associated with it – or both.

Migraine is simply defined as a benign and recurring syndrome of headache, nausea, vomiting and/or other symptoms of neurological dysfunction in varying admixtures.[1] Unfortunately, the headache associated with a brain tumour may not be totally dissimilar. And so with this in mind it is necessary for a detailed case history and examination to be taken when a patient presents with headache.

There are some important considerations to make when taking the history with respect to quality, location, duration and time course of the headache. Each

of these considerations, when viewed separately, may be of little value, but when looked at together may give a clearer picture as to the cause of the pain. Add to that information regarding predisposing, aggravating and ameliorating factors and the differential diagnosis becomes far clearer. It is not possible in a text such as this to discuss all the many and varied causes of headache and their diagnoses. As mentioned, there is a far greater likelihood that a patient presenting with a headache is safe to treat osteopathically than not; however, there are some 'red flags' to be aware of and these are detailed in Box 26.2.

OSTEOPATHIC CONSIDERATIONS

Most osteopaths at some time or other will have to treat a patient who presents with headache as their major complaint and once they are deemed 'safe' to treat, there are various options open to the practitioner. For a tension type headache, many osteopaths will concentrate on the upper cervical and suboccipital region. It goes without saying that in order for the upper spine to be working harmoniously, the rest of the spine and musculoskeletal system needs to be examined and where necessary corrected. The suboccipital region is especially important, for this is the region that makes the final minor adjustments to keep the head 'on the level'. The suboccipital muscles act very much like fine adjusters, trying to compensate for any imbalances throughout the rest of the column. They are almost like proprioceptors that will then relay the information of misalignment to the larger muscles that attach to the head, for example the splenius, the longus capitis muscles, trapezius and sternocleido-mastoids. The occipitofrontalis muscle stretching over the vertex from back to front is a frequent relay of tension from the upper neck and occipital region to the forehead. It is also capable of working in reverse, carrying tension from the front backwards. This could be as a result of eye strain or sinus trouble and so these causes would need possible investigation and rectification. It is easy to think of the head as having only a front and back, and to neglect the sides! We should be aware not only of tension from the temporal regions such as temporalis and masseter muscles but also from the temporomandibular joint as well. Many practitioners have had a lot of success treating headaches of this nature by working on the trigger points. Temporomandibular joint dysfunction is a frequently overlooked cause for headache, as is bruxism, the excessive grinding of the teeth. Nor should we neglect the possible tensions reflected from the anterior throat and cervical fascial systems, especially since it ends up rooted to the base of the skull. The stomatognathic system should be considered with respect to possible causes of headache, especially after recent dental work, whiplash type injuries or throat infections.

No self-respecting osteopath adept in the skills of working with the involuntary mechanism would pass up the opportunity to make a full cranial examination and rectify any problems discovered. Tension type headaches respond quite well to drainage techniques, cranial or otherwise, since there is usually a certain amount of congestion involved. The same goes for sinus-related problems.

As for migraine, varying degrees of success are reported. Commonly, migraine has activators; there is an endless list which includes certain foods or drinks, hunger, bright lights and fatigue. It goes without saying that the first approach to migraine is prevention by avoidance. Migraine seems to be hereditary and is far more common in women, often triggered by the menstrual cycle. It is often associated with nausea, vomiting, photophobia, scalp tenderness and light-headedness. The pathogenesis of migraine seems to have three phases and it is sufficient for this text to describe them as vasomotor, serotonergic and trigeminal.[4] The overall pattern is one of altered vascular supply to the brain and head, resulting in activation of the trigeminal nociceptive afferent nerves of the blood vessel walls, and the perception of pain.

It may well be that the success of osteopaths who treat migrainous patients is due to the 'normalization' of blood flow coupled with a reduction of tension and the effects of psychoemotional stress. It would appear that migraine sufferers are often not under any greater levels of stress than non-sufferers, but that they may be over-responsive to it. It could well be that the calming effect of osteopathic treatment may in some way restore balance to previously facilitated neural pathways and thus make the onset of an attack less likely. With this in mind, it will therefore be important to improve the overall biomechanical functioning of the body. Umanzio[5] states that 'the greatest potential benefit may derive from skilful handling of the musculoskeletal factors, for their effect on the autonomic nervous system'. Kuchera and Kuchera[6] make the link between certain gastrointestinal disorders and headaches as a 'parasympathetic dominant complaint' and regard the upper cervical region, occipitomastoid suture and occipitoatlantal articulation as important considerations.

A randomized controlled trial published in 1998[7] investigating the efficacy of chiropractic spinal manipulation in the treatment of episodic tension type headaches concluded that spinal manipulation does not have a positive effect on these types of headaches. One group received high velocity low amplitude (HVLA) and soft tissue techniques to the cervical spine and trapezius muscles; the control group received only soft tissue work and placebo laser treatment. The results showed no significant difference between the two groups in either mean daily headache hours or analgesic use. This type of study is looking at a single technique method applied to a variable population of 'individual patients'. It may have had better outcomes if the treatments were 'tailored' to the patients. With this in mind we should look at some of the thoughts of Still on the treatment of headaches. He, like the above researchers, suggested inhibitory techniques to the upper cervical region but follows these with articulation techniques 'to all the facets of all the joints of the neck, beginning with the atlas'.[8] He goes on to say 'after this is done without any twisting or wringing of the neck, which I think is not necessary, I generally stretch the neck up a little giving a slight motion to the right and left holding my fingers on any bone that is out of position. This the osteopath knows how to do.'[8] He describes treating through the whole spine correcting 'any variation from the normal between the fifth lumbar and the occiput'. His reasons for this are stated as ensuring 'good nerve and blood supply to the renal system as well as the entire excretory system'.[8] It would seem that Still respected the whole body interaction of systems with respect to headache. Finally, it should never be forgotten that headache may only be a symptom of some other dysfunction.

References

1. Raskin NH. Headache. In: Fauci AS, Braunwald E, Isselbacher KJ et al, eds. Harrison's principles of internal medicine, 14th edn. New York: McGraw-Hill; 1998: 68–72.
2. Olesen J. Headache Classification Committee of the International Headache Society: classification and diagnostic criteria for headache disorders, cranial neuralgia and facial pain. Cephalalgia 1988; 8(7):1.
3. Sanin LC, Mathew NT, Bellmeyer LR et al. The International Headache Society (IHS) Headache Classification as applied to a headache clinic population. Cephalalgia 1994; 14(6):443.
4. McCance KL, Heuther SE. Pathophysiology: the biologic basis for disease in adults and children. Missouri: Mosby; 1998: 537–539.
5. Umanzio CB. The allergic response. In: Hoag JM, Cole WV, Bradford SG, eds. Osteopathic medicine. New York: McGraw-Hill; 1969: 702–703.
6. Kuchera ML, Kuchera WA. Osteopathic considerations in systemic dysfunction, 2nd edn. Ohio: Greyden Press; 1994: 104–105.
7. Bove G, Nilsson N. Spinal manipulation in the treatment of episodic tension-type headache: A randomized controlled trial. JAMA 1998; 280(18):1576–1579.
8. Still AT. Osteopathy: research and practice. Missouri: AT Still; 1910: 359–360.

Chapter 27

Pregnancy

INTRODUCTION

Pregnancy is not an illness or disease; it is a normal state of health. However, being pregnant may, at times, seem like an illness! (Since both authors of this text are male, we have accepted this statement on good authority.)

PREPARATION FOR THE BIRTH

More and more women are turning to their osteopaths to help them prepare for the progression of their pregnancy and the impending birth. In this case osteopathy has much to offer. Naturally enough, during pregnancy the mother will go through a dramatic change in her posture but this is progressive and involves a slow adaptation, unlike the changes after the birth! Much help may be given by working with the mother's adaptations to posture using a variety of techniques that best suit the individual patient. If the mother is a patient who has been seen prior to her pregnancy, the techniques to which she has responded in the past may be used throughout the duration of her pregnancy with some obvious necessary adjustments. For example, if she has always responded well to direct techniques, then there is no reason not to continue with treatment in a similar vein, with the necessary modifications made for her present state. Likewise in the case of good prior response to indirect techniques it makes sense to continue their use. The expectant mother has enough changes of her own to contemplate without the osteopath suddenly changing tack.

During the 9-month course of a normal pregnancy a number of major changes will take place. The developing fetus will place increased demands on the mother's circulatory system and if there is an imbalance between the demands and the returns within the system, then congestion may well occur. During pregnancy the higher levels of circulating progesterone probably contribute to fluid retention and thus congestion.[1] In addition, progesterone is thought to be partly responsible for the alterations that take place in the thoracic cage. In order to accommodate the expanding uterus and growing fetus, but not to compromise respiration, the biomechanics of the thorax must alter.[2] There is a widening of the costal angle and an increase in the thoracic circumference. This, combined with an increase in diaphragmatic excursion, achieves an increase of tidal volume negating the need for an increase of respiratory rate to remain within the required physiological parameters. This effect of progesterone is most likely enhanced by the action of relaxin, a hormone produced by the corpus luteum which appears to have its major effect of relaxation on pelvic ligaments including the pubic symphysis, cervix and uterus in preparation for the birth.[1]

Without doubt, one of the more noticeable changes is the constant alteration in posture. As the fetus and its surrounding structures increase in weight and volume, the mother's centre of gravity will move anterior, resulting in an increased lumbar lordosis. This will create compensatory increases in both the thoracic kyphosis and cervical lordosis. Accompanying the increased lumbar lordosis will be an increase in the angle of pelvic tilt (Fig. 27.1). These changes will be reflected throughout the whole musculoskeletal system with resultant changes in muscular tonicity to maintain the upright posture. In short, as the size of the fetus and uterus increase, they are no longer contained within the pelvis and expand into the abdomen and begin to project even further anteriorly. This will cause the sacrum to rotate anteriorly on its horizontal axis; this movement is otherwise known as nutation. In order to maintain balance, the ilia will compensate by rotating posteriorly whilst the legs externally rotate at the hips.

Later in the pregnancy there will be relaxation of the ligaments which under normal circumstances act to limit this nutation, and they will become less effective than usual. The muscles will have to work harder still to maintain stability, notably the erector spinae, hamstrings, psoas, piriformis and levator

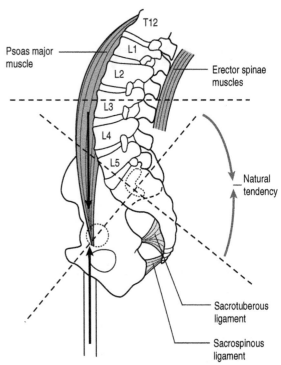

Figure 27.1 The scissors effect. (After Molinari R. Biomèchanique de la femme enceinte et adaptation posturale. Les Dossiers de l'Obstètrique 1989:163(6).)

ani muscles. If the nutation of the sacrum is pure then there is likely to be symmetrical hypertonicity but in many cases there may be an imbalance. This is further compounded by the engagement of the baby's head. Engagement is when the presenting part of the fetus, hopefully the head but sometimes the buttocks, enters the pelvic inlet in preparation for the birth. During birth the passage of the head begins with the head presented in a transverse position in the pelvic inlet. Once in the mid-cavity of the pelvis, the head begins to rotate so that the occiput contacts the ischiopubic ramus and the frontal portion and the face is cushioned on the levator ani muscle posteriorly. As the head is ready to exit the pelvic outlet, it rotates further so that the occiput lies anteriorly and the frontal towards the sacrum; in other words, it lies sagittally. The body of the baby has to follow this spiral movement and any hindrance caused by muscular or ligamentous tension creating bony restriction may make for a more difficult birth. The aforementioned nutation of the sacrum combined with the rotational spiraling of the baby will require freedom of movement around an oblique axis of the sacrum (refer to the chapter on muscle energy technique (MET)). Since rotation around an oblique axis is a physiological movement resulting in an anterior sacral torsion, the mother's pelvis should be capable of this movement; however, if there is already a restriction in one of the axes and the baby performs the opposite movement, this again may make for difficulties. Should there be a counternutatory movement around an oblique axis, a non-physiological backwards torsion, then this is far more likely to create problems. Naturally, in preparation for the birth the osteopath should be looking out for these kinds of restrictions and others discussed in the chapter on MET.

The pelvis and vertebral column need to be functioning optimally. This includes all the articulations and muscles of the pelvis including the pubic symphysis and the coccyx. With all the focus of concentration on the back and pelvis, it is easy to forget the anterior structures and especially the soft tissues. Psoas plays an important role in the descent and engagement of the head; it has been described[3] as a kind of guide for fetal descent and so should be checked for hyper- or hypotonicity and treated accordingly.

Some women complain of low back pain and associated sciatica during pregnancy. Reported incidences vary between 50 and 82%[4,5] and many are told to expect it as part of bearing a child, but by careful consideration of the above points it may be relatively easy to find the cause and treat it accordingly.

In addition, there are techniques used for working on the pregnant uterus as part of the preparation for the birth. Since the uterus is a muscular bag that will, in the end, be required to contract and expel the baby, it also needs to be in an optimal condition, as do the ligaments of the uterus. Barral[6] states 'all the uterine ligaments are distended, sometimes to four times their normal length'. Hyper- or hypotonicity of the muscles and ligaments of the uterus may be treated accordingly by visceral techniques.

More often than not the actual position of birth is not ideal for the mother; rather, it is the most comfortable position for the birth attendants, midwife and gynaecologist. The theory is that the mother only has to do this once in a while, but the attendants do it day in and day out, and so are protecting themselves, which is ergonomically a fair argument. Nowadays, mothers are beginning to stand up for their rights and squat down for the birth; this enables them to adopt a better position from a biomechanical viewpoint. However, many mothers are 'encouraged' to believe that the best position is the modified lithotomy position (supine with flexed hips and knees) and with the pressures created during labour, any hindrance to normal function will be greatly exaggerated.

The postural imbalances seen during pregnancy and birth, when combined with the increased circulatory demands, may tip the balance from the limit of normal physiological efficiency into the pathophysiological state of the continuum. In the perfectly functioning body which is very capable of compensation, this state of affairs may never arise but in an already compromised body (and whose is not?) the body's compensatory capabilities may become overloaded and dysfunction becomes apparent.

TREATMENT OF INTIMATE AREAS AND INTERNAL TECHNIQUES

As part of their preparation for birth treatment, many osteopaths feel the need to examine and, if necessary, treat the pelvic floor soft tissues and perineum (Fig. 27.2). Some treatments may involve internal techniques via the vagina and possibly rectum. Under these circumstances informed written consent should be obtained prior to treatment. Failure to do so may result in complaints and disciplinary procedures. The General Osteopathic Council of Great Britain[7] has given its members guidelines and provided consent forms for osteopaths to use in these circumstances. It is presumed that the appropriate professional registering bodies of other countries have similar procedures.

Most pregnant women will have already been examined internally, possibly on numerous occasions, by their gynaecologist or midwife, but that does not mean they expect the same from their osteopath. However, many women are happy to accept this as an important part of their treatment if the reasons for doing so are explained fully. It is often useful to have an anatomy book or some relevant anatomical charts to aid with the explanation as to why you feel it is necessary. When doing so, be professional, use simple (but not vulgar) terms that the patient can understand and allow the patient to ask any questions they wish to. It is often good practice to give the patient sufficient time to reflect if they wish to go ahead with this aspect of the treatment. It is probably good advice to suggest

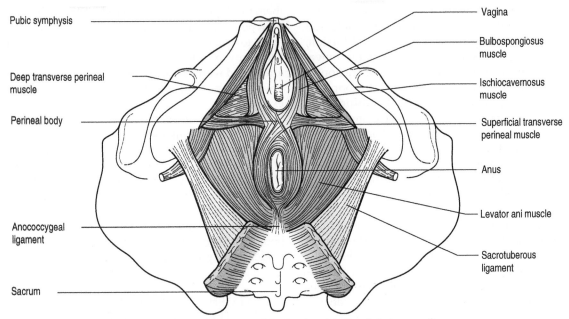

Pubic symphysis

Deep transverse perineal muscle

Perineal body

Anococcygeal ligament

Sacrum

Vagina

Bulbospongiosus muscle

Ischiocavernosus muscle

Superficial transverse perineal muscle

Anus

Levator ani muscle

Sacrotuberous ligament

Figure 27.2   The arrangement of muscles and ligaments of the female pelvic floor (inferior aspect).

that if they consent, the technique should be performed at their next appointment but that they can always decline. Always offer a suitable chaperone; many patients will feel that this is not necessary, but it is also for the protection of the osteopath should a complaint arise in the future.

Impress upon the patient that if they do not consent to these techniques, it is not the end of the treatment. Internal techniques may be the most effective way to treat a certain problem but they are most likely not the only way possible. Once written consent has been obtained, never forget the patient still has the right to stop the procedure, even while it is in progress. If the patient says stop, the osteopath stops!

In spite of all this, most women are agreeable to these techniques where indicated and much self-help advice can be given on treating the perineum in preparation for the birth. The benefits may be reduced pain and less chance for the need of instrumental assisted delivery (forceps or ventouse) or episiotomy.

COMPLICATIONS OF PREGNANCY

The aptly named morning sickness seen frequently during the first trimester of pregnancy seems to be due to hormonal changes and is of little clinical consequence unless severe, when biochemical and nutritional disturbances may ensue, a condition known as hyperemesis gravidarum.[8] Nevertheless, the nausea and vomiting of morning sickness is disturbing enough for many women to seek help, and treatment should be aimed at restoring balance within the body by whatever means are indicated, which may also include dietary advice. Important areas to be considered will include the liver with respect to its detoxification action and the upper cervicals and occipitomastoid sutures in connection with the vagus. The cerebrospinal fluid flow and thus the reciprocal tension membrane should be assessed and treated accordingly. It is common to find that gentle non-invasive techniques are preferred in this first trimester because of the fear of provoking a miscarriage. Some osteopaths prefer to only ever use these techniques on pregnant women, whilst some shy away from treating at all during the first trimester. For many reasons it is important that the osteopath is aware that the patient is pregnant or in certain cases that the patient is 'trying for a family'.

The diagnosis of pregnancy is usually made by the general practitioner or gynaecologist but most often a simple pregnancy testing kit is used by the suspicious mother to be. Most expectant mothers are alarmed to find that for pregnancy there is a list of possible complications that reads as long as the gestation period itself! However, most diagnosed pregnancies that run to term do so without major mishaps. Having stated that, it is impossible to say how many undiagnosed pregnancies are 'naturally terminated'; these may be retrospectively diagnosed or not even noticed as a real pregnancy. Impey[9] states that spontaneous miscarriage may occur in up to 50% of all conceptions. Many women may bear a fertilized embryo and for whatever reason, the body decides against running to term and a spontaneous abortion occurs, resulting in a slightly delayed period. The woman may not have even been aware of it.

It is quite well accepted that most spontaneous abortions or miscarriages occur during the first trimester and 15% of diagnosed pregnancies spontaneously abort.[9] Some reports[10] state that weeks 12 and 16 are the most dangerous weeks. There is a fear that overtreatment may well induce miscarriage. Sandler[10] states 'there has not been one reported case in the literature of miscarriage caused by the use of manipulation during pregnancy'. It has to be agreed that 'overtreating' may well be risking miscarriage but then an osteopath should never overtreat! Still is supposed to have told us, 'find it, fix it and leave it alone'. All treatment should be adapted for the individual patient (a constantly recurring theme of this text) and so, if in our preparation for the birth we decide to really strongly articulate the lumbar spine and pelvis and perform direct visceral techniques on the uterus of a woman who has been pregnant for only 8 weeks, then we are in danger of overtreating and as such, risk provoking a miscarriage. On the other hand, we probably would not suggest she begins her day with fifty sit-ups in order to prepare her abdominal musculature for the big day. Everything needs to be kept in proportion: there are many osteopaths who will articulate the lumbar spine in these early stages without problems, but they do so respectfully of the patient's condition. Let us not forget that if we choose to use involuntary mechanism techniques as a form of 'gentle approach' to the patient, these 'subtle' techniques may also be very potent in their physiological effects (if not, why do we learn them in the first place?). There are many women who have an active and fulfilling sex life throughout the whole duration of their pregnancy. The very act of coitus is likely to be far more traumatic on the developing fetus nestled in the uterus than osteopathic articulation of the lumbar spine. Many women continue their aerobics classes or other sporting activities well past the end of the first trimester. Impey[9] states that 'exercise, intercourse and emotional trauma do not cause miscarriage'. However, there is a growing body of evidence that high enough levels of stress or repeated stressors can certainly induce miscarriage in animals and probably in humans too.[11,12,13]

In terms of energy expenditure, becoming pregnant is one of the most 'costly' things a woman can do to her body. The physiological changes that take place when under chronic or acute stress are aimed at the utilization of energy for defence or escape – fight or flight. And so the body may 'decide' to abort the fetus under exceptional circumstances. Hippocrates[14] is supposed to have advised pregnant women to avoid excessive emotional disturbances and so maybe the 'old wives' tales' that get passed down from mother to daughter do have some truth in them.

However, if by chance a woman should miscarry the day after an osteopathic treatment, the possibility that it may have been about to happen anyway, regardless of the treatment, is still a hard pill to swallow for the patient and osteopath alike. So, if there is any doubt in your mind, do not do it! If, for example, a woman has a history of miscarriage or if there are signs of threatened miscarriage then caution should prevail and an immediate referral should be made.

If all of these aspects are discussed openly and honestly with pregnant patients at the initial consultation, then most are quite happy to proceed confidently in the hands of their practitioner.

Later on in the pregnancy, the previously mentioned congestive states may result in the formation of haemorrhoids which may be very painful. Aside from the general considerations given above, specific techniques such as functional inhibition to the perineum may be helpful. The kneeling position with the upper body flat on the floor or bed may aid drainage and reduce pelvic congestion but this may be contraindicated if the patient is suffering from gastric reflux or heartburn. In this case, treatment aimed at normalizing the diaphragm and the autonomic balance of the stomach, intestines and lower oesophagus may be of use.

It is not the purpose of this text to list or describe in detail all the possible complications of pregnancy, but it is prudent for the osteopath treating pregnant women to be aware of the major considerations. On accepting a pregnant woman for treatment, an osteopath is assuming some responsibility for her well-being. Of course, the osteopath is not taking on the roles of midwife, gynaecologist and obstetrician all in one, but we should still be on the lookout for signs of ill-health. Any signs of infection, hyper- or hypotension (measure the blood pressure at every consultation) or reported vaginal discharge, blood or otherwise are considered 'red flags' and should result in immediate referral to the gynaecologist. It is prudent to check the blood pressure at every visit since the onset of eclampsia may be very rapid. Some complications of pregnancy are life threatening for mother, child or both and early detection may reduce or completely avoid these risks.

Pregnancy is a normal state of health with modified homeostatic parameters to accommodate a transient productive change. There are possibilities of ill-health resulting from a number of causes should the normal compensatory homeostatic mechanisms be unable to adequately adapt. The osteopath can offer much help to the pregnant patient provided that the complications are ever-present considerations in the osteopath's mind. The final word on this subject goes to Simon Fielding:

One must never lose sight of the fact that one has a responsibility not only to the mother, but to the unborn child and also to the father. It is important to involve the whole family in the pregnancy as this will encourage a more supportive environment for both mother and child.[15]

References

1. Carr BR, Bradshaw KD. Disorders of the ovary and female reproductive tract. In: Fauci AS, Braunwald E, Isselbacher KJ et al, eds. Harrison's principles of internal medicine, 14th edn. New York: McGraw-Hill; 1998: 2097–2102.
2. Tettambel MA. Obstetrics. In: Ward R, ed. Foundations for osteopathic medicine. Baltimore: Williams and Wilkins; 1997: 349–361.
3. Molinari R. Biomèchanique de la femme enceinte et adaptation posturale. Les Dossiers de l'Obstètrique 1989: 163(6).
4. Moore K, Dumas GA, Reis JG. Postural changes associated with pregnancy and their relationship to low back pain. J Clin Biomech 1990; 5:169–174.
5. Bullock JE, Jull G, Bullock MI. The relationship of low back pain to the postural changes of pregnancy. Aus J Physio 1987; 33:11–17.
6. Barral JP. Urogenital manipulation. Seattle: Eastland Press; 1993: 128.
7. General Osteopathic Council of Great Britain. Pursuing excellence. June 2002:9–13.
8. Douchar N. Nausea and vomiting in pregnancy: A review. Br J Obstet Gynaecol 1995; 102:6–8.
9. Impey L. Obstetrics and gynaecology. Oxford: Blackwell Science Oxford; 1999: 94–101.
10. Sandler SE. The management of low back pain in pregnancy. Man Ther 1996; 1(4):178–185.
11. Sapolsky RM. Why zebras don't get ulcers: an updated guide to stress, stress-related diseases and coping. New York: WH Freeman; 1998: 120–123, 372–373.
12. Berger J. Induced abortion and social factors in wild horses. Nature 1983; 303:59.
13. Myers R. Maternal anxiety and foetal death. In: Ziochella L, Pancheri P, eds. Psychoneuroendocrinology in reproduction. New York: Elsevier; 1979.
14. Huisjes H. Spontaneous abortion. Edinburgh: Churchill Livingstone; 1984: 108.
15. Fielding S. Osteopathic care in pregnancy. J Soc Osteopath 1982; 11:26–30.

Chapter 28

Otitis media in the infant

INTRODUCTION

Babies and children are not smaller versions of adults, they have differences in their anatomy and their physiological mechanisms may differ from those of an adult. Paediatrics and paediatric osteopathy could well be considered as specializations in their own right and many paediatric osteopathic courses are offered at a postgraduate level. (The subject of specialisms in osteopathy will be addressed in Ch. 34.) Much has been done to advance the knowledge of treating children osteopathically over the last 20 years but certain names amongst many deserve particular mention. One is that of Viola Frymann, of the Osteopathic Center for Children in San Diego, USA. In the UK, Stuart Korth founded the Osteopathic Centre for Children in London in 1991. Due to the success of this venture, he and his co-workers have opened a second centre for children in Manchester. Jane Carreiro[1] of the University of New England, author of *An Osteopathic Approach to Children,* has done much lecturing throughout the world in association with the highly respected anatomist Frank Willard. Another key player is Sue Turner, the founder and first director of the Children's Clinic within the European School of Osteopathy. All the aforementioned have helped in their own ways to promote the knowledge of paediatrics throughout the osteopathic world.

OTALGIA

Otalgia or ear pain is a common condition, especially during childhood. It is mostly an indication of an infection of the external auditory meatus, the middle ear or the mastoid air cells. Of these, by far the most common in children is otitis media. It has been estimated that 85% of children will have at least one episode of acute otitis media by the age of 3 years.[2] Moreover, those who do develop it in their early years are at increased risk of recurrent acute attacks or development of chronic otitis media.[3] With such an alarmingly high incidence it is quite likely that an osteopath will see a child suffering from otitis media, although this may not be the main reason for consultation. Numerous mothers bring their child along for other reasons and have the impression that nothing can be done for the ottis media other than antibiotics. However, this bewilderment of mothers is slowly changing as the enlightenment that osteopathy may be able to help is spread. The standard medical treatment is to prescribe antibiotics and although this is often effective, many mothers are reluctant to repeatedly dose their children up with drugs each time the problem recurs and risk the problem of antimicrobial resistance. Having said that, the orthodox medical profession is actually now changing its ideas on the widespread use of antibiotics. Many prefer to seek 'alternative' methods which aim to treat the root of the problem rather than the symptoms produced.

The usual presentation of acute otitis media is otalgia, fever and hearing loss of acute onset in a child who has recently suffered an upper respiratory tract infection.[4,5] Most episodes of acute otitis media result from bacterial infection and so examination reveals an inflamed, possibly bulging tympanic membrane with a yellowish white effusion deep to it. The mobility of the membrane will be reduced and this can be simply tested by using a pneumatic otoscope. Further testing may include tympanometry but often the diagnosis will have already been made by the paediatrician. In spite of this it is still necessary for the osteopath to be aware of possible complications[4] that may arise should the treatment be ineffective. These include chronic suppurative otitis, mastoiditis, adhesive otitis and acquired cholesteatoma, any of which could lead to further infection and hearing loss. There is always the danger that infection from the middle ear could lead to intracranial complications and so this should always be borne in mind. In addition, it is also possible that the middle ear infection may have arisen from a suppurative intracerebral complication[4] and so a neurological examination should be carried out and if any positive signs are found, immediate referral made.

PATHOGENESIS

The middle ear is connected to the nasopharynx by the Eustachian (pharyngotympanic or auditory) tube. It has a bony portion within the temporal bone and a cartilaginous portion extending to the nasopharynx. It has a dual role: it permits equilibration of the pressures between the middle ear and external atmosphere, and secondly, it provides a drainage route for middle ear secretions into the pharynx. Should it become blocked it obviously cannot perform these functions normally. Consequently the secretions of the middle ear can build up whilst at the same time a negative pressure is created within the cavity of the middle ear. This negative pressure further hinders the drainage and is coupled with a reduced functioning of the mucociliary system. Should the Eustachian tube be only partially blocked then there is a danger that the negative pressure could aspirate nasopharyngeal secretions, or that they may enter the middle ear cavity by reflux or insufflation.

As already mentioned, the Eustachian tube is composed of bony and cartilaginous sections. Under normal circumstances the patency of the Eustachian tube is maintained by a number of factors: the stiffness of the cartilage and the actions of salpingopharyngeus muscle and tensor veli palatini muscle, the latter being the only true active opener of the tube[6] (Fig. 28.1). Evidently, the anatomy of the child and adult differ in many ways but never more so than in the head. The shape of the head, and in particular the craniofacial base ratio (Fig. 28.2), creates a situation in the child whereby the mechanical advantage of the tensor veli palatini muscle is compromised. This unlikely disadvantage due to the differing anatomy is made up for in other ways; for example, the shape of the pharynx in the neonate permits suckling and respiration to occur simultaneously. Furthermore, in the child, the bony part of the tube is relatively shorter and the cartilaginous part is more horizontally placed. So, add together the increased nasopharyngeal mucus due to the recent upper respiratory tract infection with the impaired opening mechanism and the result is acute otitis media. Once this has recurred a few times, there is a greater chance of a reduction of stiffness in the cartilage of the tube and the chances are that the problem is on its way to becoming chronic.

A

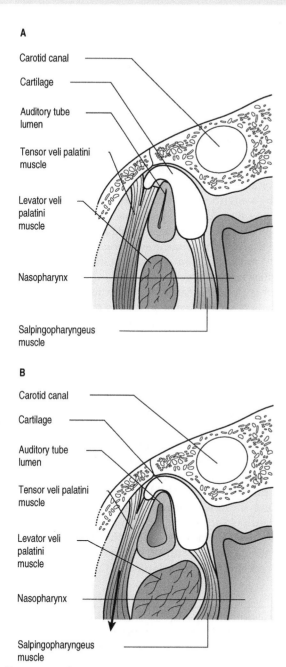

Carotid canal

Cartilage

Auditory tube
lumen

Tensor veli palatini
muscle

Levator veli
palatini
muscle

Nasopharynx

Salpingopharyngeus
muscle

B

Carotid canal

Cartilage

Auditory tube
lumen

Tensor veli palatini
muscle

Levator veli
palatini
muscle

Nasopharynx

Salpingopharyngeus
muscle

Figure 28.1   Opening and closing of the Eustachian tube.
(A) closed. **(B)** Open.

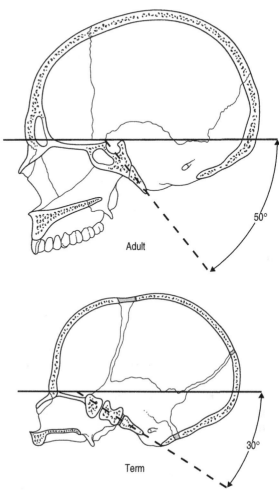

Adult

50°

Term

30°

Figure 28.2   Diagrams comparing the orientation of the newborn and adult cranial base as measured in relation to the axial
plane passing through glabella and inion. (Reproduced with permission of the Willard & Carreiro collection.)

OSTEOPATHIC CONSIDERATIONS

So if it is normal to have this inefficient opening
mechanism, then it follows that it is normal to suffer
otitis media – but not all children suffer. The ones
who do not suffer are lucky, but luck is backed up
by the presence of good vitality and an optimally
working pharynx and immune system.

It goes without saying that the primary aim of the
treatment would be to examine and treat as necessary any dysfunction found in the pharynx,
Eustachian tube and related structures. The bony
part of the tube lies within the temporal bone and
ends at the junction of the squamous and petrous
portions. Though the cartilaginous portion in the
adult is twice as long as the bony part, in the newborn it is comparatively longer still. It passes to the
tubal elevation of the nasopharynx and is fixed to
the basicranium in a groove between the petrous
portion of the temporal bone and the greater wing

of the sphenoid, the groove ending near the medial pterygoid plate.

The cartilaginous part of the tube is an 'inverted J' shape in section with a mucous membrane lining that is continuous at either end with that of the pharynx and the tympanic cavity. The tube is narrowest at the osseocartilaginous junction and it is easy to imagine how with excess mucus and an inefficient opener the walls could become stuck together. Carreiro[7] states 'in the new born and infant, the petrosphenoid junction is cartilaginous and vulnerable to mechanical stress. Tissue strains transferred from the cartilaginous structures into the fascial tissues of this area may influence Eustachian tube function'.

An osteopath faced with treating this type of problem would naturally look to the cranial base and temporal bones. The soft tissues of the pharynx and the cervical fascia may well be compromised especially when remembering that most episodes of otitis media follow on from upper respiratory tract infections. It would be prudent to examine the tongue and to check for imbalances of muscle tension on suckling which could provide a means for fluid aspiration. It is interesting to note that almost all children with cleft palate develop chronic otitis media.

Do not forget that the patient is a 'child' with otitis media and so we need to consider treating the 'rest' of the child as well. We should be aware that the child may have suffered a number of recurrent respiratory infections and so the immune system may need 'boosting'. Lymphatic drainage will be important in this condition and so the lymph routes from the head down through the cervical region and back into the venous circulation will need to be free from restrictions. This includes any restrictions to cervical mobility, especially the occiput–atlas–axis complex which may be compromised as a result of birth trauma. The use of forceps as a means to aid birth may well create vertebral restrictions in the upper cervical region and, in the same way, ventouse-assisted births are seen to create their own problems osteopathically, including cranial articular restrictions and associated soft tissue dysfunctions. Children born by Caesarean section are not free of insults either. In the case of emergency sections after labour has begun, the rapid change of the baby's environmental pressure from the high pressure of the uterine contractions to the low pressure of the external world may create a rebound effect in the tissues.[7] It may mean working with the involuntary mechanism in order to restore balance and reduce facilitation.

It is possible that the children who escape otitis media or other similar problems could well be the ones who are free from upper cervical or cranial articular restrictions. To our knowledge there are no studies to date that have researched the cervical connections with otitis media but it is an interesting possibility for future research. However, Degenhardt and Kuchera[8] reported an association between cranial strain patterns and the incidence of otitis media in children.

It would appear from the above that the most useful means of treating the infant with this problem is by using involuntary mechanism approaches. In practice, young children are often best treated using these techniques, but that does not mean exclusively so. There are many conditions that can be treated equally as well with other methods; as in the case of treating the pregnant patient, they may well need to be adapted to suit the patient.

References

1. Carreiro JE. An osteopathic approach to children. Edinburgh: Churchill Livingstone; 2003.
2. Pomeranz AJ, Busey SL, Sabnis S et al. Pediatric decision-making strategies. Philadelphia: WB Saunders; 2002: 2–4.
3. Durand M, Joseph M, Sullivan Baker A. Infections of the upper respiratory tract. In: Fauci AS, Braunwald E, Isselbacher et al, eds. Harrison's principles of internal medicine, 14th edn. New York: McGraw-Hill; 1988: 179–182.
4. Behrman RE, Vaughan VC, Nelson WE. Nelson's textbook of pediatrics, 13th edn. Philadelphia: WB Saunders; 1987.
5. Seller RH. Differential diagnosis of common complaints, 3rd edn. Philadelphia: WB Saunders; 1996.
6. Williams PL, Warwick R. Gray's anatomy, 35th edn. Edinburgh: Churchill Livingstone; 1980: 1197.
7. Carreiro JE. An osteopathic approach to children. Edinburgh: Churchill Livingstone; 2003: 129–139.
8. Degenhardt BF, Kuchera ML. The prevalence of cranial dysfunction in children with a history of otitis media from kindergarten to third grade. J Am Osteopath Assoc 1994; 94: 754.

Chapter 29

Sports injuries

INTRODUCTION

The treatment of sports injuries is an area that could well become a specialization, and a growing number of osteopaths do consider themselves specialists in this field. It is a subject that requires some clarification. Consider for a moment two patients of the same age and past medical history who consult their osteopath complaining of knee pain. One patient describes the onset as occurring after a twisting movement during a game of tennis, and the other twisted his knee whilst running for the bus. The first example is clearly a sports injury, the second is clearly not, although the injuries may be identical. Now add a third patient with an identical problem, also sustained playing tennis. We now have two patients with sports injuries but one of the tennis players is professional whilst the other is an occasional player who twisted his knee playing tennis with his son in the park. Clearly, they are both sports injuries but of a different nature – do they both need to consult a specialist? The professional relies on his game for his livelihood whilst the other may not give two hoots if he never plays again! He simply wants to get out of pain and will find another activity to occupy his son. It is considerations like these that make the distinction of specializations a difficult area.

In 1978 the Health Education Council of Great Britain[1] launched the 'Look After Yourself' campaign which encouraged people to exercise but more importantly to exercise correctly. Spurred on by slogans such as 'You would enjoy sex better if you wore running shoes!', many people took to the streets using running as a means of looking after themselves and the marathon boom began in the UK. The idea was not that running was any better than any other form of endurance exercise but more that running is a relatively cheap, freely available and easy means of getting or staying fit. Inevitably, with many novice runners out on the streets there were soon to be many injured novice runners seeking help.

Endurance exercise in general has positive effects on the cardiovascular and respiratory systems, affects the endocrine and metabolic function of the body and to those who enjoy it, has some very pleasing psychological effects too. The musculoskeletal system is the primary machinery of life and although distance running is associated with a low incidence of disabling injuries when compared to some of the other more traumatic sports, it can certainly place a heavy load on the musculoskeletal system. In fact, it is truer to say that it places a heavy load on the articulations and mainly on the articular surfaces of the lumbar spine, hips, knees and ankles in particular.

When a serious sportsperson becomes injured, one of the first questions asked will be 'Will it stop me from doing my sport?'. Perhaps they are a professional sportsperson and need to get back to 'work' quickly. It could be that although they only play for fun there is a tournament or cup match coming up soon that they want to be ready for. Or it could be, as was the case so often with the runners in the 70s and 80s, that they are planning to run a marathon for charity and already have many sponsors pledging money to their chosen cause. Finally, they could just wish to get back to their sport as soon as possible because they enjoy it so much! Regardless of the reason, it places an extra psychological load onto the injured sportsperson. This is not to say that the non-sporty person with a medial collateral ligament strain that came on after slipping on wet leaves whilst getting out of a taxi does not want to get better too. It means that to a keen sportsperson, an aspect of their lifestyle that is held very important to them has been altered. So does this make a difference to treatment? Well, yes, in some ways it does, and luckily in most cases it is a positive difference. For example, on the whole, if we recommend a particular exercise to aid a patient's recovery, some patients will do it a few times for a few days and then forget it. If we tell a keen sportsperson to do an exercise ten times a day, most will do it ten times a day until they are told to stop. It may just be that they are accustomed to a routine from their sport but nevertheless they are keen to be a part of their own treatment and return to their chosen sport as soon as possible.

TYPES OF INJURY

Most sports injuries fall into one of the following three categories:

- Traumatic injuries, involving an external force exerted on the body that creates the damage.
- Degenerative injuries, which are caused by wear and tear, often of the weight-bearing joint surfaces, although any tissue might be affected.
- Overuse, which is the most common cause of injuries and is generally caused by overloading the body and by repeated microtrauma.

Injuries are most frequent after a long injury-free period when caution may be cast aside. Overuse and degeneration, though not limited to endurance sports, are seen more often as a result of them. Trauma is a misfortune that can happen to anyone.

Most sports people are aware that the first aid treatment for most sports injuries is 'RICE':

- R – rest the affected part
- I – ice to reduce inflammation
- C – compression of the affected region in order to reduce tissue swelling and to stabilize the region
- E – elevation of the part in order to promote drainage and help reduce swelling.

For most injuries, especially of an acute nature, the sooner this regimen is begun the better. Injuries that are ignored or left untreated may develop into chronic problems and thus become far more difficult to resolve completely.

INFLAMMATION

The Roman writer on medicine, Aulus Aurelius Cornelius Celsus,[2] was the first to formulate the physical characteristics of inflammation in the 1st century AD. He gave four distinct characteristics: rubor, calor, tumor and dolor.

- Redness (rubor). When a tissue is acutely inflamed it has a red appearance which is due to vasodilatation of the injured tissues.

- Heat (calor). Accompanying the redness is an increase in temperature, which locally is again due to the vasodilation. There may be a systemic rise of temperature due to fever but in the case of most sports injuries this is not a significant factor.
- Swelling (tumor). Initially this is due to the accumulation of fluid at the site of injury or oedema. It may become augmented by the infiltration of inflammatory cells and later by production of new connective tissue as healing begins.
- Pain (dolor). The site becomes painful due to the engorgement of the tissues increasing pressure and in addition, by some of the biochemical products of inflammation.

Rudolf Ludwig Karl Virchow,[2] a Berlin pathologist, added 'loss of function' (functio laesa) to the picture. This may be due to inhibition of movement by pain or by physical restriction as a result of the swelling.

During acute inflammation a number of physiological processes take place.[3] Firstly, alterations in blood vessel diameter cause vasodilatation and thus changes in blood flow. This is followed by changes in the permeability of the blood vessels resulting in outflow of fluid into the extravascular spaces creating oedema. Finally, there is migration of the phagocytic neutrophils into the extravascular space where they ingest bacteria, dead cells and cellular debris. This response is further strengthened by the chemotactic mediated influx of more neutrophils. Other cells including lymphocytes and macrophages are also involved in the response. All of these processes seem to be initiated by the stimulation of mast cell degranulation, which itself may be initiated by physical, chemical or immunological means. The ideal end result of these processes is that the irritant stimulus is taken care of and tissue repair or resolution can take place. That is fine for most cases but in the case of physical injury as in many sports injuries, this irritant may well still be present and so a state of chronic inflammation ensues.

CHRONIC INFLAMMATION[3]

The term 'chronic' has changed somewhat in its medical usage with time and is usually applied, somewhat vaguely, to a process that has 'lasted a long time'. The period of time is somewhat indeterminate but in the case of inflammation, it is termed chronic when the cellular processes that take place are different to that seen in the acute stage. In chronic inflammation there is a more active lymphocyte, macrophage and plasma cell action. In both the acute and chronic phases there is the formation of scar tissue but it is proliferate in chronic inflammation. In most cases, chronic inflammation is preceded by an acute stage but in certain instances there may be no acute stage; the term primary chronic inflammation is then applied. However, in the case of sports injuries this is not the normal scenario and so it will not be discussed in detail here.

FIBROSIS[3]

Fibrosis takes place at the site of tissue injury and involves two stages: firstly, proliferation of fibroblasts and secondly, the laying down of extracellular matrix by the fibroblasts. The major part of connective tissue formed at the injury and thence repair site is in the form of fibrillar collagens. After the deposition of the extracellular matrix there is a stage of remodelling in which there is maturation and organization of the fibrous tissue.

COMPLICATIONS

Abnormalities of any of the aforementioned repair processes may result in complications of wound healing and repair. The major complications are:

- Inadequate scar formation
- Excessive scar formation
- Contracture formation.

These processes of tissue injury and healing and their possible complications may occur in a number of musculoskeletal problems as a result of a sports injury. Sprains and strains are amongst the most common injuries in sports and may be associated with inflammatory changes in specific structures such as the common extensor origin of the forearm resulting in lateral epicondylitis (tennis elbow) or Achilles tendinitis. It is generally accepted that a sprain is a stretching or tearing that takes place in a ligament whilst the same injury in a muscle or tendon is named a strain.[4]

Muscle and ligament injuries vary from mild strains where there is disruption and tearing of some of the fibres, through avulsion of the structure from the bone to complete rupture. Bursae are synovial lined sacs that serve as protective cushioning or have a lubricating function. They may become inflamed as a result of overuse or friction resulting in a painful bursitis. It is commonly seen at sites where a tendon passes over a bony prominence such as at the hip, elbow or knee. They may become infected resulting in a septic bursitis. Prompt effective treatment of these conditions may prevent any complications and further recurrence of the injury. A recurrent injury is likely to lead to chronic tissue changes and, in the case of muscle injuries, myositis ossificans. This is a condition in which the repetitive tearing of the muscle tissue has created scar tissue that begins to calcify and later ossifiy.

It must be stressed that these injuries need not arise as a result of a sporting injury. Many patients present with 'tennis elbow' but have never played tennis in their lives. It is not the remit of this text to describe all the possible sports injuries but rather to consider how an osteopath may be of use when they do occur specifically to the sportsperson.

OSTEOPATHIC CONSIDERATIONS

One of the first considerations the osteopath has to make is to decide if the injury is treatable by osteopathic means alone. In the example of a fracture it is obvious that referral should be made to the appropriate department. Having stated that, some sports-induced injuries come about as a result of overuse, resulting in a 'stress fracture' that may not require a plaster cast and immobilization – in these cases the osteopath may be of great value to the patient. The osteopathic approach to the biomechanical aspects of optimizing the structure/function relationship may be invaluable in the rehabilitation and recovery of the injured sportsperson. But it does not require a fracture in order for osteopathic treatment to be of value. For example, tendinitis is commonly seen in sports and as with lesser sprains and strains the treatment approach to acute and chronic problems will naturally differ.

In the acute stage the aim of treatment will be to assist the healing process and so the emphasis will be on good tissue perfusion and drainage with minimal derangement. In short, there is an avoidance of excessive movement; however, it has been seen that a certain amount of movement actually aids recovery. On the other hand, in chronic problems that have passed through the acute stage, there will be tissue changes that will require time and possibly much treatment to resolve. Furthermore, in the chronic condition it is quite likely that there are compensatory patterns set up that may well have become chronic themselves. And so the planning of treatment becomes ever more important since changes to the compensations will need to be made hand-in-hand with those of the presenting complaint. This will require a good understanding of the particular case in order to make the changes stabilize, whereas in the acute condition this problem may not arise as treating the immediate problem may allow any recently set up compensations to resolve on their own.

In certain cases, the osteopathic treatment will necessitate an inflammatory response. In other words, we want to create the normal inflammatory response in order to make the local physiological changes necessary to promote a healing response within the tissues and thus give a second chance at resolution. This may then create a 'paradoxical' situation in which the osteopath is provoking an inflammatory response but the patient is still taking anti-inflammatory medication. In this case it is necessary to educate the patient that this is a normal response and to only take the medication should the reaction be too great. A well planned and calculated treatment tailored for the individual will not create too great a reaction. It may involve a treatment that is aimed at restoring biomechanical balance throughout the whole body but with specific soft tissue techniques such as neuromuscular or balanced membranous techniques to create the local changes. As ever, this will be dictated by the individual's problem and general state of health. On the whole the average sporty person will have good physiological status that aids quick response and recovery.

As for choice of techniques, the situation will depend on individual patients and their individual injuries. In the acute stages, the tendency will be to use the more indirect techniques such as balanced ligamentous tension and functional approaches to the specific structure injured. Conversely, in order to make an effective change in chronic cases, the choice may be to use more direct techniques such as high velocity low amplitude, articulation or neuromuscular technique. This is only a guideline and not a rule.

It was mentioned earlier that the osteopath may be of use in the recovery and rehabilitation of the injured sportsperson and this is where the idea of being a specialist gains some credence. All sports people have a common interest when they become injured: they want to return to their sport quickly and not to lose all the efforts they have made in training prior to the onset of the injury. Under these circumstances the 'sports osteopath' has to have a fairly if not highly detailed knowledge of the particular sport and what the training for it entails. The osteopath needs to know how to advise a patient when to return to their sport, at what level they should return and what they can do in the meantime. Many sports people when injured will be able to perform some other sporting activity that will help to maintain their level of fitness but not hinder the recovery of the injured part. For example, a rock climber who has an injured wrist resulting in a tendinitis may be able to maintain cardiovascular efficiency by running or swimming, and strength by specific weight training that avoids using the injured tendons. Likewise, a footballer with an injured knee may use a rowing machine to keep up cardiovascular system capabilities and do certain exercises in water to maintain strength in the legs. In many cases, common sense will be enough to ensure the right advice is given but in certain cases it will require in-depth knowledge beyond the experience of the average osteopath.

Allen[5] writes: 'athletes are people in motion' and cites Sheehan,[6] the late cardiologist and marathon runner, as stating 'everyone is an athlete – only some of us are in training and some not'. This topic of discussion opened with exactly that thought in mind: you do not have to be a sports person to sustain a knee injury. But if you are, and it affects your ability to participate in your chosen sport, then it requires an adapted type of treatment approach to deal with it.

References

1. Health Education Council of Great Britain. Look after yourself. London: HMSO; 1978.
2. Weissman G. Inflammation: historical perspectives. In: Gallin JI, Haynes BF, Snyderman R eds. Inflammation: basic principles and clinical correlates, 3rd edn. Philadelphia: Lippincott Williams and Wilkins; 1999: 5–13.
3. Cotran RS, Kumar V, Collins T. Robbins pathologic basis of disease, 6th edn. Philadelphia: WB Saunders; 1999: 51–87.
4. Underwood JCE, ed. General and systematic pathology, 3rd edn. Edinburgh: Churchill Livingstone; 2000: 201–222.
5. Allen TW. Sports medicine. In: Ward RC, ed. Foundations for osteopathic medicine. Baltimore: Williams and Wilkins; 1997: 285–287.
6. Sheehan G. Sports medicine renaissance. Physician Sportsmed 1990; 18(11):26.

Chapter 30

Blood pressure

INTRODUCTION

The term blood pressure means 'the force exerted by the blood against any unit area of the vessel wall'.[1] Conventionally it is measured in millimetres of mercury and expressed as two figures, the first representing the systolic reading and the second, the diastolic reading. If there is such a thing as a normal blood pressure, then the accepted value for a resting, healthy adult is 120/80 mmHg. However, there may be significant deviation and the values may increase or decrease with various circumstances, for example age, physical exertion, psychoemotional stress and certain pathological disease states.

The above description of blood pressure and normal values are of the arterial blood pressure. Since the cardiovascular system is a closed system, theoretically it is possible to measure the pressure at any point throughout the whole system. Naturally enough, since the heart is the driving force and also since the aorta and its major branches are the first of the vessels in the system, it is here that we find the highest pressure. As the blood passes around the systemic circulatory system the blood pressure drops and the pulsatile effect diminishes. By the time the blood leaves the arterioles and enters the capillary beds, the pressure has dropped to about 30 mmHg and there is almost no perceivable pulsation. Throughout the capillary beds the pressure drops further and on reaching the venules it has reduced to about 10 mmHg; by the time it reaches the vena cavae and returns to the heart again it is at about 0 mmHg.[1]

Another consideration to be made is that of the hydrostatic pressure placed upon the blood in the venous system. In the normal adult, the blood pressure of the veins varies from about 10 mmHg to zero. In the normal adult standing absolutely still, the pressure varies from the head to the feet as a result of the hydrostatic effect. Pressure in the venous sinuses of the head will be about −10 mmHg and in the feet about 90 mmHg, an appreciable variation due simply to the weight of the fluid in the system.[1] This would tend to create a pooling of the blood in the lower extremities and so to minimize this effect the veins are equipped with a one-way valve system, directing the blood back to the heart. Muscular contraction, on walking or moving, puts pressure on the veins and literally squeezes the blood back to the heart. Failure of this system for too long a period of time may result in varicose veins. Furthermore, in the case of standing still, fluid leaks from the circulatory system into the surrounding tissues and creates oedema and thus swollen ankles or legs. It is the relative immobility leading to a reduction of the muscular pumping action that is the culprit, and so the same phenomenon may occur during long periods of sitting, as is commonly seen in travelling. Air travel makes the problem even worse due to reduced cabin air pressure.

The pulmonary system is a law unto itself; it requires a certain amount of blood pressure to drive the blood through the lungs for gaseous exchange to take place but not too great a pressure to create leakage or extravasation of the fluids into the interstitial spaces or the alveoli resulting in pulmonary oedema. Normal resting pulmonary blood pressure varies from about 22 mmHg at systole to about 8 mmHg at diastole.[1] Once again in the standing adult at rest there is a variation due to the hydrostatic pressure of about 3 mmHg in the apex of the lungs and 21 mmHg at the bases, indicating a variation in the blood flow throughout different regions of the lungs.[1]

CONTROL OF BLOOD PRESSURE

The term 'mean arterial pressure' refers to the average pressure throughout each cycle of the heart and is 'approximately' equal to the average of the systolic and diastolic blood pressures. In fact, it is usually a little below this average due to the longer phase of diastole. Mean arterial pressure is dependent on the product of the cardiac output and the peripheral resistance.

Arterial pressure = cardiac output × total peripheral resistance

The regulation of the mean arterial blood pressure is carried out by two different but related mechanisms, one for short-term regulation and the other for long-term regulation. It should also be remembered that there is a system of local blood flow regulation carried out at a tissue level by merely dilating or constricting the arterioles as required by the organ concerned. Short-term regulation is controlled by the nervous and hormonal systems whilst longer term regulation is by regulating the blood volume and involves the kidney.

The fast acting mechanisms for control of blood pressure are mediated by the baroreceptor reflex (Fig. 30.1). Baroreceptors are stretch receptors located in the walls of major arteries but notably in the carotid sinus at the bifurcation of the common carotid arteries and in the arch of the aorta. Increased pressure creates increased stretch which is then transmitted as nervous impulses via Hering's nerve to the glossopharyngeal nerve (from the carotid sinus) and vagus nerve (from the aortic arch) and thence to the nucleus of the tractus solitarius. From there, fibres pass to the reticular formation of the brain stem in a region known as the cardiovascular centre. The efferents from this centre then pass to the nucleus ambiguus and then by the vagus nerve to reduce the chronotropic and inotropic function of the heart, i.e. to reduce the rate and strength of contraction and thus cardiac output. Other fibres pass to the vasoconstrictor centre in order to inhibit the action of the sympathetics via the intermediolateral cell column of the spinal cord. The net effect is a reduction of mean arterial pressure. Naturally enough, should there be a drop in the blood pressure being monitored in this way, the opposite sequence of events will occur.

These mechanisms are sufficient for the rapidly adapting needs of the body in response to short-term changes in pressure such as that seen in going from lying to standing, onset of exercise and loss of blood. The higher centres can have an influence on this system, for example, the response of increased blood pressure during the fight/flight response. However, this mechanism is not only rapidly acting but also fairly rapidly adapting, and so the baroreceptors become less sensitive and adapt to a sustained higher or lower blood pressure within a few days.

Aside from the above described neural mechanism for rapid control of blood pressure is the

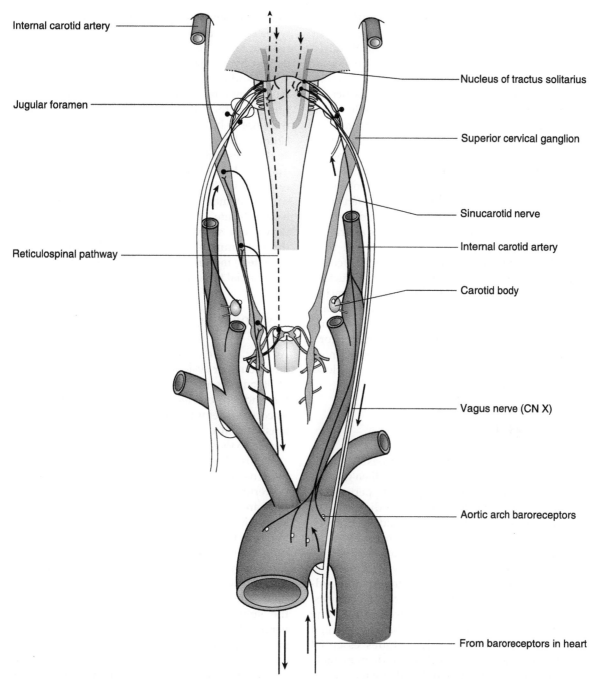

Internal carotid artery

Jugular foramen

Reticulospinal pathway

Nucleus of tractus solitarius

Superior cervical ganglion

Sinucarotid nerve

Internal carotid artery

Carotid body

Vagus nerve (CN X)

Aortic arch baroreceptors

From baroreceptors in heart

Figure 30.1 The baroreceptor reflex nervous pathways. (Reproduced from Wilson-Pauwels L, Stewart PA, Akesson EJ. Autonomic nerves. Hamilton: BC Decker; 1997:205.)

relatively slower acting hormonal mechanism, principally the adrenaline-noradrenaline system and the renin-angiotensin system. Though the hormones take a little longer to effect a change they back up the neural mechanism.

Adrenaline and noradrenaline are two of the neurotransmitters utilized by the sympathetic nervous system which quite simply when activated stimulate a rise in blood pressure due to their vasoconstrictive action. Regulation of these hormones in the blood gives a certain amount of control over blood pressure. However, the renin-angiotensin system utilizes angiotensin II which until fairly recently was considered the most powerful vasoconstrictor known in the body. Nowadays it is considered 'one' of the most powerful vasoconstrictors. Nevertheless its mechanism is a very potent one involving (as is the case in most hormonal mechanisms) a cascade reaction. In a very simplified version of the whole response, a reduction of blood pressure results in the release of renin from the kidney; this then activates the release of angiotensin I which is converted in the lungs to angiotensin II. Angiotensin has a short half-life but a rapid effect, notably causing a vasoconstriction of the arterioles, which increases peripheral resistance and thus raises the blood pressure. Furthermore, it effects a response in the kidneys; firstly it causes a reduction in the excretion of salt and water, thus increasing blood volume, and secondly it promotes the release of aldosterone that further reinforces this same effect. These latter effects are important in the short- to mid-term regulation of blood pressure but, more importantly, it is this system that controls the blood pressure in the longer term.

HYPERTENSION

Butterworths Medical Dictionary[2] describes hypertension as 'high arterial blood pressure': it then goes on to describe sixteen different types of hypertension! Aetiologically, hypertension can be divided into two major groups: primary and secondary. Primary hypertension is sometimes known as essential hypertension and is defined as that which arises from no known cause. Secondary hypertension may be due to numerous causes ranging from kidney disorders to tumours to iatrogenic causes. Hypertension is also classified according to the pathological changes it creates in the body. Benign hypertension, which usually includes essential hypertension, may create little or no demonstrable system or organ damage. On the other hand, malignant hypertension results in serious damage and an increased risk of death from numerous causes.

HYPOTENSION

Butterworths Medical Dictionary[2] describes hypotension as 'a fall in blood pressure below the normal range'; it then goes on to describe four different types of hypotension. It is evident that the greater risks to health come from hypertension but nevertheless, hypotension is potentially deleterious to the health and as such deserves a mention. By far the most commonly seen form of hypotension is postural or orthostatic. This is due to an inefficient response to blood pressure changes on going from sitting or lying to the standing position. It manifests as dizziness, blurred vision or even syncope. It is due to a lack of the normal autonomic responses required in the short-term changes as mentioned earlier. It may be transient or persistent and is named 'acute' or 'chronic' accordingly. Its causes vary from starvation and physical exhaustion, through immobility, to specific diseases such as diabetes mellitus, adrenal insufficiency and intracranial tumours.

OSTEOPATHIC CONSIDERATIONS

As may be seen from the above discussion, there are two major systems of importance in the control of blood pressure, the nervous control and that of the endocrine effect on the kidneys. Thus any osteopath attempting to treat a patient with hypertension will need to check for any dysfunctions related to these two systems.

Firstly, the kidneys are to be found in a 'nest' of perirenal adipose tissue on the internal aspect of the posterior abdominal wall. Their anatomical relations are numerous and varied[3] (Fig. 30.2). The right kidney is related anteriorly to the suprarenal gland, the liver, the second part of the duodenum and the right colic flexure. Posteriorly it is related to the diaphragm, the costodiaphragmatic recess of the pleura and the twelfth rib, the psoas, quadratus lumborum and transversus abdominis muscles and the subcostal, iliohypogastric and ilioinguinal nerves. The left kidney is related anteriorly to the suprarenal gland, spleen, stomach, pancreas, left colic flexure and jejunum. Posteriorly its relations are to the same but contralateral structures as the right kidney with the addition of the eleventh rib – this is due to the left kidney lying slightly higher in position. Evidently, with all these anatomical relations, there is always the possibility of dysfunction that may compromise normal function of the kidneys. The anatomical arrangement is that of visceral structures anterior to the kidneys and with that goes all the 'sliding surfaces' necessary for normal

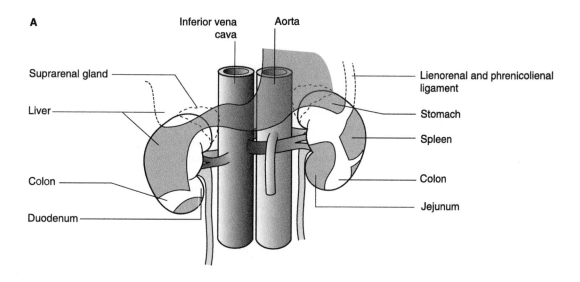

A

Inferior vena cava

Aorta

Suprarenal gland ——

Liver ——

Colon ——

Duodenum ——

—— Lienorenal and phrenicolienal ligament

—— Stomach

—— Spleen

—— Colon

—— Jejunum

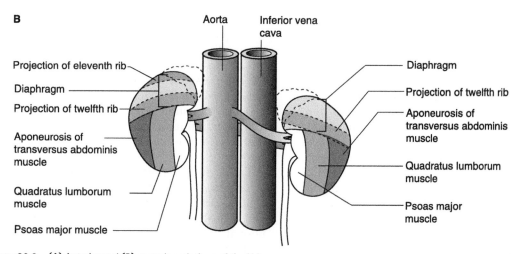

B

Aorta

Inferior vena cava

Projection of eleventh rib —

Diaphragm ——

Projection of twelfth rib —

Aponeurosis of transversus abdominis muscle

Quadratus lumborum muscle ——

Psoas major muscle ——

—— Diaphragm

—— Projection of twelfth rib

—— Aponeurosis of transversus abdominis muscle

—— Quadratus lumborum muscle

—— Psoas major muscle

Figure 30.2   (A) Anterior and (B) posterior relations of the kidneys.

mobility. However with all the musculoskeletal elements posteriorly, and the effect of the diaphragm, there are many non-visceral aspects to be considered. So no matter which 'direction' the osteopath is coming from, there is the possibility to treat dysfunction. It should also not be forgotten that the kidneys receive their sympathetic supply from the T10–L2 spinal cord levels thus making the dorsolumbar junction a very important area in the consideration of these types of problems.

Barral[4] writes that kidney mobility and motility are important considerations in hypertensive patients and thus should be checked for any dysfunction and

treated accordingly. Kidney 'ptosis' may occur, in which the kidney descends or slips down within its fascial sheath that is lying on the psoas major muscle. Athletes and serious runners are especially susceptible to this type of problem due to the repetitive jarring from training coupled with the fact that a serious runner probably has a minimal amount of fat acting as a support for the kidneys. Barral[4] cites the case of an extremely hypertensive young lady who was diagnosed as having idiopathic hypertension. She was treated osteopathically for a left renal ptosis and her blood pressure reduced quite rapidly. It is his thought that osteopathic treatment does not restore the ptosed kidney to its correct position, rather the treatment is successful due to 'stimulation, dynamization and revitalization of the organism'. In other words, the kidney is given the space in which to restore its normal homeostatic functions.

William Baldwin Jnr[5] writes in the classic text *Osteopathic Medicine* edited by Hoag, Cole and Bradford, that 'renal function must be involved in the hypertensive process, sooner or later' and that 'the longer optimum renal function can be maintained, the better the patient's chances for avoiding the extreme complications'. He goes on to say that 'one of the best hypotensive agents is sedation' and that 'generalised manipulative therapy has just such an effect'. This underlines the oft-neglected principle that there should be a treatment of the person and not merely the pathological condition.

Since stress is often implicated in hypertension, a general treatment that may result in the reduction of circulating stress hormones to normal levels may be considered as a means of approaching hypertension either directly or indirectly. Pain is associated with higher levels of catecholamines and thus higher blood pressure. The osteopathic means of pain reduction is likely to result in a reduction of blood pressure. The relationship between pain, range of joint motion and stress is quite significantly correlated and it is the osteopathic approach which may have the beneficial effect.[6]

The baroreceptor reflex has been the subject for some osteopathic studies with respect to blood pressure but as mentioned, this reflex is more important in the short term and although important will be less so in the longer term control. However, this reflex is coordinated via the circulatory centres of the brain stem which are lying just deep to the floor of the fourth ventricle. It is with this in mind that many osteopaths direct part of their treatment to this region. Magoun[7] states that 'persistent use of compression of the fourth ventricle to influence the centers for blood pressure in its floor, as well as vault lift for better venous drainage, is often of help in altering tissue chemistry and stagnation sufficiently to maintain the pressure at a safe level'.

Unfortunately, as is often the case in osteopathy, there are numerous anecdotal accounts of a reduction in blood pressure in patients treated osteopathically but few controlled trials. However, a recent study[8] concluded that long-term manipulation to the T2–3 and T11–12 may provide decreases in both systolic and diastolic blood pressures in hypertensive patients. Unfortunately the subject population was very small and, as is often stated, further investigations with larger populations are required and in the case of this particular research, a longer-term study and follow-up.

In the 1955 *Yearbook of the Applied Academy of Osteopathy*, Northup[9] describes his method for management of hypertension and although he recognizes the necessity to work on any vertebral restrictions, notably those related to kidney or liver, he also describes 'cranial technique'. It involves releasing all the tissues around the suboccipital region and the cervical fascia, followed by easing restrictions of the temporal bones and especially the occipitomastoid sutures. He states the importance of the meninges and their attachments within the cranial vault. A major part of his treatment approach is aimed at relaxation of the tissues and of the person as a whole, two important factors known to aid in the reduction of mean arterial pressure. Northup cites a modification of his technique used by Dr Paul C Snyder that 'has had outstanding results' and which involves a type of mild but sustained traction to the cervical fascia (Northup used a rocking motion in this region). Snyder felt that the success of the technique was due to a stretching of the carotid sheath and inhibitory influence on the carotid sinus, a claim that is quite feasible when considering short-term changes.

Earlier still, McCole[10] wrote in the 1951 *Yearbook of the Applied Academy of Osteopathy* that the suboccipital triangle is important, as are the first, second and fifth thoracic segments, in order to maintain normal autonomic balance. He also makes mention of the importance of the kidney and of psychosocial aspects of the patient's lifestyle including: alcohol, tobacco and coffee consumption.

It would seem that osteopathy does have something to offer towards the treatment and management of hypertensive patients. The anatomical regions highlighted earlier are undoubtedly of importance and the osteopathic holistic approach will further reinforce this effect. The management of a person with hypertension will necessitate examination of diet and lifestyle in addition to the physical side of treatment. Osteopathic treatment and management of the hypertensive patient should not be considered as an alternative to medication but as an adjunct to it which may result in shorter-term medication or possibly a reduced dosage.

References

1. Guyton AC, Hall JE. Textbook of medical physiology, 10th edn. Philadelphia: WB Saunders; 2000.
2. Butterworths Medical Dictionary, 2nd edn. London: Butterworths; 1989.
3. Williams PL, Warwick R. Gray's anatomy, 36th edn. Edinburgh: Churchill Livingstone; 1980.
4. Barral JP. Visceral manipulation II. Seattle: Eastland Press; 1989.
5. Baldwin W. Hypertension. In: Hoag JM, Cole WV, Bradford SG, eds. Osteopathic medicine. New York: McGraw-Hill; 1969:519–528.
6. Marcer N. Osteopathy in the treatment of stress. Abstract. J Ost Med 2003; 6(1):34–42.
7. Magoun HI. Osteopathy in the cranial field. Boise: Northwest Printing; 1976.
8. Morden J, Gosling CM, Cameron M. The effect of thoracic manipulation on blood pressure in pharmacologically stable patients with hypertension: a pilot investigation. Abstract. J Ost Med 2003; 6(1).
9. Northup TL. Manipulative therapy in the osteopathic management of hypertension. Applied Academy of Osteopathy Yearbook; 1957.
10. McCole G. Clinical aspects of blood pressure determination. Applied Academy of Osteopathy Yearbook; 1951.

Chapter 31

Whiplash

INTRODUCTION

Whiplash has been under a lot of scrutiny for some time within the medical and medico-legal worlds. The main reason for this is that by far the most common reason for a whiplash injury is as a result of a 'road traffic accident'. With this often goes a claim for compensation which, according to some, may lead to exaggeration of the severity of symptoms on the part of the patient. In 1990 the Society of Automobile Insurers of Quebec formed a committee of physicians, researchers and epidemiologists to carry out a literature review and to make recommendations as to the prevention and treatment of whiplash. The Quebec Task Force,[1] as it became known, is probably the world's foremost authority on whiplash and whiplash-related disorders. It is behind the International Congress for Whiplash that is held every 2 years at different sites throughout the world and has contributed, in collaboration with numerous world-renowned experts, many advances in our understanding of this controversial problem.

In 1995, the Quebec Task Force proposed a definition of whiplash:

> Whiplash is an acceleration-deceleration mechanism of energy transfer to the neck. It may result from rear end or side-impact motor vehicle collisions, but can also occur during diving or other mishaps. The impact may result in bony or soft tissue injuries (whiplash injuries), which in turn may lead to a variety of clinical manifestations (whiplash-associated disorders).[1]

The word whiplash is quite descriptive of the events that take place in this type of injury. It gives the image of the relatively mobile neck and head being rapidly flicked back and forth on the relatively inert lower body. This 'lash of the whip' may create a wide variety of problems both in the short and long term.

By far the most common reason for a whiplash injury is as a result of a 'road traffic accident' (RTA). The most common type of accident to produce this type of injury occurs when a stationary vehicle is hit from behind.[2,3] The occupant of the stationary vehicle will receive an 'acceleration type' whiplash but the occupant of the vehicle running into the stationary vehicle will suffer a 'deceleration type' whiplash. These two types of whiplash may present different problems with respect to the injured tissues. However, a whiplash injury may also result from a head-on collision, or a collision from the side. To further complicate the matter, avoiding action may result in an offset glancing blow to the car which may again create a different symptomatology.

It is the inability of the body, and in particular the cervical muscles, to withstand this rapid increase or decrease of velocity which causes injury. It may cause injury in numerous different tissues, see Table 31.1.

Table 31.1 The types of tissues and possible injuries that may occur as a result of whiplash type injury

Type of tissue	Possible injuries
Muscle	Anterior cervical musculature
	Scalenes
	Posterior cervical musculature
Ligament	Anterior longitudinal ligament
	Posterior longitudinal ligament
	Intervertebral ligaments
	Zygapophysial ligaments
Articular	Zygapophysial joint sprain or fracture
	Intervertebral disc herniation
Nerve	Cervical nerve root
	Sympathetic chain
	Brachial plexus
Other	Oesophageal, tracheal or laryngeal damage
	Retropharyngeal haematoma
	Vertebral artery ischaemia
	Temporomandibular joint dysfunction
	Thoracic outlet syndrome
	Concussion
	Traumatic brain injury

Naturally, the healing time will vary greatly depending on which tissues are affected. Animal studies[1] have shown that in the case of musculoligamentous healing there is an initial acute inflamed stage which may last up to 72 hours, followed by a period of repair and regeneration which can last from 3 days to 6 months, and then a period of rematuration and remodelling which may last up to a year. It is this long-term healing process that creates the problem of scepticism in the medico-legal situation of litigation. It is assumed by some that patients are merely malingering in order to boost their claims for compensation.

The common picture of whiplash is that of cervical pain and immobility. It is usually associated with headache and thoracic pain, and further symptoms may include dizziness, tinnitus, blurred vision and numerous psychological sequelae such as anger, depression, irritability, lack of concentration, nervousness and anxiety.

Symptoms do not generally begin immediately after the accident, and this is another reason for scepticism; the patient may go home or back to work and then find over the course of some hours that the symptoms establish themselves.[4] On the whole, as the clinical picture develops over the course of a few days it also worsens. This delay, followed by an intensification of the symptoms, is probably due to the time required for oedema and haemorrhage to build up in the soft tissue structures affected. It is these soft tissue structure changes that will then create the reduced mobility and pain so characteristic of an acute whiplash syndrome. A patient taken to hospital after a car accident may show few symptoms and be found to be radiologically normal with respect to their age, etc. However, radiographic examination is often performed to rule out bony injuries such as fractures or subluxations.

The normal medical approach to the management of whiplash was to prescribe non-steroidal antiinflammatory drugs (NSAIDs) and a soft collar to be worn until the pain subsides; indeed, this is still the case in many emergency departments. The effectiveness of both of these forms of treatment is dubious with respect to the true goal of treatment which should be a return to normal. A return to normal does not mean pain reduction or abolition; it means a return to normal function. The use of a cervical collar for too long may result in disuse atrophy, with shortening and thickening of the cervical soft tissues.[5] Although NSAIDs most certainly do have a beneficial effect in the acute stage their use should not be allowed to develop into an abuse with all the potential risks and side-effects. They will probably be most useful in pain control and less so in their antiinflammatory action.[6] According to a recent study[7] on the initial assessment of whiplash patients, once major injury has been ruled out there are four key points to remember with respect to treatment:

1. Reassurance about the evolution of the problem
2. No soft collar
3. NSAIDs
4. Early mobilization.

Number four on the list indicates how views have changed. As was the case with low back pain, there is a trend towards early mobilization and away from the previously prescribed rest and immobilization.

If a stationary car is struck from behind by a moving car, a rear-end collision, the driver of the stationary car will undergo a complex movement pattern that can be divided into two simple, distinct phases. The first is of a forced extension to the spine and in particular the cervical and upper thoracic regions. This is then followed by a forced flexion, once again, predominantly in the cervical and thoracic regions. The structures at risk of injury may also be divided into two distinct groups. In the extension phase, the anterior structures are subjected to a rapid stretching, whilst the posterior structures are at risk of a compression type injury. This may result in tearing of the soft tissues anteriorly, notably tearing of the muscles and avulsion of the ligaments, whilst posteriorly, there is risk of facet joint damage due to compression which may even extend to possible fracture. In the extreme it is possible to fracture the spinous processes. The flexion phase creates the opposite potentially damaging forces; compression anteriorly and stretching of the posterior structures. Although rare, there is risk of disc herniation, anterior vertebral body compression and possible fracture. The risk is increased with higher impact velocity and predisposing factors such as increased age, osteoporosis and degenerative change. The stretching of the posterior structures in the flexion phase places soft tissues at risk for tearing and avulsion.

Until the fitting of head restraints was made compulsory, the limiting factor in the extension phase was the impaction of the bony structures posteriorly and the contraction of the anterior muscula-

ture. The limiting factor for the flexion phase was the contact made between the mandible on the sternum. With the advent of airbags, the range of flexion should be considerably reduced.

There is also risk of brain tissue injury. The inertia of the brain within the fluid environment of the cranial cavity causes it to move differently to its surrounding structure. In the extension phase, as the head moves backwards, naturally enough so will the brain, but the brain does so at a slower velocity resulting in the possibility of contact between the brain on the inside of the cranial cavity anteriorly. Obviously, the reverse will happen during the flexion phase with the brain making cranial contact posteriorly. However, research aimed at evaluating brain injury as a result of whiplash is varied in its conclusions. EEG studies vary wildly in the reported incidence of brain injury, ranging from 4% to 46%.[8,9,10] It has been suggested that neuropsychological assessments may be more reliable in their measurements, but in the studies that draw these conclusions, the subjects have usually been drawn from a selective population.[11] Until a properly controlled prospective study is performed the outcomes will remain clinically inconclusive.

OSTEOPATHIC CONSIDERATIONS

In the case of whiplash injury, it is doubly important that the case history examination is recorded in fine detail and accurately. Should there be the need to stand as an expert witness in a court of law, poorly taken notes are of no use to anyone. That does not mean to say that it is only for the benefit of the courts that detailed notes should be kept. The case history should reveal as much information as possible regarding the accident. Was the impact anticipated, or did it come completely out of the blue? Was the person looking into the rear view mirror? The rotation component of the trauma will vary from left hand to right hand drive vehicles under these circumstances, as would the restraint provided by a seat belt as it passes over the shoulder. Did the driver have a foot on the brake? Was the patient the driver or a passenger? Consideration should be given to the fact that the driver would be likely to have their hands on the steering wheel, whereas a passenger would not. This difference in the position of the pectoral girdle may give a drastically different lesion pattern. Nevertheless, all this information (and much more not even mentioned here) will have to be integrated and interpreted by the osteopath. Do the palpatory findings support the reported information? In the end it is the skill of the osteopath as a palpator that will finally guide them to the correct treatment approach.

Despite all the agreement amongst osteopaths that the treatment should be directed at the patient as a whole, there are still differences in the treatment approaches. Since its inception into the 'osteopathic armoury', specific adjusting technique (SAT) has long been favoured by its followers as the best approach to reverse the traumatic components of a whiplash injury. However, it has not been accepted by all. Barral[12] scotches the idea that a single manipulative thrust will suffice. He views whiplash as a 'superposition of articular, neuromuscular, fascial and fluid disorders which interconnect like series of Russian dolls one inside the next'. He feels that 'restoration of craniosacral harmony should be considered as the ultimate goal of treatment'.

The flaw in the medical management of whiplash (or any other condition for that matter) is the symptomatic viewpoint. Osteopaths look at the person as a whole. Teasell and Shapiro[6] sum it up perfectly in the text *Clinical Anatomy and Management of Cervical Spine Pain*, in the chapter on whiplash injuries. Under the heading of 'future directions' they state:

> … patient-focused care, the so-called art of medicine which focuses on the person and not simply the injury. Such an approach deals with the physical, psychological, social and spiritual aspects, and sees the person as greater than the sum of his or her parts.

If this is the recommendation for 'future directions', and if there are clinicians and practitioners open-minded enough to take heed of this advice, then maybe they should turn to any osteopathic text for guidance – this approach has been used in osteopathy since day one! It was always Still's vision for the future (and it is a recurring theme of this book) to look to the patient as a whole and recognize the problem as part of their overall make-up. With this in mind, whiplash loses its impact as a trauma resulting in a cervical problem, but becomes a whole body problem.

References

1. Quebec Task Force on Whiplash-Associated Disorders 1995. Spine 20:1S–72S.
2. Bogduk N. The anatomy and pathophysiology of whiplash; Clin Biomech 1986; 1:92–101.
3. LaRocca H. Acceleration injuries of the neck. Clin Neurosurg 1978; 25:205–217.
4. Deans GT, McGailliard JN, Kerr M et al. Neck pain is a major cause of disability following car accidents. Injury 1987; 18:10–12.
5. Lieberman JS. Cervical soft tissue injuries and cervical disc disease. In: Leek JC et al, eds. Principles of physical medicine and rehabilitation in the musculoskeletal diseases. New York: Grune and Stratton; 1986: 263–286.
6. Teasell RW, Shapiro AP. Whiplash injuries. In: Giles LGF, Singer KP, eds. Clinical anatomy and management of cervical spine pain. Oxford: Butterworth-Heinemann; 1998: 71–86.
7. Gunzberg R, Szpalski M, Goethem JV. Initial assessment of whiplash patients. Pain Res and Manag 2003; 8:124.
8. Gibbs FA. Objective evidence of brain disorder in cases of whiplash injury. Clin Electroencephalogr 1971; 2:107–110.
9. Jacome DE. EEG in whiplash: a reappraisal. Clin Electroencephogr 1987; 18:41–45.
10. Torres F, Shapiro SK. Electroencephalograms in whiplash injury. Arch Neurol 1961; 5:28–35.
11. Radanov BP, Dvorak J. Impaired cognitive functioning after whiplash injury of the cervical spine. Spine 1996; 21:393–397.
12. Barral JP, Croibier A. Trauma: an osteopathic approach. Seattle: Eastland Press; 1999.

Chapter 32

Geriatrics

CHAPTER CONTENTS

INTRODUCTION

In Chapter 28, we looked at a case of middle ear infection in the infant. Now we swing to the other end of the age scale and the study of the older generations. Gerontology is defined by *Butterworths Medical Dictionary*[1] as 'the branch of medical science which is concerned with the physiological and pathological phenomena of senescence', whilst geriatrics is defined as that branch 'concerned with the clinical study and treatment of old age and its manifestations'. By and large they are the same thing.

Humankind is the only species that makes such a great fuss about ageing and death. Furthermore, not all humans view the process with such fear and trepidation; it is only the 'westernized' world that views it this way. Some societies see death as a springboard to a new life, whilst others consider older people to be in the prime of life, a time to be a respected and worldly elder. The fact that people are living longer, and that the proportion of elderly people in the community is increasing, has created some discussion within the world of healthcare. If only people could age healthily, they would cost less to keep! It is only fairly recently that much time and expense has been poured into studies to find out what goes wrong in the ageing body and how to slow the deterioration and postpone the 'final call of nature', death. A number of studies have begun that look into the subject of 'successful ageing'. One major ongoing study performed in the USA, the MacArthur Successful Aging Study,[2] has highlighted the impact of stress on ageing. It seems that the more stress we are exposed to, the more there is wear and tear on our body systems that leads to the pathological changes associated with mortality.

There are a number of theories as to what actually happens in the body as we age. Some feel that it is a gradual breakdown of our immune system whilst others go for the theory that free radicals create cellular damage.[3,4] The discussions and proposition of new theories continues. According to Warner,[5] from 1923 to 1977 13 different theories of ageing have been proposed, none of which seem to satisfactorily explain the whole story. These theories may be grouped into three major areas: genetic and environmental mechanisms, alterations of cellular control mechanisms and degenerative extracellular changes.[6] Selye[7] says that people never die of old age but of ageing of a vital part or organ. He feels that if it were possible to die of old age, then all the parts or organs would have aged proportionately. Another concept to consider is the differences between chronological and physiological age. We all know of someone who had a grandparent who lived to 94 years old and died only as a result of being knocked off his bicycle. Who knows, if he had been slightly more alert and a little freer in his neck, he might have seen the car coming and lived to be 100! Nevertheless, there may be a wide range of differences between chronological and physiological ages. Why do some people age more quickly than others? Why do some physiologically young but chronologically old people suddenly and rapidly deteriorate? Is it a possibility that they just 'throw in the towel'?

As the body ages, many different processes and homeostatic mechanisms begin to alter their rate and efficiency of functioning; the digestive, cardiovascular, respiratory, genitourinary and nervous systems to name a few. We live in fear of poor bowel function, heart attacks, breathlessness, incontinence, dementia and so on, the list is endless. Many different systems of assessing ageing have been used; decreased immune function, increased blood pressure, decreased respiratory parameters, slowed reaction times and impaired visual acuity have all been used as biological markers for ageing.[6] One of the frequently overlooked, although often accepted parts of growing old is our musculoskeletal deficiencies. The wear and tear and its associated degenerative changes in our bones, joints and muscles is often seen as a normal part of old age and wanes in its importance when seen alongside more life-threatening changes such as atherosclerosis or coronary artery disease. However, the musculoskeletal system is the main consumer of energy within the body and, when compromised and inefficient, will tax the body's resources further.

The musculoskeletal system, comprised of bones, joints and muscles and their associated connective tissues, undergoes changes with ageing. The bones become weaker, stiffer and brittle whilst the muscles reduce in strength and bulk, although their ability to be trained may remain to quite advanced ages. The joints undergo a reduction in their range of motion that is attributable to the reduced flexibility of their associated ligaments, capsules and muscles. The cartilage becomes stiffer and more fragile. All of these changes are deemed to be 'normal' with age because ageing is not a disease. Having said this, it is difficult to define when the transition from normal ageing to disease occurs; it is the change from physiology through pathophysiology and into pathology that escapes definite borders, it is a continuum. The problem with these 'normal changes' associated with ageing is that they predispose the musculoskeletal system to trauma-related microinjury which then leads to pathological change.

One of the major pathological changes that may take place, and which is of particular interest to the osteopath, is osteoporosis. In osteoporosis there is a reduction in the density or mass of bone. It may be general or regional and has certain risk factors associated with it. There appears to be a genetic disposition, and a positive family history of osteoporosis places a person at higher risk for developing it. It is more common in white populations than black, and most common in those with fair skin and smaller, thinner stature. Obesity and osteoarthritis appear to lower the risk of osteoporosis, but naturally they increase the risk of other diseases. The hormonal risk factors are the most notable, with men being at lower risk than women. Furthermore, in women, late menarche, early menopause and nulliparity increase the risk. Low dietary calcium and excess protein increase the risk, whilst a sedentary lifestyle, smoking, caffeine and alcohol consumption are all related to an increased risk. However, excessive exercise in women, to the point of inducing amenorrhoea, may increase the risk of osteoporosis, whilst excess alcohol consumption has been associated with both an increase and a decrease in bone density, and so the picture is not always so clear. Certain conditions in the body that disrupt the homeostatic balance of the endocrine system have also been considered risk factors. Lowered testosterone levels in men may create male osteoporosis. Altered calcitonin levels as in hyperparathyroidism, cortisol levels in Cushing's syndrome, growth hormone levels in acromegaly and thyroid hormone levels in hyperthyroidism all seem to increase the risk of osteoporosis. Certain drug-induced states of osteoporosis may occur, for example prolonged high doses of cortisol or excessive heparin therapy may result in an osteoporotic state that is usually reversible. Regional osteoporosis is usually attributable to known causes such as immobilization of a region after a fracture or limb disuse due to paralysis.

As the bone weakens the trabeculae become fewer and the compact bone more porous which results in lowered ability to resist the mechanical stress. Over time, bone deformity and pain may ensue with a risk for bone collapse and fracture. In the aged, the picture of the greatly kyphosed elderly lady is the classic image of advanced osteoporosis. The risk of vertebral collapse and the degenerative change result in the so-called 'dowager's hump'. Although there is the possibility of pathological fractures within the spine due to osteoporosis, it is more common to find fractures of the long bones, and especially fracture of the neck of the femur, giving the 'fractured hip'. This is usually brought about as a result of a fall and for many aged persons may be the beginning of the decline towards death. Death may ensue as a result of surgical complications or due to the decreased mobility further compromising the already 'at risk' body systems. Pneumonia and other respiratory or cardiovascular complications are the commonest reasons for the decline, although nowadays most patients benefit from a physiotherapy and occupational therapy programme aimed at reducing these risks.

It is not necessary to have a fracture in order to be at risk for respiratory or cardiovascular decline; chronic degenerative change in the joints is very common among the aged. The mere act of walking consumes a certain amount of energy in all persons, whether healthy or not. Fusion of a lower extremity joint such as the hip, knee or ankle increases the energy requirements quite dramatically. Fusion at the ankle requires 3% more energy to maintain the customary walking speed, whilst fusion at the knee increases energy consumption by 23% and at the hip by 32%.[8] The figures quoted are for joint fusion but it may be assumed that any reduction in the normal function of a joint will compromise the gait mechanism to some extent, resulting in increased energy requirements. It is often seen in elderly patients that more than one joint of the lower extremity may be affected to a greater or lesser

extent and it can only be assumed that this summation of reduction in efficiency will result in further energy requirements in order to function normally. A well-planned treatment will improve function and in doing so will reduce the patient's energy requirements. In an elderly patient with a compromised cardiovascular or respiratory system this improvement may represent a significant change to the quality of their lives.

The lumbar spine, as the weight-bearing section of the vertebral column, is subject to a number of age-related changes.[9] The intervertebral discs tend to 'dry out' with age and there is a change in the ratio of fibrin and elastin components; elastin decreases and fibrin increases in content. The distinction between the two parts of the disc, the annulus fibrosus and the nucleus pulposus, becomes blurred as their younger different structures become more homogenized. Thus the discs become stiffer and less able to change shape with respect to the everyday turning and twisting forces applied to them. The result is a reduction of mobility to the lumbar spine as a whole.

It was always thought that age-related loss of disc height was the norm, but in the light of more recent research[10] it now appears that discs do not reduce in height. Disc height is maintained, but it is the vertebral body that loses height. This, combined with a relative weakening of the bone with age, results in a concavity of the bony end plates of the vertebral body and an overall reduction in the height of the aged individual. It is the loss of the horizontal trabeculae of the vertebral body, especially in the central portion, that permits this intrusion of the disc into the substance of the body. It appears that loss of disc height is not a feature of ageing but of some other process that may or may not be concurrent with ageing.[10,11,12]

Other processes attributed to ageing include osteophyte formation around the zygapophyseal joints of the vertebrae. Osteophytes generally develop as a result of tension on the attachments of the capsular ligaments which results in osteoblastic activity and the laying down of new bone. This probably reflects an attempt to extend or increase the surface area of the joints, and the joints frequently become covered with an extension of the articular cartilage. However, experiments on cadavers[13,14] that involve sectioning of the posterior ligaments or removal of the zygapophyseal joints does not increase flexion to any significant extent. It appears to be the dehydration and fibrotic changes of the intervertebral discs associated with ageing that are responsible for the decreased mobility.

The changes that take place in the joints of the lumbar region have been described as 'spondylosis' if they occur within the disc and 'degenerative joint disease' if they occur at the zygapophyseal joints. Nikolai Bogduk,[15] one of the foremost researchers and authors on the study of the lumbar spine in health and disease argues that these are 'natural consequences of the stresses applied to the spine throughout life' and 'not some aggressive disease that seemingly attacks the body'. It may be purely semantics to label them age-related changes or degenerative changes but as stated earlier the changes at the zygapophyseal joints appear to be an attempt to adapt to the biomechanical disturbance and not a true pathological change. Bogduk goes on to discuss the fact that these so-called diseases are infrequently associated with symptoms and disease. From an osteopathic viewpoint, it may be considered that those patients exhibiting symptoms have merely failed in their compensatory mechanisms to fully adapt to these biomechanical alterations, whereas the asymptomatic patients have succeeded. This will be important for the osteopath to recognize when making a treatment plan for the patient. A patient showing no symptoms of low back dysfunction may well be hiding a degenerative or aged back that is well compensated and that may well be upset by injudicious treatment.

In the above discussion we have looked quite closely at the lumbar spine in particular, but it must be remembered that similar principles will apply to the rest of the musculoskeletal system. The cervical spine, although not subject to the same stresses of weight-bearing, will nevertheless be subject to stresses due to its greater mobility. It goes without saying that the integration of the pectoral and pelvic girdles with the vertebral column should also be considered. In the case discussion of low back pain, we have already seen the importance of the self-bracing mechanism and it may be assumed from its importance in normal gait that a compromise of function may not be attributable solely to one joint or region of the spine.

OSTEOPATHIC CONSIDERATIONS

An article on geriatric technique by Hadden Soden[16] in the 1941 *AAO Yearbook* states 'The ideal technic, giving the maximum results, is one whereby each articulation or the articulations are put through their normal physiological articular ranges of motion with the least possible effort or muscular action'. It is certain that any treatment of the elderly (or for that matter, even a young but compromised patient) should be minimally invasive and non-taxing for the patient. That does not just apply to the time spent during the treatment. For the treatment to be effective, there should be some changes that take place following the treatment and this will also require a certain amount of energy expenditure by the patient in order to 'pay' for those changes. Most of us who have experienced treatment may have felt a sense of tiredness and possible minor aches or pains as a result of the treatment as the body adapts to the input. Aged persons are at risk due to the likelihood of reduced vitality and the treatment needs to be gauged accordingly to prevent a serious reaction. Having stated that, when administered appropriately, osteopathy does have a lot to offer the geriatric patient.

From our earlier discussions it may be seen that good mobility and range of motion in joints is important for optimum efficiency. However, it is not sufficient to merely improve ranges of motion within joints. Efficiency of energy expenditure requires a coordinated balance between mobility and stability. A hypermobile joint will require greater energy expenditure in the form of muscular action in order to maintain stability. It is with this in mind that the planning of treatment is even more important in the elderly; it is very easy to decompensate the aged person. The adaptations made by the ageing body have much less room for error: a slight biomechanical change made by treatment may result in a reaction that prevents restoration afterwards. Imagine walking a tightrope with a long pole to help us balance. The aged body has a very short pole with less ability to react accordingly should an input be too great. Nevertheless, a well-planned treatment that addresses the biomechanical dysfunctions will improve efficiency by reducing excessive energy expenditure. Moreover, the 'normalization' of the musculoskeletal system may well improve proprioceptive feedback. A major fear and problem for the elderly is that of falling. With the heightened risk of osteoporosis, there will be a concurrent, heightened risk of fracture. A fracture of the wrist will be hindrance enough for any elderly person, especially if they live alone. Worse still would be a fractured hip or leg which will necessitate hospitalization. An improvement in proprioceptive feedback should reduce the risk of losing balance and falling, whilst better musculoskeletal function may make the reaction times quicker, thus avoiding potential falls. It must always be remembered that falls may result from some underlying pathology and the necessary tests should be carried out and further investigations made as required.

Let us take the example of a patient who has fallen and suffered a fractured hip, or even a patient who has undergone an operation for a hip replacement. The obvious first approach to treatment is to aid in the restoration of mobility of the patient. This does not mean taking over the role of the physiotherapist who will have an important and valuable role to play in the patient's recovery and rehabilitation. The role of the osteopath may be to support that of the physiotherapist. By using techniques to reduce muscle tensions and balance muscle functions to improve mobility and stability, the osteopath may help in restoring normal gait as efficiently as possible. A risk in the elderly and relatively immobile patient is that of respiratory complications such as pneumonia and so special attention should be paid to the thorax and rib articulations to optimize the breathing mechanism. Hand-in-hand with this is the possibility of fluid retention and so drainage techniques for the thorax and the lower extremities may well be indicated. Another complication of immobility is the reduction of gastrointestinal function leading to constipation which may be worsened by the use of codeine-based pain-reducing medication. The above considerations are part of the 'whole patient' approach to treatment and require a certain amount of patient cooperation. The patient should be encouraged to help themselves as much as possible with the osteopathic intervention as an adjunct to their recovery and not as the sole means of treatment.

Aside from the obvious improvements in biomechanical and musculoskeletal function there are numerous other possibilities for osteopathy to protect the quality of life of the aged patient. It should be noted that many of the problems encountered in the elderly can also be found in younger patients and so the techniques may well be the same with the proviso regarding the complications mentioned earlier. For example, postural hypotension is common, as is hypertension, and the important regions and approaches to treatment were discussed in the chapter on blood pressure.

Incontinence in the elderly is a common problem and with it goes the risk of bladder and urinary tract infections. Once again, pelvic function should be optimized and the judicious use of visceral techniques where indicated may well assist in these problems.

Techniques used on elderly patients tend to be gentler than those used on their younger counterparts, and there is often a complete avoidance of high velocity thrust techniques. Involuntary mechanism, functional, articulatory and myofascial techniques are used much more, and with good effects.

Osteopathy has much to offer the elderly patient but the complications and risks should never be overlooked. These encompass a wide variety of conditions, from osteoporosis to the possibility of thromboembolism, and so treatment should be aimed at restoration of function with the minimum of input. Changes in the elderly patient take time and will not be achieved sooner by stronger treatment – this will put the patient at risk of greater reaction, or worse still, a life-threatening complication.

References

1. Butterworths Medical Dictionary, 2nd edn. London: Butterworths; 1989.
2. MacArthur Successful Aging Study. MacArthur Foundation, Chicago, USA.
3. Dwyer J. The body at war. London: Unwin-Hyman; 1988.
4. Pauling L. How to live longer and feel better. New York: Freeman; 1986.
5. Warner HR, Butler RN, Schneider EL. Modern biological theories of aging. New York: Raven Press; 1987.
6. McCance KL, Heuther SE. Pathophysiology: The biologic basis for disease in adults and children. Missouri: Mosby; 1998.
7. Selye H. The stress of life. New York: McGraw-Hill; 1956.
8. Waters RL, Mulroy S. The energy expenditure of normal and pathological gait. Gait Posture 1999; 3:207–231.
9. Adams M, Bogduk N, Burton K et al. The biomechanics of back pain. Edinburgh: Churchill Livingstone; 2002.
10. Nachemson AL, Schultz AB, Berkson MH. Mechanical properties of human lumbar spine segments. Spine 1979; 4:1–8.
11. Eriksen MF. Aging changes in the shape of the human lumbar vertebrae. Am J Phys Anthropol 1974; 41:477.
12. Eriksen MH. Some aspects of aging in the lumbar spine. Am J Phys Anthropol 1975; 45:575–580.
13. Twomey L, Taylor J. Sagittal movements of the human lumbar vertebral column: a quantitative study of the role of the posterior vertebral elements. Arch Phys Med Rehab 1983; 64:322–325.

14. Twomey L, Taylor J. Flexion creep deformation and hysteresis in the lumbar vertebral column. Spine 1982; 7:116–122.

15. Bogduk N, Twomey LT. Clinical anatomy of the lumbar spine. Edinburgh: Churchill Livingstone; 1991.

16. Hadden Soden C. Geriatric technique. AAO Yearbook; 1941.

Chapter 33

Treatment planning

CHAPTER CONTENTS

INTRODUCTION

It is the experience of the authors after several years of study, practice and teaching, that diagnosis, treatment planning and application of treatment are very individual things! There are many factors to be considered, some arising from the osteopath's perspective and some from the patient's: for example the influence of the environmental and psychosocial factors on patients and their complaints; the osteopath's own abilities and osteopathic and philosophical predilections; the dilemma of wanting to make an osteopathic treatment in the true holistic sense of the word, when the patient may have come expecting only quick symptomatic relief. Taking factors such as these into consideration can result in the need to find a balance between theory and practice. Considerations like these arise in practice every day and this introduction to treatment planning will try to allay some of the fears that a neophyte osteopath may have by discussing a basic plan which can be adapted as the need arises.

THE CONSULTATION

The initial meeting is normally the first contact made between the patient and practitioner, although in certain cases some patients will speak with the osteopath by phone about their problems prior to making an appointment. Whenever the first contact or meeting is made, initial impressions will be made by both parties. Paulus[1] states 'the conscious act of becoming a patient is not seen as a failure, but is the honest recognition of the continuity of connection between fellow human beings'. This should be borne in mind by all aspiring osteopaths; our role is to support that of patients and their inherent healing mechanisms and not to try to take over that role single-handed. A major part of treatment is reassurance: patients need to know that they are confident in asking this particular person for help with their problems. For this reason, the 'welcome' made by the osteopath needs to be professional, caring and efficient. This applies to the whole 'practice set-up', from the waiting room, receptionist, and treatment room, right through to the osteopath's demeanour. A clean, tidy practice with appropriate magazines in the waiting room and thoughtfully provided facilities will relax patients and give them confidence. A stark, messy or dirty practice speaks for itself and no matter how skilled the osteopath may be, the initial impression will diminish the patient's confidence and most probably influence the outcome.

Consideration should be made for the individual's needs. Elderly patients, children, patients with disabilities and pregnant women are amongst the many variables encountered in normal everyday practice life.

The initial meeting between the patient and practitioner is a key point of the process of understanding patients and their concerns, and establishing a healing relationship that will be further developed as the course of examination and treatment progresses. It may appear somewhat facile to state this, but if you remember that you are first and foremost a human being, and *then* that you are an osteopath, you will be able to draw on the innate human skills that are present, to a lesser or greater extent in us all, those of being able to assess people's emotional state – to observe their anger, fear, sorrow, love, hate, in fact all of the emotions; reading this in their eyes, their faces and their bodies, and also 'feeling' their energy. This will give one a subjective hypothesis as to the patient's state.

It is perhaps of interest to reflect on the fact that this is in fact a two-way process, and that the patient is assessing you in the same way that you assess the patient. This stage results in the unconscious relationship forged between the two individuals from which future interactions will evolve.

It should be remembered that osteopaths are primary care practitioners so that as well as making an 'osteopathic' assessment of each patient, it is also necessary to make a pathological differential diagnosis. Some individuals differentiate between the allopathic and osteopathic procedures, others do not. This is a moot point, as the culmination of these processes should arrive at a diagnosis that is relevant for the osteopath, be it a functional or pathological diagnosis. The diagnosis then should lead to an appropriate management plan. Functional problems are obviously candidates for osteopathic treatment, but in fact so are many 'pathological' problems. Few pathological processes require referral to a GP or hospital prior to giving some treatment (though there are some cases that necessitate this). Even so, for clarity within this text, some differentiation between tests designed to diagnose pathological changes (allopathic) and those designed to assess functional changes (osteopathic) has been made. The process of objective hypothesis testing to discover the diagnosis, as with the subjective analysis mentioned earlier, also begins at the point of initial contact.

The gender of the individual should be noted. Many conditions have a gender bias; for example, two young adults, one female and the other male, complaining of low back pain, some abdominal bloating and associated nausea will have one key diagnostic difference between them – men are not able to become pregnant. This is an extreme example but other examples are that: women have a greater incidence of rheumatoid arthritis (3 : 1), systemic lupus erythematosus (9 : 1) and hypothyroidism (3 : 1), whereas males have a greater incidence of gout (20 : 1) Perthes' disease (5 : 1) and ankylosing spondylitis (8 : 1).[2]

Similarly the age of the individual affects the differential diagnosis, both allopathic and osteopathic. Thus the differentials included for someone complaining of hip pain will be dramatically different for a child in comparison to that of an elderly individual. The same applies with trends that occur within different races.

Of a debatably less objective viewpoint it is also possible to make note of the individual's biotype. This offers further possible hypotheses based on the studies of biotypologists, such as Sheldon, Goldthwait, Vannier, Kretschmer and numerous others. They have related various features on both a physical and psychological or emotional level, to each of the specific biotypes. Having assessed the patient's biotype, those features attendant on that biotype can then be proposed as possible further differential hypotheses. Mixtures of biotypes could be expected to present a proportionate mixture of various aspects of each biotype represented in the specific individual. This is not imposing concepts onto a patient but offering potential hypothetical considerations regarding the patient that can be tested in subsequent aspects of the consultation and accepted or rejected as necessary.

Having made these initial observations even before saying anything to the patient, it is now time to engage verbally, introducing yourself and generally putting the patient at ease. Many patients consulting an osteopath for the first time have preconceived ideas of what to expect of the initial consultation which may well be incorrect; or they may have no idea at all. So a brief summary of what will take place may be of use. Moreover, they might have seen other osteopaths in the past who have a different approach to the initial consultation and may feel 'lost' in this new approach.

THE CASE HISTORY

The next stage is the case history examination. This involves taking a detailed account of the patient's presenting complaint in order to ascertain the true root of the patient's concerns. Again, body language will be important here. Some practitioners prefer to distance themselves slightly from their patients by using the barrier of the desk and white coat. Others prefer the informality of no white coat and easy chairs for case history taking. Whilst taking the details from the patient, the osteopath needs to be attentive; eye contact is important – listening and constantly scribbling notes without looking at the patient does not create confidence. Patients should be given the time to give their account of the problem. If they, however, appear to be straying from the point too much the osteopath may be required at times to gently (and sometimes more firmly) steer the patient 'back on track'. Specific details that patients may not regard as important to their particular problems may need to be drawn from them and should they seem unsettled by this, then a brief explanation as to their importance will normally restore confidence. It is necessary to be aware of hidden concerns that patients may have but that they feel inhibited to mention or that they feel are inappropriate. Throughout the whole case history taking, the osteopath must be aware of the need to identify with patients as to their underlying needs and to believe them. Trust is a major part of the two-way interaction between the patient

and the practitioner and will undoubtedly influence the outcome.

Questioning is a very delicate area that can either be fully productive or of no use to anyone. Asking open-ended questions allows patients to give their own accounts and leaves the discretion to the patient as to what information to offer. Leading questions are at times dangerous, such as: 'You don't have any other pains then?'. It is easy to miss valuable information should the patient be led to respond to such a question as expected to. (That question is, in fact, a closed, negative and leading question! It is not one to be employed often.) Direct or closed questioning is generally employed to obtain specific information, to perhaps complete the information gained from the more open questions, or to ask about specific features associated with a particular condition to aid inclusion or exclusion of the condition in the differential diagnosis. For example, if you suspect ankylosing spondylitis (AS), and have asked the general open questions about other systemic problems, it is then useful to ask specifically if they have experienced the associated problems, which are in the case of AS, Achilles tendonitis, gastrointestinal disturbance (ulcerative colitis or Crohn's disease) or eye pain (iritis). A balance of open and closed questions will usually be used, and though space is created for the patient to express themselves, ultimately it is the role of the osteopath to ensure that as much of the relevant information as possible is obtained, and therefore the osteopath necessarily needs to be in control of the situation.

This process is often perceived as an information gathering process, which it is in part. But this stage is much more dynamic than just receiving information. It is an active process where initial hypotheses are tested and, as more information is brought into the equation, progressively more complex and hopefully accurate hypotheses are tested. This stage is one that demands active engagement with patients and the information that they are offering, following hypotheses to an end-point, be it inclusion or exclusion.

To facilitate this there needs to be an order; 'random approaches often result in random solutions, seriously limiting the likelihood of successful outcomes'.[3] The consultation needs to have direction and an aim but the route taken to achieve this aim need not be fixed; flexibility should be used as necessary. Furthermore, it should not be performed as a series of questions merely to be answered or boxes ticked on a sheet. Facilitation may be required in order to provide the true goal of the question. Repeating or reflecting answers to patients will enable them to confirm what they have just offered and may result in clearer answers or further detail. Having stated that the consultation needs to be flexible, most osteopaths do use some kind of format in their note taking and the following list is included as a guide:

- personal details
- presenting complaint
- past medical history including accidents, illnesses, surgery and medications
- family history
- personal and social history; sports and exercise, nutrition and tobacco and alcohol use and abuse
- review of the body systems.

With respect to the presenting complaint, in order to evaluate the condition fully a number of details need to be clarified:

1. When did it begin?
2. How or why did it begin?
3. How has it progressed since the onset?
4. Exacerbating and relieving factors?
5. Past history of similar problems?

In many cases the patient will be consulting the osteopath because of pain but this is not always the case; it may be for a reason of dysfunction that is not pain-related. Heinking et al[4] offer the 'PQRST mnemonic for investigating pain':

P = position/palliation
Q = quality
R = radiation
S = severity
T = timing

The severity of pain is very subjective but a useful indication may be achieved by using a visual analogue scale which is a 10 cm line with 'no pain' indicated at one end and 'worst pain ever' at the other end. The patient is instructed to mark on the scale where they feel their pain level lies. It is also a useful method for measuring the progression of treatment.

The review of the systems is to determine whether there are other problems that the patient may not be aware of, or that they feel is not relevant to the osteopath. It usually involves asking some screening questions for each of the body systems and should positive indicators be found then fur-

ther questioning and possible referral will be necessary. The list of systems includes:

- integumentary
- musculoskeletal
- cardiovascular
- respiratory
- gastrointestinal
- genitourinary
- neurological
- endocrine.

Once all of the above information has been gathered, the osteopath should reflect and satisfy himself that the requirements of the case history interview have been satisfied for both parties. With all the information the osteopath should now consider the possibilities for the underlying causes of the patient's problem. In certain cases the cause will be blatantly obvious but in others there may be a number of possibilities. The possibilities or hypotheses need to be recognized before passing to the next stage in order to construct an examination plan. Considerations should be given to both the tissues and the processes involved. The tissues involved are:

- skin
- fascia
- muscle
- tendon
- ligament
- joint
- bone
- blood vessels
- nerves
- viscus.

With respect to the processes, Collins[5] offers the mnemonic VINDICATE to assist in the screening procedures:

V = vascular
I = inflammatory
N = neoplastic
D = degenerative
I = intoxication
C = congenital
A = autoimmune
T = trauma
E = endocrine

The above system is not infallible and 'infectious' should be included and of particular interest to the osteopath, 'mechanical'. A variation on the same theme is to use DR VITAMIN C:

- D = degenerative
- R = referred
- V = vascular
- I = inflammatory and infectious
- T = trauma
- A = autoimmune
- M = metabolic (endocrine) and mechanical
- I = intoxication
- N = neoplastic
- C = congenital

Smith[6] used a system known as the osteopathic sieve and a modified version is shown in Figure 33.1. It provides an 'at a glance' indication of the tissues and processes involved and, especially for the neophyte osteopath, serves as a useful memory tool. For example, if a trauma such as a whiplash has occurred then there may be damage to the muscles of the neck and so the relevant boxes would be marked. However, there may be a pre-existing degenerative change in the facet joints of the neck with a mechanical irritation of the adjacent spinal nerves; once again, the relevant boxes would be marked.

The examination will be used in order to confirm or deny the hypotheses and in addition to rule out any other pathology not related to the presenting complaint.

Before moving on to the physical examination, it is wise to explain clearly to the patient what that will involve. Since it will be necessary for the patient to undress to the underwear, irrespective of the fact that the patient eventually ends up standing semi-clothed in front of the osteopath, many patients prefer to undress in privacy. This may mean undressing in a changing room or that the osteopath leaves the room whilst the patient undresses. It has been suggested by some that to watch patients undress may give valuable information as to how they move their bodies with respect to pain avoidance manoeuvres but all of this information may be gained from a well-planned examination without the need for what some patients may consider as voyeurism.

THE PHYSICAL EXAMINATION

The physical examination that is followed is dictated, to a large extent, by the hypotheses arising from the case history stage. Should the individual

	Skin	Fascia	Muscle	Tendon	Ligament	Joint	Bone	Vessel	Nerve	Organ
Degenerative										
Referred										
Vascular										
Inflammatory										
Infectious										
Trauma										
Autoimmune										
Metabolic										
Endocrine										
Mechanical										
Intoxification										
Neoplastic										
Congenital										

Figure 33.1 The Osteopathic Sieve. (Modified after Smith.[6])

present with possible pathological problems, such as a cardiovascular, neurological or an articular pathology, these can be explored via the relevant tests, which can be found in any decent clinical medical text. Having performed these tests, or in the absence of any suspected pathology, the osteopathic assessment should then be done. (With experience it is possible and in fact preferable to combine the allopathic and osteopathic tests to minimize the inconvenience to the patient, so that all tests performed standing are done together, and then similarly for sitting, prone and supine.) Certain hypotheses may require exclusion before any other testing, e.g. fracture, and very rarely may require referral without further assessment, i.e. any medical or surgical emergency.

Assuming no pathological possibilities the osteopathic examination can be performed. The osteopathic examinations will not be discussed fully within this text, but it is perhaps worth quoting Oschman again[7].

Body shape and patterns of movement simultaneously tell three stories, each relating to the way we experience gravity:

- *An evolutionary history, representing the millions of years that our ancestors adapted to life in the gravity field of our planet.*
- *A shorter history of personal traumas and adaptations during our lifetime.*
- *The history of our present emotional state, including the effects of our most recent experiences.*

The authors feel strongly that not enough attention is paid to the act of looking at the patient intelligently. As a result of good observation (and with the results of a well-taken actively questioned case history) the examination routine is there to confirm or refute the current possible hypotheses. This is in contrast to entering the examination phase knowing that you want to assess certain areas but not knowing specifically why.

Armed with the information from the case history and that of the physical examination, the osteopath is usually now in a position to make a diagnosis or evaluation and to decide whether or not to proceed with treatment. The primary decision to make is necessarily one of safety, are there any 'red flags' contraindicating treatment? It may be the case that the osteopath decides not to treat until further information can be obtained through, for example, radiographic examination,

blood tests or prior medical history records. It may be that osteopathy is not the most appropriate treatment for the patient's problem. This may mean that the patient may require other treatment first and then the osteopath may be of help, or that there is nothing that the osteopath can do to help this particular person. Should the osteopath consider that referral is the required course of action then it should be the responsibility of the osteopath to assist the patient in finding a suitable practitioner and not to merely abandon the patient. There is the possibility that the patient's expectations of treatment do not agree with that of the osteopath; for example, the patient wants a symptomatic treatment merely to alleviate a painful condition and is not prepared to undergo treatment that is not primarily aimed at that goal. In this case the osteopath must decide firstly, if he/she is prepared to treat in this manner and secondly, if he/she is capable of doing so. There may be a complex lesion pattern that requires a sufficient level of experience and understanding in order to remove the acute level of the pattern without upsetting the compensatory mechanisms that have been set up, thereby exacerbating the problem. Another consideration will be the osteopath's own preferences and prejudices: does he/she honestly feel that his/her preference for cranial, high velocity low amplitude techniques or otherwise is the best suited mode of treatment for a particular patient's presenting problem? Contraindications to treatment do not include just the 'red flags'; the osteopath's capabilities, experience, and knowledge of what is going on with a particular patient all become matters of safety if overlooked, due to disregard, ignorance or egoism.

However, if the osteopath is satisfied that they can safely proceed then they need to formulate a treatment plan with both short- and long-term goals and to establish an expected prognosis. The plan needs to reflect the wishes of the patient and the capabilities of the osteopath. The prognosis should include an awareness of the psychosocial factors that may influence the rate of recovery. The psychosocial risk factors have been termed 'yellow flags', in contrast to the 'red flags' which are physical risk factors (see Ch. 5). Once this has been discussed and fully understood by the patient, it acts as an informal management contract. When this has been agreed the treatment may begin.

The above series of events leading up towards the treatment are summarized in Figure 33.2.

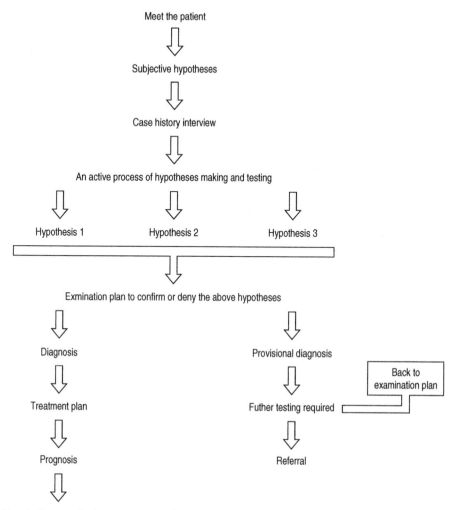

Figure 33.2   Steps in the consultation process towards treatment.

TREATMENT

Although the plan in Figure 33.1 appears linear in fashion it may be adapted at any stage and needs to remain flexible in order to accommodate new findings or information. For example, in the case of a patient forgetting or neglecting to mention that they had had abdominal surgery, this would naturally be picked up during the physical examination and should be added to the case notes. In doing this, rethinking of the situation may be necessary, and a new hypothesis may be developed or one of the original ones rejected. Furthermore, in the summary given in Figure 33.1, there are three hypotheses; this is just an example and there may be more or less in number.

Once the treatment plan has been made and the treatment begins, it also may be subject to change; flexibility remains throughout the whole patient/practitioner relationship in order to optimize the treatment best suited for the patient and their condition. It is here that another possibility for discussion arises: many osteopaths feel that mixing of certain modes of treatment is not acceptable whilst others disagree. The authors feel that it is perfectly acceptable to mix treatment modes provided that it is done in a manner which reflects an intelligent thought process with respect to the individual patient being treated. An example could be that structural type techniques have been used on a patient throughout the body but that it has been decided for reasons of safety that they would be contraindicated in the cervical region. In this case, it would be acceptable to use a more gentle functional type approach solely in this region. Some osteopaths would be horrified at the thought of using cranial and structural type techniques in the same treatment session. A good example of doing exactly that would be in the case of childhood asthma where it may well be indicated to use cranial type approaches in order to balance the autonomic nervous system but equally importantly, it may be indicated to use structural type articulation techniques to release possible thoracic restrictions and prevent chronic tissue change. Using both these approaches within the same treatment session is perfectly valid though it is probably better to finish the treatment with the gentler cranial techniques. So this then becomes an important part of treatment planning. It should not be forgotten that if a practitioner does not feel confident in certain modes of treatment then using them cannot be justified; however, as was mentioned earlier, if the practitioner forces their preferred type of treatment onto a patient when the problem clearly requires a different approach, then the practitioner is doing the patient a disservice.

For the reader who has diligently read every page of this book there will be a sense of an underlying message. The crux of the matter is that there is no strict protocol to follow with respect to treatment planning or how to treat. Osteopathy is not a prescriptive medicine, there are no magic formulae to follow and any osteopath who says there are is not aware of the principles and philosophy of osteopathy as proposed by Andrew Taylor Still. Having stated that there are no magic formulae does not mean that it is all down to chance. Each patient should be looked at individually as a whole human being, with a mind, body and spirit, and existing in a particular environment at a certain time. When this is analysed with respect to the information gained from the case history, the anatomical palpatory findings made on examination and the knowledge of physiology in health and disease, and with an understanding of the essential principles of osteopathy and a degree of self-awareness, the plan of treatment will then become apparent. Still[8] wrote 'when you fully comprehend and travel by the laws of reason, confusion will be a stranger in all your combats with disease'. Osteopathy will then work.

References

1. Paulus S. The six stages of an osteopathic treatment. Inter Linea 2002; 4(1):9–14.
2. Huskisson EC, Dudley Hart F. Joint disease: all the arthropathies. Bristol: Wright; 1987.
3. Seidel HM, Ball JW, Dains JE et al. Mosby's guide to physical examination, 4th edn. St Louis: Mosby; 1999: 15–35.
4. Heinking K, Jones JM, Kappler RE. Pelvis and sacrum. In: Ward RC, ed. Foundations for osteopathic medicine. Baltimore: Williams and Wilkins; 1997:601–622.
5. Collins RD. Differential diagnosis in primary care, 2nd edn. Philadelphia: Lippincott; 1987.
6. Smith A. Osteopathic diagnosis. London: The British School of Osteopathy; 1984.
7. Oschman JL. Energy medicine. Edinburgh: Churchill Livingstone; 2000: 173–174.
8. Still AT. Osteopathy, research and practice. Missouri: Still; 1910: 39.

Chapter 34

Specialisms in osteopathy

CHAPTER CONTENTS

INTRODUCTION

There has been much discussion recently in osteopathic circles regarding the subject of specialisms in osteopathy. In the UK, much of the debate has been floored through the forum of the General Osteopathic Council (GOsC). In an article published in the October 2001 issue of *The Osteopath*, the official journal of the General Osteopathic Council, the subject was broached and a survey made.[1] Three months later in *The Osteopath* the results of the survey were published.[2] Of the 3000 plus members of the GOsC only 228 responded, 147 considering themselves specialists and 81 not. By far and large the field of osteopathy that contained the major number of specialists in this particular survey was cranial. This was followed by paediatrics, sports, veterinary, visceral, research and 'others'. Since the number of respondents and the number of specialists did not tally (147 respondents and 206 specialists), it may be assumed that a number of osteopaths considered themselves to be specialists in more than one field. The 'specialists' gained their expertise variously, ranging from educational establishments to being self-taught, or from other osteopaths. A letter published in the same issue from Stuart Korth,[3] founder and director of the Osteopathic Centre for Children (OCC), highlighted the point that until the GOsC validated a particular course, the GOsC should not allow its members to state that they are a specialist in any particular field of osteopathy. At the time of writing, the GOsC has not as yet made provisions for validation of any particular specialty but with the pending inception of a programme of continuing professional development it is quite likely that this will eventually follow.

There are two points of view to this problem. One view is that the osteopath is a generalist and by applying his/her knowledge and principles of osteopathy he/she should be capable of treating the patient before him/her. The opposite view is that as the knowledge in a particular field increases, that particular osteopath does become 'more qualified' to work in that particular field than someone who has not pursued that particular route. Korth[3] gives the example that treating a '24 week gestation preterm baby on full life support' does require 'special skill and knowledge'. It goes without saying that veterinary osteopathy also requires extra knowledge to that learned in an undergraduate osteopathy degree course and there are a number of postgraduate courses offering training in veterinary osteopathy. A problem arises with the distinction of the 'sports osteopath'. What is it that actually constitutes a sports injury? A professional sports player may well require specialist treatment whereas the 'injured dad' playing football in the garden may not. Is the important criterion the onset of the injury, the fact that the injury was brought about by a sport, or the fact that the patient relies on their sport for their livelihood? What about the linesman at a football match who slips over and injures his knee? It may seem like semantics but this is a problem requiring a great deal of thought.

There are a number of osteopathic practices that go under the name of 'back clinics' or 'pain clinics' or 'neck and back pain clinics'. It may be argued that these practitioners are not treating osteopathically and are undermining the reputation and the principles upon which osteopathy is based. Nevertheless, these practitioners are providing a valid service to their patients using the skills they have learned during their osteopathic education. But do they consider themselves specialists? And if so, how did they gain their title of 'specialist'?

Then we have the problems of treatment approaches. The majority of respondents in the survey considered themselves specialists in cranial osteopathy. Is cranial not just a mode of treatment, a method used by osteopaths to treat their patients? Should there also be muscle energy technique, functional or high velocity low amplitude specialists? Is the cranial specialist imposing his/her preference for technique onto the unsuspecting patient rather than deciding the true needs of the patient's condition? Instead of labelling ourselves 'cranial osteopaths', perhaps we could equally say that we are 'limited to cranial approach' (or whatever our chosen approach may be). It has been suggested by some that to proclaim oneself as a cranial osteopath is merely jumping on the bandwagon and profiteering from public knowledge. As the public awareness of osteopathy increases, so does the idea that there is a difference between osteopathy and cranial osteopathy. The danger is that this creates a rift and may serve to divide a profession that is, at present, trying to unify its body of members and thus its acceptance in the medical and public worlds. Naturally enough the same may be said for the specialism of visceral osteopathy and we, the authors, ask 'cranial specialists' or any others for that matter, not to take umbrage at these observations. The foregoing discussions are a collation of information taken from the GOsC survey and personal communications from numerous osteopaths, both 'specialists' and 'generalists'.

At the moment the profession (in the UK at least) is undecided as to how to approach this problem. It is evident that in order to be a specialist in any given profession, one needs a certain amount of special training over and above that of the initial qualification: this means postgraduate education. This education needs to be assessed and validated externally to the educational body providing the course. Until that state of affairs is reached it is unreasonable and probably unprofessional to publicize oneself as anything other than a 'self-proclaimed specialist'.

References

1. Specialisms. The Osteopath 2001; October.
2. Specialisms. The Osteopath 2001; December.
3. Korth S. Letters to the editor. The Osteopath 2001; December.

INDEX

Abbreviations used: CNS, central nervous system; CSF, cerebrospinal fluid; ERS, extension, rotation, side bending lesion; FRS, flexion, rotation, side bending lesion; NMDA, N-methyl-d-aspartate
Page numbers in italics refer to figures, tables or illustrations

Printed and bound by CPI Group (UK) Ltd, Croydon, CR0 4YY

03/10/2024

01040364-0006